Rapid Review of
Radiology

Shahid Hussain
MA, MB, BChir, MRCP, FRCR
Consultant Radiologist
Heart of England NHS Foundation Trust, Birmingham, UK

Sherif Aaron Abdel Latif
MB, ChB, MRCS, FRCR
Consultant Radiologist
Dudley Group of Hospitals NHS Foundation Trust, West Midlands, UK

Adrian David Hall
MB, ChB, MRCP, FRCR
Consultant Radiologist
Dudley Group of Hospitals NHS Foundation Trust, West Midlands, UK

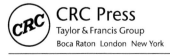

CRC Press is an imprint of the
Taylor & Francis Group, an **informa** business

Dedications

S.H. – To my mum

S.L. – To my mum and dad, my wife Darine and baby Danny

A.H. - For my parents, my wife Kirstie and my sons Oliver, Tristan and Seb

CRC Press
Taylor & Francis Group
6000 Broken Sound Parkway NW, Suite 300
Boca Raton, FL 33487-2742

© 2010 by Taylor & Francis Group, LLC
CRC Press is an imprint of Taylor & Francis Group, an Informa business

No claim to original U.S. Government works

ISBN-13: 978-1-84076-120-7 (Paperback)

This book contains information obtained from authentic and highly regarded sources. While all reasonable efforts have been made to publish reliable data and information, neither the author[s] nor the publisher can accept any legal responsibility or liability for any errors or omissions that may be made. The publishers wish to make clear that any views or opinions expressed in this book by individual editors, authors or contributors are personal to them and do not necessarily reflect the views/opinions of the publishers. The information or guidance contained in this book is intended for use by medical, scientific or health-care professionals and is provided strictly as a supplement to the medical or other professional's own judgement, their knowledge of the patient's medical history, relevant manufacturer's instructions and the appropriate best practice guidelines. Because of the rapid advances in medical science, any information or advice on dosages, procedures or diagnoses should be independently verified. The reader is strongly urged to consult the relevant national drug formulary and the drug companies' and device or material manufacturers' printed instructions, and their websites, before administering or utilizing any of the drugs, devices or materials mentioned in this book. This book does not indicate whether a particular treatment is appropriate or suitable for a particular individual. Ultimately it is the sole responsibility of the medical professional to make his or her own professional judgements, so as to advise and treat patients appropriately. The authors and publishers have also attempted to trace the copyright holders of all material reproduced in this publication and apologize to copyright holders if permission to publish in this form has not been obtained. If any copyright material has not been acknowledged please write and let us know so we may rectify in any future reprint.

Except as permitted under U.S. Copyright Law, no part of this book may be reprinted, reproduced, transmitted, or utilized in any form by any electronic, mechanical, or other means, now known or hereafter invented, including photocopying, microfilming, and recording, or in any information storage or retrieval system, without written permission from the publishers.

For permission to photocopy or use material electronically from this work, please access www.copyright.com (http://www.copyright.com/) or contact the Copyright Clearance Center, Inc. (CCC), 222 Rosewood Drive, Danvers, MA 01923, 978-750-8400. CCC is a not-for-profit organization that provides licenses and registration for a variety of users. For organizations that have been granted a photocopy license by the CCC, a separate system of payment has been arranged.

Trademark Notice: Product or corporate names may be trademarks or registered trademarks, and are used only for identification and explanation without intent to infringe.

Visit the Taylor & Francis Web site at
http://www.taylorandfrancis.com

and the CRC Press Web site at
http://www.crcpress.com

Second impression 2011

A CIP catalogue record for this book is available from the British Library.

Design: Cathy Martin, Presspack Computing Ltd
Colour reproduction: Tenon & Polert Colour Scanning Ltd, Hong Kong
Printed by: Replika Press Pvt Ltd, Kundli, Haryana, India

Contents

Preface	4
Contributors	5
Abbreviations	5
General Introduction	7
Chapter 1 – Chest Imaging	11
Chapter 2 – Abdominal Imaging	71
Chapter 3 – Central Nervous System, Head and Neck Imaging	147
Chapter 4 – Musculoskeletal Imaging	205
Chapter 5 – Paediatric Imaging	289
Chapter 6 – Breast Imaging *by Professor Iain Lyburn*	331
Further Reading	343
Index of Differential Diagnoses	344
General Index	346

Preface

As in all specialties, learning in radiology is a lifelong process. Yet the rate of learning is undoubtedly highest in the trainee years, when there is a vast amount of information to assimilate. There are many excellent, comprehensive radiology texts available to facilitate this, yet learning for most of us is a more haphazard process than reading such a text from cover to cover. More commonly, we learn initially unrelated pieces of information from multiple sources and these gradually join together like the pieces of a jigsaw, using the comprehensive textbook as a reference along the way. The practical aspects of image recognition and formulating a differential diagnosis become ever more important, especially as postgraduate exams loom! Again, there are already excellent radiology atlases and text-based differential diagnosis guides that become standard reading for the trainee.

Our aim in writing this text was to bring together the images with the differential diagnosis information, adding some practical advice along with it. Such a book cannot be comprehensive without becoming another large general text. Instead, we have tried to compile a selection of cases covering many aspects of radiology, particularly the types used in radiology vivas. These include the so-called 'Aunt Minnie' cases, where a classic image becomes simple pattern recognition, and also the cases where findings need to be pieced together along with the clinical history to formulate a differential diagnosis. This selection of cases will thus provide image and factual learning material for a broad sample of disorders that will intertwine with material learnt elsewhere. The format is intended to help the trainee starting out with practical issues such as how to approach films and the vocabulary to use; the trainee approaching exams with a means of self-testing and rehearsing cases; and also the nonradiologist to practise some more challenging material. The selection of cases is hopefully broad enough to provide an introduction to some 'exam favourites' for the beginner, but also more testing cases for those in later stages of training.

In order for the candidate to test him- or herself, we have presented each case as an image (or set of images) together with the pertinent clinical details. Over the page is a description of the images as would be given to an examiner in a long case or a viva situation. This is perhaps the most important part in getting to the correct diagnosis since the description contains the relevant positive and negative imaging findings, and will help to identify the correct diagnosis as well as narrow down the differentials. The correct diagnosis for the film is given, followed, in most cases, by a differential diagnosis list, which contains the best diagnoses to fit with the images and history. A discussion of the underlying diagnosis is then presented; this includes teaching points and main imaging findings regarding the diagnosis and any other important conditions that emerge in the course of the discussion. Each case concludes with practical tips and notes on further management.

We have tried to include as many plain radiograph images as possible, since these still constitute the primary investigation performed in radiology departments. Subsequent investigation is usually based on these initial images and therefore their correct interpretation cannot be understated. In the abdominal chapter, we have also included many barium contrast images, which are often poorly performed on in examinations. Subsequent multi-modality images have been included – ultrasound, CT, MRI, interventional radiology and nuclear medicine. In this way, we have presented the imaging cases as they would appear in both exam situations and in the real world. For example, chest disease would be initially investigated with a chest x-ray, with subsequent investigation with a CT. CNS disease is usually initially investigated with CT/MRI. We have therefore tried to follow the clinical investigation pathway as closely as possible to present trainees with the images in the order in which they would expect to see them, in exams and clinical situations.

The lists of differential diagnoses, radiological signs and practical tips are often presented in 'bullet point' list format to allow for rapid revision just before the exams. We have also indexed the differential diagnosis lists allowing for easy and quick referral throughout training, and when it comes time to revise. Hopefully, we have provided a book that can be referred to throughout the radiologist's training, through various levels of ability.

Shahid Hussain, Sherif Latif and Adrian Hall

Contributors

Professor Iain Lyburn, Consultant Radiologist, Gloucestershire Hospital NHS Foundation Trust for the breast imaging chapter.

Dr Bernd Wittkop, Consultant Radiologist, Worcestershire Acute Hospitals Trust for the nuclear medicine cases.

For the contribution of images: Dr Anne Gregan, Consultant Radiologist, Dudley Group of Hospitals NHS Trust; Dr Peter Oliver, Consultant Radiologist, Dudley Group of Hospitals NHS Trust; Dr Ruth Shave, Consultant Radiologist, Dudley Group of Hospitals NHS Trust; Dr Katharine Foster, Consultant Radiologist, Birmingham Children's Hospital NHS Foundation Trust; Dr Umesh Udeshi, Consultant Radiologist, Worcestershire Acute Hospitals Trust; Dr Dee Dawkins, Consultant Radiologist, Sandwell & West Birmingham Hospitals NHS Trust; Dr Hong Gap-Teo, Consultant Radiologist, Sandwell & West Birmingham Hospitals NHS Trust; Dr Colin Walker, Consultant Radiologist, University Hospital Birmingham NHS Foundation Trust; Dr J Reynolds, Consultant Radiologist, Heart of England NHS Foundation Trust; Dr M Djearaman, Consultant Radiologist, Heart of England NHS Foundation Trust; Dr A Pallan, Consultant Radiologist, Heart of England NHS Foundation Trust; Dr S Roy-Choudhury, Consultant Radiologist, Heart of England NHS Foundation Trust; Dr S Cooper, Consultant Radiologist, Heart of England NHS Foundation Trust.

We would especially like to thank Dr L Arkell for the film library she collated over the course of her career and passed on at retirement, many cases from which have been used in the course of this text.

Abbreviations

ABC	aneurysmal bone cyst
ABPA	allergic bronchopulmonary aspergillosis
AD	autosomal dominant
ADC	apparent diffusion coefficient
ADEM	acute disseminated encephalomyelitis
ADPKD	autosomal dominant polycystic kidney disease
AF	atrial fibrillation
AIDS	acquired immunodeficiency syndrome
ANA	antinuclear antibodies
AP	anteroposterior
ASD	atrial septal defect
AVM	arteriovenous malformation
AVN	avascular necrosis
AXR	abdominal x-ray
BP	blood pressure
CAD	computer-aided detection
CAM	cystic adenomatoid malformation
CC	craniocaudal
CDH	congenital diaphragmatic hernia
CF	cystic fibrosis
CFA	cryptogenic fibrosing alveolitis
CMV	cytomegalovirus
CNS	central nervous system
COP	cryptogenic organizing pneumonia
CP	cerebellopontine
CRM	circumferential resection margin
CSF	cerebrospinal fluid
CT	computed tomography
CVA	cerebrovascular accident
CWP	coal worker's pneumoconiosis
CXR	chest x-ray
DCIS	ductal carcinoma *in situ*
DWI	diffusion weighted imaging
EAA	extrinsic allergic alveolitis
ECG	electrocardiogram
ECMO	extracorporeal membrane oxygenation
ENT	ear, nose and throat
ERCP	endoscopic retrograde cholangiopancreatography
FAP	familial adenomatous polyposis
FDG	18 fluoro-2-deoxyglucose
FFDM	full-field digital mammography
FLAIR	fluid attenuated inversion recovery
FNA	fine needle aspiration
FNH	focal nodular hyperplasia
GBM	glioblastoma multiforme
GCT	giant cell tumour
Gd-BOPTA	gadolinium benzyloxypropionic-tetra-acetate
Gd-EOB-DTPA	gadolinium-ethoxybenzyl-diethylenetriamine penta-acetic acid

Abbreviations

GI	gastrointestinal	OPG	orthopantomogram
HIV	human immunodeficiency virus	PA	posteroanterior
HMD	hyaline membrane disease	PCA	posterior cerebral artery
HPOA	hypertrophic pulmonary osteoarthropathy	PCP	*Pneumocystis carinii* pneumonia
HRCT	high-resolution computed tomography	PD	proton density
HRT	hormone replacement therapy	PDA	patent ductus arteriosus
HSP	Henoch–Schönlein purpura	PET	positron emission tomography
HSV	herpes simplex virus	PICA	posterior inferior cerebellar artery
HU	Hounsfield units	PIE	pulmonary interstitial emphysema
IAC	internal auditory canal	PMF	progressive massive fibrosis
IDC	invasive ductal carcinoma	PNET	primitive neuroectodermal tumour
ILC	invasive lobular carcinoma	PSC	primary sclerosing cholangitis
IPF	idiopathic pulmonary fibrosis	PVL	periventricular leukomalacia
ITU	intensive treatment unit	RA	rheumatoid arthritis
IV	intravenous	RTA	renal tubular acidosis
IVC	inferior vena cava	SACE	serum angiotensin converting enzyme
IVU	intravenous urogram	SAH	subarachnoid haemorrhage
LP	lumbar puncture	SBC	simple bone cyst
MCA	middle cerebral artery	SI	superioinferior
MCUG	micturating cystourethrogram	SLE	systemic lupus erythematosus
MEN	multiple endocrine neoplasia	SMV	superior mesenteric vein
MIBG	meta-iodobenzylguanidine	STIR	short tau inversion recovery
MIP	maximum intensity projection	SUFE	slipped upper femoral epiphysis
MISME syndrome	multiple inherited schwannoma, meningioma and ependymoma	SVC	superior vena cava
		TB	tuberculosis
		TCC	transitional cell carcinoma
MLO	mediolateral oblique	TE	time to echo
MRA	magnetic resonance angiography	TIA	transient ischaemic attack
MRCP	magnetic resonance cholangiopancreatography	TIPS	transjugular intrahepatic portosystemic shunt
MRI	magnetic resonance imaging	TME	total mesorectal excision
MS	multiple sclerosis	TNM	tumour–node–metastases staging
MSK	musculoskeletal	TOF	tracheoesophageal fistula
NAI	non accidental injury	UBOs	unidentified bright objects
NEC	necrotizing enterocolitis	UC	ulcerative colitis
NF1	neurofibromatosis type 1	US	ultrasound
NG	nasogastric	UTI	urinary tract infection
NOS	not otherwise specified	VAD	vacuum assisted device
NSAIDs	nonsteroidal anti-inflammatory drugs	VATS	video assisted thorascopic surgery
OA	osteoarthritis	VHL	von Hippel–Lindau syndrome
OKC	odontogenic keratocyst	VSD	ventricular septal defect

GENERAL INTRODUCTION

This book has been written primarily for senior radiology trainees preparing for final radiology exams and in particular for trainees studying for the Fellowship of the Royal College of Radiology. With this in mind, the cases presented herewith have been presented in the exact manner that the cases are presented in the Royal College of Radiology FRCR 2B exam. In the exam, long cases and viva cases are presented with a very minimal but highly relevant history and the required response is expected to be presented in a particular way. This format of reporting[1] involves giving a Description/Interpretation of the images; Diagnosis; Differential Diagnosis; and advice on Further Management. We have laid out the answers here in exactly this manner and have included a Discussion to give in-depth further information about each condition which will enable the student to answer any questions directed to him or her in the viva situation. By following the RCR exam format, the candidate should be ideally prepared for this exam and for the future as a Consultant Radiologist.

FILM TECHNIQUE

Whatever the imaging modality, the radiologist interprets images using all the information and clues available, to produce a differential diagnosis and/or advise on further investigation and management. Above all else, this must be done in a SAFE manner, and this often requires one to be systematic in approach. Secondly, this process must be done in a SENSIBLE manner – it is easy to quote endless lists of differential diagnoses but if these are not refined for each individual case, the radiologist's input is of little value. The following discussion concentrates in particular on performing these tasks in the examination viva scenario. However, much of the advice is applicable to everyday practice too, in particular the emphasis on a safe and sensible approach.

TYPES OF FILM

The types of film one may encounter in an exam/viva are as follows:

The 'Aunt Minnie'

There are certain disorders that have a characteristic appearance on imaging that allows one to make an instant 'spot diagnosis'. It will be assumed the candidate has come across it before, and thus the best preparation here is exposure to as many of these cases as possible. Radiological atlases and film libraries provide ready access to many of these classic cases, which can then be committed to memory. You can prepare a ready-made description of these cases for the viva. If you are sure of the diagnosis, dispatch the film promptly with your preprepared 'speech' so that you can progress to the next case as soon as possible. Of course there may be 'Aunt Minnie' cases that you haven't seen and this may present a problem. Such cases are often not amenable to working out the diagnosis – you either know it or you don't. The only thing to do is be methodical in your analysis and description of the findings so that at the very least you can suggest whether you feel an abnormality is likely to be longstanding and benign or otherwise, and make appropriate suggestions on how you would proceed.

The 'test of observation'

Here, there is an abnormality present that once seen, may well lead to an easy diagnosis. The abnormality is subtle or hidden however, such that it tests the candidate's perception and approach to a case. Perceptual ability, however, is variable, not only between people but also in the same observer on different days (this is particularly true in examinations where anxiety levels are high). You must therefore be systematic in analysing each film if there is no obvious abnormality to see on first inspection. There are many different systematic approaches and it is beyond the scope of this discussion to be more prescriptive. However, make sure you have a system and use it. Moreover, describe the process you are going through aloud in the viva so that the examiner knows that you are practising safe radiology.

The 'jigsaw puzzle'

This type of case presents several findings that once identified and considered together, lead to a specific or differential diagnosis. This not only tests perceptual skill and systematic approach, but also the ability to mentally 'cross-reference' several differential diagnosis lists for the various abnormalities identified, to find the 'best fit' diagnosis. Whenever producing a differential diagnosis in an examination or real life, it is vital to produce a sensible list, not just a recital of long lists learnt from books. To do this, you must use all clues available from the clinical history and film, and combine this information with knowledge of the incidence of each possibility in a given patient population.

General Introduction

The 'discussion'
In the real world, there are many abnormal radiological studies that have no specific 'best fit' diagnosis, but rather a differential diagnosis that cannot be narrowed down without further investigation. It is easy to assume that all cases used to test an examination candidate will have a single correct answer but this is a dangerous assumption – these 'real world' cases with no specific diagnosis are clearly a good test of how a radiologist will operate in daily practice. As always, a safe and systematic approach to film analysis is vital, together with a sensible approach to a differential diagnosis. Such cases, in particular, also assess the other role of the radiologist – advising on further investigation and management.

ANALYSING THE CASE
As already emphasized, have a system of analysis for all types of film. More specific advice on possible approaches will be given in further chapter introductions.

Use all clues available to you. Background clinical information is most important when interpreting radiological studies, so listen very carefully to any information the examiner provides with the case. Make a note of the age and sex of the patient if possible using either identification data on the film or anatomical information – many disorders can be eliminated or suspected from the differential diagnosis list on the basis of such simple information. Specific features on the film may also help narrow down the differential diagnosis – the presence of central venous cannulae and airway intubation immediately indicates a seriously ill patient for example.

Examiners will often try to help you. For example, they may offer further information, affirm your suggestions or perhaps suggest you might like to reconsider something you have said. It is fairly safe to assume they are not trying to mislead you deliberately, so do not ignore their hints. If their hints lead you to reconsider previous statements as erroneous, do so graciously and honestly – you cannot fool them that you knew all along.

PRESENTING THE CASE
When presenting any radiological film in an exam or as a report in clinical practice, the approach should be the same. The Royal College of Radiology has given guidance on the required format that reports in the long cases/viva should take and this is as we have presented the cases in this book. After briefly looking at the film, present the:

Description
Relevant positive and negative radiological findings in a systematic manner, summarizing the findings at the end of the description.

Diagnosis
Try to identify relevant information in the history/patient data/radiological findings/other investigations which narrows the differential list down.

Differential diagnosis
Give a list of differentials for the findings.

Further management
Suggest further investigations to confirm the diagnosis or suggest further clinical management.

Obviously, the description is presented dynamically at the same time as evaluating the film and this requires some mental 'multitasking'. You can afford a brief pause when the case is presented to make an initial assessment, but after a few seconds, further silence does not create a good impression. Introductory statements such as 'This frontal chest radiograph of an adult male…' or 'this AP radiograph of the humerus in an unfused skeleton…' are not only appropriate, but also buy you another brief moment to think. In the initial stages of assessing an abnormality prior to reaching a conclusion, be careful not to use specific terminology that implies a specific diagnosis.

Even when you are completely unsure of what the abnormality is, it is still important to keep talking thus providing evidence that you continue to approach a film systematically and safely, even when you are uncertain. Summarizing your negative findings can often be as important as the positive ones and even if you remain oblivious to any abnormality after considered review of the case, verbally excluding acute life-threatening possibilities in your analysis shows, at the very least, a degree of safety in your practice.

Asking questions of the examiner to help interpret the film is usually acceptable, but only after you have made a considered assessment of the film and have either offered some thoughts or made it clear that you are merely seeking final confirmation of a particular possibility you have in mind. Asking questions early on, before you have made a systematic analysis of the case, however, only points to desperation.

The final stage of suggesting further investigation or management is vital in illustrating that you are a safe and valuable practitioner. If you have identified a life-threatening emergency on a film, statements such as 'I would contact the referring doctor immediately' are essential. Finally, when considering whether further investigation should be suggested, you may well note that the examiner already has a film ready to show you.

It is useful to practise ways of ending a case because there is danger in continuing to talk and talk about a case when you have already reached the limit of what you can interpret from it – it is all too easy to 'dig yourself into a hole' in this situation, making comments that appear indecisive. If you have already suggested a differential diagnosis, likely diagnosis and suggested further management options, you have naturally provided a conclusion – just make sure you look at the examiner when doing so to clearly make the point that you have finished.

If you are uncertain about what the film shows, it can be more difficult. However, if you have reached an impasse and cannot proceed any further, options available include presenting a summary of your observations, suggesting further investigations, asking for more information, etc. (always looking at the examiner).

General Introduction

GENERAL VIVA CONSIDERATIONS

- **Practice makes perfect.**
  Practice sessions in groups where you get to watch your colleagues being tested are particularly useful as you can learn much from their errors and successes. As well as honing your radiological skills, take note of irritating personal habits that might be better resolved before your real examination (e.g. fidgeting). Practise your descriptive findings for the classic exam-type cases so that you can dispatch these cases quickly and with confidence.

- **See as much material as possible.**
  Time spent looking through film libraries and radiological atlases will build up a knowledge base of classic exam-type cases, whilst time spent looking at endless 'everyday' studies not only fosters sensible 'real world' practice, but will also turn up pathology and build up your mental database of 'normal appearances'.

- **Don't give up.**
  Anxiety levels are high during examinations and can lead to foolish errors. However, never assume that a particular case has gone so badly that overall failure is inevitable. There are no doubt many candidates who have failed an exam, not because of the single case they thought they had failed, but because of the cases they failed thereafter because of this presumption and altered mental state. Every case is a new opportunity to demonstrate your ability, irrespective of how badly the previous case went.

- **Be thorough.**
  At the same time, however, it is advantageous to get through as many cases as you can. Thus, when you are presented with an 'Aunt Minnie' case of which you are confident, proceed quickly and confidently through it using your preprepared 'speech'.

- **Do not miss life-threatening or serious conditions.**
  Make sure you check for conditions such as a fracture and pneumothorax when you have failed to identify any other abnormality.

- **Be safe.**
  Most of all, show that you are safe and sensible in your practice.

Reference
1. Royal College of Radiology Guidance on Format of Reporting Session Reports for FRCR Part 2B; http://www.rcr.ac.uk/content.aspx?PageID=713

SUMMARY

Use the same structured format for reporting radiology cases, which consists of:

DESCRIPTION
Give your OBSERVATIONS on the films including relevant positive and negative findings and then give your INTERPRETATION of these findings.

DIAGNOSIS
Give the 'best fit' diagnosis for the image findings.

DIFFERENTIAL DIAGNOSIS
Give a limited number of possible differential diagnoses for the image findings.

FURTHER MANAGEMENT
Give suggestions for relevant further investigations and immediate management which need to be undertaken.

Chapter 1

CHEST IMAGING

The approach to plain chest radiographs and to chest CT scans is essentially the same and it requires a systematic approach to the images presented. A suggested approach to these images is presented here, though it is worth finding a systematic approach that works best for you, covering all of the important areas and that you find easy to remember. Ensure that whichever approach you take, it is well practised and well rehearsed, since it becomes rapidly obvious to examiners whether or not you have looked at and regularly reported this type of film before. As always, you should be able to modify the specific order in which you carry out your systematic analysis depending on the most apparent findings.

THE PLAIN CHEST RADIOGRAPH
Initial assessment
There are three vitally important things to do when first presented with a chest radiograph:

1. Make a quick mental note of any technical inadequacies that might influence further interpretation, e.g. suboptimal exposure, rotation. Remember that in an exam situation the examiner will have brought their best example of a given case, so although it is worth noting the flaws in the film, vocalizing these would not be advised unless they are significantly hampering your ability to make a diagnosis.

2. 'Unforgivable misses': there are a few conditions that you must simply never miss:
- Pneumothorax – in particular tension pneumothorax is a medical emergency requiring an immediate chest drain.
- Free gas under the diaphragm, indicating perforation of an abdominal viscus.

In real life the clinical history will often guide you to these, but in a viva, it is worth making a rapid exclusion of such conditions early on in your own mind before you become immersed in detailed evaluation and discussion of the case. Missing such serious abnormalities is unacceptable and only spotting them after several minutes of evaluation doesn't inspire confidence!

3. In a viva, you have about 10–15 seconds to make your initial evaluation before you need to start speaking – any information that can be gained about the patient's sex, age and ethnicity will be useful in making a diagnosis, so look for this information on the film.

Lines
Comment on the additional lines that you can see on the film – these may include ECG leads, oxygen tubing, NG tube, central venous catheters, chest drain and pacemakers/wires. These are important, first because you should assess that they are in the correct place and that their insertion has had no complications, e.g. ensure the NG tube is in the stomach, that there is no pneumothorax associated with the jugular central line. Secondly, identifying lines is important in assessing how unwell the patient is – your differential diagnosis is clearly going to be different if the chest radiograph is from an intubated ITU patient than if it is from an outpatient.

Lungs
First assess the chest to ensure that the general opacification in both lungs is the same – if not, then you need to determine which is the abnormally hyper or hypo transradiant lung and determine what the cause is. Mastectomy is one obvious cause that must not be missed as a history of breast cancer means the film must be checked carefully for evidence of metastatic spread.

Once you have decided what/where the abnormality is then describe the findings using a common vocabulary that is understood by all and which leaves no room for confusion. Accordingly, abnormalities can be described as:
- Focal or diffuse.
- Located in upper/middle/lower zones (avoids the difficulty of assessing lobes at the outset).
- Central or peripheral.
- Single or multiple.
- Exhibiting calcification or cavitation.

Broadly speaking lung abnormalities consist of:

Focal pulmonary lesion
You need to assess whether there are single or multiple lesions. Is there calcification? Is there cavitation? The differential diagnosis will depend on these patterns and useful information that will help you to narrow down the diagnosis can be sought from the examiner, such as a history of pyrexia, weight loss, haemoptysis, etc.

Diffuse pulmonary opacity
First, make a distinction between alveolar (airspace) and interstitial opacity. The former has a poorly defined, fluffy, cottonwool-like appearance, while the latter consists of reticular opacities, nodular opacities or a combination of both. The differential diagnosis will often be very different, as explained in subsequent cases in this chapter.

Chest Imaging

Hila
Assess the hila for position (left should be slightly higher than the right), shape (a V-shape made by the angle of the superior pulmonary artery and inferior pulmonary vein) and size.
- A change in the position of the hilum suggests volume loss. Accompanying interstitial opacity suggests fibrosis, whereas airspace opacity might suggest atelectasis, for which there are many causes, in particular obstructing masses.
- If there is change in the hilar angle or size then this would suggest a hilar mass such as enlarged nodes or central tumour.

Mediastinum
Comment on the heart size – is it enlarged or small? If there is any doubt from observation alone, state that you would like to formally measure it. Assess the mediastinal contour, including the cardiac contour itself and the great vessels. Ensure the trachea is central, that there is no pneumomediastinum or pneumopericardium. Large mediastinal masses will be readily evident but check that there is no loss of the paratracheal stripe due to smaller masses such as lymphadenopathy.

Pleura
Pleural lesions form an obtuse angle with the chest wall, as compared to a lung parenchymal lesion, which forms an acute angle. A differential list for pleural lesions should be easily brought to mind. Check for underlying rib destruction as a sign of a malignant nature. Always consider a pleural origin for opacities projected over the lungs but with unusual appearance, e.g. the typical 'holly leaf' pattern of pleural plaques.

Bones
Check the ribs, looking for:
- Lytic/sclerotic lesions to suggest metastases.
- Fractures – if present look for a pneumothorax or other signs of trauma. Certain fractures, such as those of the upper three ribs, suggest significant trauma and a high index of suspicion for other injuries is required.
- Rib resection from a previous thoracotomy.

Check the thoracic spine, not forgetting to pay attention to the paravertebral soft tissues that may point to underlying bony abnormalities. The cervical spine may be partly seen – look for a cervical rib.

Bony abnormalities around the shoulders present some favourite cases for vivas, so don't forget to check these areas towards the edge of the film!

Review areas
Everyone will have particular areas on certain investigations that they forget to evaluate well. These areas vary for each individual, but there are certain recurring patterns of missed abnormalities on the chest radiograph. So know your own perceptual 'blind spots'. In general, it is useful to check:
- Behind the heart – to look for a hidden mass or left lower lobe collapse.
- At the lung apices – is there a Pancoast tumour there?
- Beneath the diaphragm – is there free gas/splenomegaly/liver lesion?
- At the edges of the film – for a bone abnormality.

General tips
- Comparison with previous films is very useful in everyday practice. A solitary pulmonary nodule measuring 2 cm but not present on a film taken just a few months ago may well be neoplastic, whereas a stable appearance over many years makes this unlikely.
- Once you have described the film and given a differential diagnosis, only then ask for other studies or more clinical information if it will help narrow down the list of possibilities or aid management – it shows that you are able to make a differential list with no clinical information and then narrow this down in line with the clinical scenario. This is radiology in practice!

CT THORAX
Just as for the plain radiograph, one must systematically evaluate lungs, mediastinum, pleura, bones, peripheral soft tissues, etc. In doing so, it is of course important to utilize soft tissue, bone and lung 'windows' if available. Make a note of whether IV contrast has been given.

Lungs
Focal lesions may well be obvious but don't forget to check for more subtle abnormalities. Look carefully for interstitial abnormalities, paying particular attention to any relation to the secondary pulmonary lobule. Is the overall lung density normal and homogeneous? Poor inspiration will cause an artefactual increase in lung attenuation but will be evident by inward bowing of the posterior wall of the trachea. Don't forget to check the airways both large and small. Modern multidetector CT scans provide excellent visualization of the pulmonary vasculature when IV contrast is given – check for emboli.

Mediastinum
Check for normal patency and anatomy of great vessels, excluding aneurysm, dissection flaps, etc. Assess for abnormal lymphadenopathy. Assess heart for size, morphology, normal myocardial enhancement, filling defects, etc. Modern CT scans often demonstrate the proximal coronary arteries even without specific cardiac gating techniques. Don't forget to follow the superior mediastinum into the lower neck and supraclavicular fossae.

Pleura
Small pleural nodules and plaques can be easily missed if not specifically evaluated. Pneumothorax may well only be evident on lung windows.

Bones
Bone windows are essential. Multiplanar reformats made possible by multidetector CT scanners make assessment of the spine and ribs much easier than axial images alone.

Soft tissues and the 'periphery'
Just as with the chest radiograph, check the soft tissues of the chest wall, breast, neck, axillae and the upper abdomen on the lowest scans for hidden or incidental pathology.

CASE 1

History
A 34-year-old Caucasian male presented to his GP with a dry cough and shortness of breath for 3 months. He was otherwise fit and well.

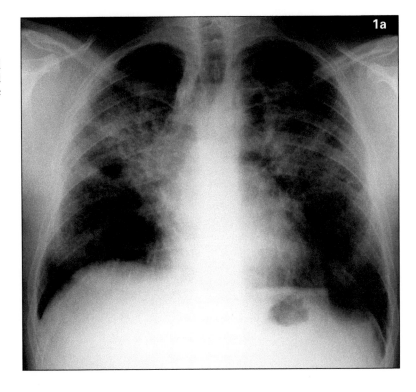

CASE 2

History
A 32-year-old Asian male presented with productive cough, shortness of breath and night sweats.

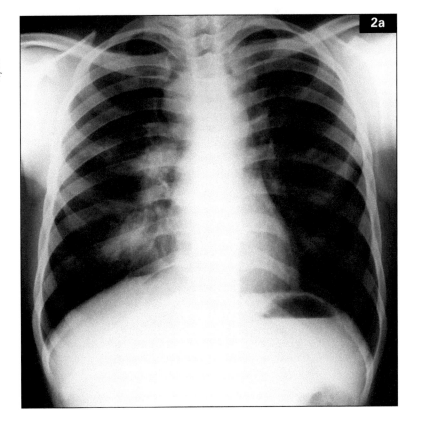

ANSWER 1

Observations (1a)
This chest radiograph shows bilateral reticulonodular shadowing predominantly affecting the mid and upper zones with sparing of the absolute apices. The nodules are small, ~3–4 mm in diameter, and appear ill defined, and form confluent airspace opacities centrally. There is hilar enlargement more obvious on the right, and also widening of the right paratracheal soft tissues due to lymphadenopathy. Given the clinical details, sarcoidosis is the most likely diagnosis.

Diagnosis
Pulmonary sarcoidosis.

Differential diagnosis
For hilar node egg shell calcification:
- Sarcoid.
- Silicosis.
- Lymphoma following radiotherapy.

For bilateral hilar enlargement:
- Sarcoid.
- Lymphoma.
- TB.

For perilymphatic nodules:
- Sarcoid.
- Silicosis.
- Coal worker's pneumoconiosis (CWP).
- Lymphangitis carcinomatosa.
- Lymphoma.

Discussion
Sarcoidosis is a systemic disorder characterized by the presence of noncaseating granulomas within several organs. It most commonly presents in young adults in the 3rd–5th decades, and is more common in women and in black populations. Multisystem involvement can result in uveitis, bilateral parotid enlargement, erythema nodosum, lupus pernio, arthralgia, heart block, cardiomyopathy and bony changes most commonly seen in the phalanges.

Radiological features of pulmonary sarcoidosis are as follows:
- Lymphadenopathy (70–80%) is characterized by bilateral, symmetrical hilar lymph node enlargement and paratracheal lymphadenopathy. Egg shell calcification of the nodes (1b) is seen in ~5% of patients. Lymphadenopathy without pulmonary changes has a more favourable outcome. Figure 1c shows bilateral hilar lymphadenopathy with no parenchymal disease.
- The most common form of parenchymal change is multiple small pulmonary nodules within the mid and upper zones of both lungs – the distribution described in this case is classical. Presentation with larger nodules measuring 1–5 cm, possibly with central cavitation and calcification, account for ~5% of cases. Airspace opacities are seen in 2–10%.
- End stage disease results in upper zone fibrosis with associated traction bronchiectasis.

- Chest radiograph changes have been classified from 0–4 as follows:
  Stage 0 – Normal film.
  Stage 1 – Lymphadenopathy only.
  Stage 2 – Lymphadenopathy and pulmonary infiltrate.
  Stage 3 – Pulmonary changes without adenopathy.
  Stage 4 – Pulmonary fibrosis.

Diagnosis is usually confirmed by HRCT of the thorax. The classical finding is of very small pulmonary nodules

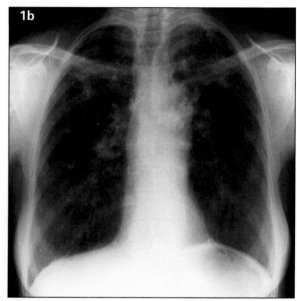

1b Chest radiograph shows bilateral hilar enlargement with hilar lymph node egg shell calcification.

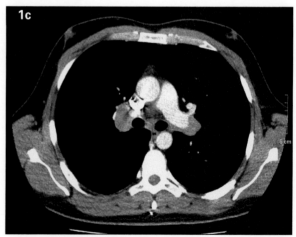

1c Axial CT image shows bilateral hilar lymphadenopathy.

distributed in a perilymphatic manner, i.e. along the bronchovascular bundles, the interlobular septae and subpleural region (**1d**).

Practical tips
- Whenever there is evidence of adenopathy and abnormal pulmonary opacities, always consider sarcoidosis in the differential diagnosis.
- The features described above are largely the classical appearances. However, sarcoid can have almost any appearance on a chest radiograph, so be wary of categorically dismissing the diagnosis when the chest film shows abnormal pulmonary parenchyma. Conversely, it will often be a reasonable condition to list in the differential diagnoses because of its protean appearances.
- HRCT is very useful for further evaluation. Look for nodularity along the bronchovascular bundles, interlobular septae and pleura. Pleural nodularity due to subpleural lymphatic spread is often easiest to appreciate at the interlobar fissures where multiple layers of pleura make the changes more apparent.

Further management
- Gallium scanning is now rarely used in diagnosing the condition and in assessing disease activity. Recognized patterns of activity include the 'lamda' sign (paratracheal and bilateral hilar uptake) and the 'panda' sign (uptake in the parotid, salivary and lacrimal glands gives appearance of a panda face).
- Elevated serum angiotensin converting enzyme (SACE) levels may provide further supportive evidence of the diagnosis and the degree of disease activity.

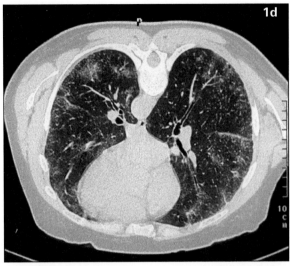

1d HRCT axial image demonstrates multiple nodules distributed along the bronchovascular bundles and subpleural regions with nodular thickening of the interlobular septum.

ANSWER 2

Observations (2a)
The chest radiograph shows consolidation in the medial segment of the right middle lobe. There are right hilar and right paratracheal nodular, soft tissue density opacities consistent with lymphadenopathy. No pleural effusions are seen.

Given the clinical details and radiological appearances, pulmonary TB is most likely.

Diagnosis
Primary tuberculosis (TB).

Differential diagnosis
For consolidation and lymphadenopathy:
- TB.
- Sarcoid.
- Lymphoma.
- Other infective organisms: histoplasmosis, mycoplasma, varicella.

Discussion
Although primary TB usually presents in children, there is now increasing incidence in adults. Primary TB now accounts for 23–34% of all adult cases of TB.

Unlike post-primary pulmonary TB that usually manifests in the upper lobes, primary TB affects lower lobes, middle lobes and anterior segment of the upper lobes. Presentation is with:
- Parenchymal airspace consolidation.
- Lymphadenopathy – the patterns of distribution are usually unilateral hilar +/– right paratracheal lymphadenopathy or isolated right paratracheal lymphadenopathy. Bilateral lymphadenopathy is unusual and when it does occur, is usually asymmetric.
- Miliary tuberculosis.
- Pleural effusion – seen in 23–38%.
- Tuberculoma.

(*cont.*)

Complications of TB include:
- Progressive primary TB – due to a failed immune response with subsequent disease progression.
- Miliary TB – massive haematogenous dissemination.
- Post-primary/reactive TB – presents in adults, with reactivation of dormant organisms after several asymptomatic years. Usually the apical and posterior segments of the upper lobes are involved (85–95%), the superior segment of the lower lobes being less commonly affected. Radiological presentation is with cavitation, fibrosis, empyema, miliary TB, tuberculoma, mycetoma. Adenopathy is not a major feature.

HRCT can be useful for further evaluation and TB presents with nodules in a centrilobular distribution due to endobronchial spread. This gives a 'tree in bud' appearance. The differential diagnosis for centrilobular nodules includes TB, endobronchial metastases, allergic bronchopulmonary aspergillosis (ABPA), obliterative bronchiolitis and hypersensitivity pneumonitis. Figures **2b** and **2c** show axial CT images demonstrating multiple poorly defined centrilobular nodules giving a 'tree in bud' appearance in a young male Asian patient with TB. Note that there is sparing of the subpleural areas with no nodules seen within 5 mm of the pleural surfaces or fissures.

Practical tips
TB is a multisystem disorder with haematogenous spread to multiple other sites. On a chest radiograph look for TB discitis and TB affecting shoulder joints. The most commonly affected joint is the hip with features of monoarticular involvement. Radiographic changes of loss of joint space, peripheral bone erosions and juxta-articular osteoporosis are seen, which can lead to ankylosis of the joint and limb shortening (**2d**).

Further management
Respiratory referral with a view to sputum cytology/bronchoscopy to identify the acid fast bacilli.

Further reading
Harisinghani MG, McLoud TC, Shepard JO, *et al.* (2000). Tuberculosis from head to toe. *RadioGraphics* **20**: 449–470.

Kim HY, Song KS, Goo JM, *et al.* (2001). Thoracic sequelae and complications of tuberculosis. *RadioGraphics* **21**: 839–858.

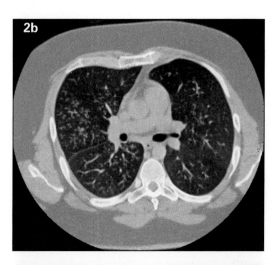

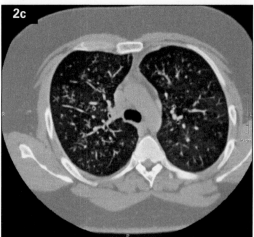

2b, 2c Axial CT images of the chest showing widespread centrilobular nodules giving a 'tree in bud' appearance.

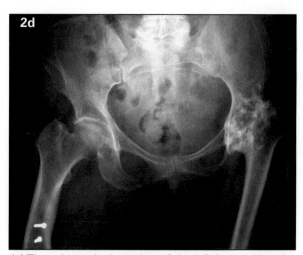

2d There is marked erosion of the left femoral head with ankylosis of the hip joint. Marked limb shortening is the consequence.

CASE 3

History
A 65-year-old male presented with progressive dyspnoea and weight loss.

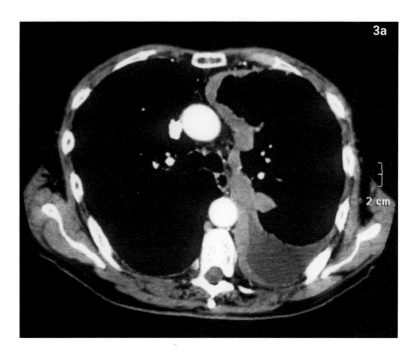

CASE 4

History
A 68-year-old male presented with haemoptysis.

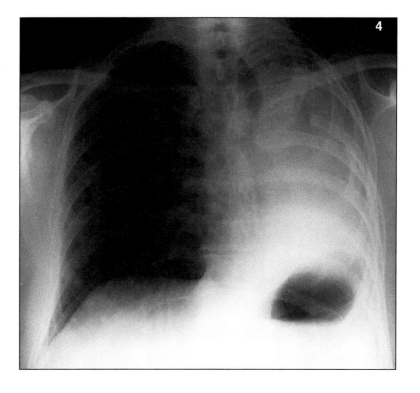

ANSWER 3

Observations (3a)
CT image of the thorax shows diffuse, irregular and nodular pleural thickening in the left hemithorax. This measures upwards of 1 cm in thickness and also involves mediastinal pleura. No focal intraparenchymal pulmonary abnormality is seen on these soft tissue window settings and there is no visible mediastinal mass. Taken together with the clinical history, the features are suspicious of mesothelioma, though metastases cannot be excluded. With regard to the former, the rest of the CT scan should be examined for features of asbestos-related pleural disease and asbestosis. An occupational history should also be taken.

Diagnosis
Malignant mesothelioma.

Differential diagnosis
For diffuse pleural thickening:
- Malignant mesothelioma.
- Pleural metastases – usually from adenocarcinoma primary, e.g. breast, lung.
- Empyema.
- Pleural fibrosis from infection – tuberculosis, fungal.

Discussion
Malignant mesothelioma is a rare primary tumour of the pleura, seen more commonly in men, with a peak incidence in the 7th–8th decades. Aetiology is strongly associated with asbestos exposure, and underlying lung changes from asbestos are often seen in association. Between 5 and 10% of asbestos workers will develop mesothelioma with a latent period of up to 45 years. The parietal pleura is usually involved and spread is locally to the chest wall, mediastinum, diaphragm and peritoneum; there is lymphatic spread to the hilar and mediastinal nodes and haematologically to lungs, liver and adrenals. Unilateral pleural effusion is commonly seen, but with no mediastinal shift due to the tumour creating a 'fixed' or 'frozen' hemithorax.

Prognosis is poor, with life expectancy of 12 months after diagnosis. Treatment including radiotherapy, chemotherapy and radical surgical pleurectomy produces universally poor results.

Practical tips
- Pleural thickening involving the mediastinal pleura is a very good sign for mesothelioma.
- Bilateral, calcified pleural plaques are characteristic of asbestos exposure. (Figure **3b** is a single axial CT image showing calcified pleural plaques, which are characteristic of asbestos exposure.) When identified, examine the CT closely for evidence of asbestosis as this may have greater immediate implications for the patient in terms of morbidity (and in the UK at least, financial compensation).

Further management
- Pleural biopsy is required to confirm the diagnosis and to differentiate mesothelioma from pleural metastatic disease, which can show some response to chemotherapy.
- Discussion within a lung cancer multidisciplinary team is required.
- A detailed occupational history needs to be taken since asbestos-related disease may entitle the sufferer to compensation.

Further reading
Wang ZJ, Reddy GP, Gotway MB, *et al.* (2004). Malignant pleural mesothelioma: evaluation with CT, MR imaging, and PET. *RadioGraphics* **24**: 105–119.

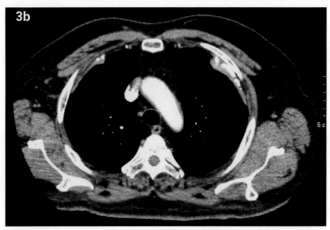

3b Axial CT image shows bilateral anterior calcified pleural plaques characteristic of previous asbestos exposure.

ANSWER 4

Observations (4)
This chest radiograph shows complete opacification of the left hemithorax with mediastinal shift to the left as evidenced by the displaced trachea and elevated left hemidiaphragm. There is a defect in the posterior aspect of the left 5th rib in keeping with a previous thoracotomy and presumed left pneumonectomy. In the right lung, there are multiple small miliary nodules seen throughout the lung. With evidence of previous pneumonectomy, these most likely represent miliary metastases from a previously resected bronchogenic tumour.

Diagnosis
Miliary metastases from previous bronchogenic carcinoma.

Differential diagnosis
For miliary nodules:
- Miliary metastases.
- TB.
- Sarcoid.
- Chronic extrinsic allergic alveolitis.
- Coal worker's pneumoconiosis (CWP).
- Histoplasmosis.

Of a completely opaque hemithorax:
- Total lung collapse.
- Pneumonectomy – looks like total collapse but there will be evidence of thoracotomy.
- Huge pleural effusion – volume expansion rather than volume loss, i.e. the mediastinum will be displaced away from the side of opacity.

Discussion
Thyroid cancer is classically described as a primary carcinoma likely to produce miliary metastases (others include melanoma and sarcoma). However, breast and lung cancer can less typically produce this pattern, but because they are more prevalent, may well be seen more often.

Practical tips
- This fairly straightforward case illustrates how films used to test candidates in postgraduate exams will often require 'piecing together of the pieces' rather than being presented with miliary shadowing alone and being asked for a differential.
- As always, look for other clues on the film. A primary malignancy may be evident as a mastectomy, a thyroid mass in the neck, a bony sarcoma on the edge of the film or signs of previous lung cancer, as in this case.
- Check the patient data for likely ethnicity to help predict likelihood of TB.

Further management
- Comparison with previous chest radiographs to look for new features is very useful and should be done in both clinical and exam situations.
- A chest CT will characterize these changes in greater detail.

CASE 5

History
A 40-year-old male presented with haemoptysis and renal impairment.

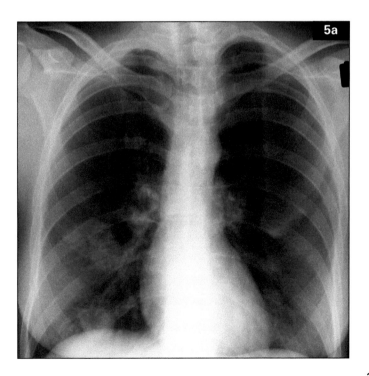

ANSWER 5

Observations (5a)
This frontal chest radiograph shows multiple relatively thick walled cavitating nodules throughout both lungs. Mediastinal contours are normal with no evidence on the film of hilar or mediastinal lymphadenopathy. No pleural effusion can be seen. Appearance of the shoulder joints and the lateral ends of the clavicles is normal.

Diagnosis
Wegener's granulomatosis.

Differential diagnosis
For multiple cavitating lung nodules:
- Neoplasia: metastases – in particular, squamous cell, sarcoma, melanoma and colorectal tumours.
- Infection: bacterial septic emboli, TB, aspergillosis and other fungal organisms.
- Collagen vascular disease: Wegener's granulomatosis, rheumatoid nodules.
- Granulomatous disease: histiocytosis X and sarcoidosis.
- Vascular: pulmonary emboli with infarction.

Discussion
This is a systemic condition characterized by necrotizing granulomata and a necrotizing vasculitis affecting medium to small vessels. Pulmonary Wegener's granulomatosis has a variety of presentations, which include:
- Widespread nodules that typically cavitate, have varying sizes (up to several centimetres) and show no zonal predilection. Figure 5b is a single axial CT image showing left lower lobe pulmonary nodules that are relatively thick walled and some of which are demonstrating cavitation. A coronal reformat of the same patient is also shown (5c).
- Patchy alveolar infiltrates/consolidation/'ground glass' opacity.
- Lymphadenopathy is a rare feature.
- Pleural effusions can be seen.

Upper respiratory tract involvement is always seen in Wegener's and features include destruction of nasal cartilage and bone, nasal mucosal ulceration, paranasal sinus mucous membrane thickening, tracheal inflammation and sclerosis resulting in stridor.

Other organ features include: glomerulonephritis, migratory polyarthropathy and skin nodules.

Practical tips
- There is a long differential for cavitating lung nodules so look for clues on the film to point towards an underlying diagnosis and also be guided by the history. Check the bones for evidence of rheumatoid arthritis and primary/secondary bone malignant lesions.
- A history of haemoptysis and renal impairment with pulmonary abnormalities on the chest radiograph brings to mind the diagnoses of Wegener's granulomatosis and Goodpasture's syndrome. Renal failure causing fluid overload may also result in pulmonary oedema that may be blood tinged.

Further management
Initial management should be referral to a respiratory physician to exclude malignant/infective causes for cavitating nodules.

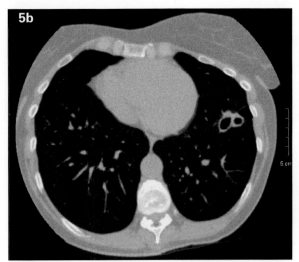

5b Axial CT image showing two thick walled nodules in the left lower lobe consistent with but not specific for Wegener's granulomatosis.

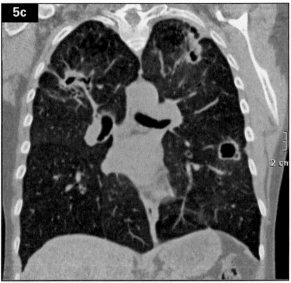

5c Coronal reformatted CT image showing bilateral cavitating nodules.

CASE 6

History
A 45-year-old female presented with progressive dyspnoea and an inflammatory arthropathy.

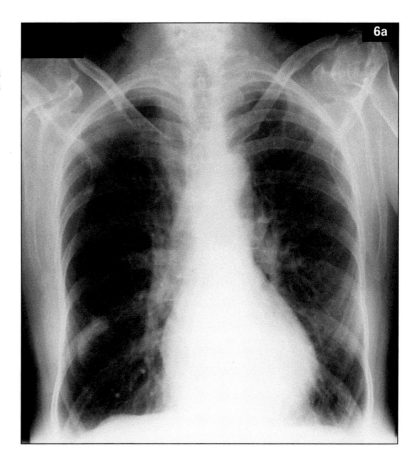

CASE 7

History
A 70-year-old factory worker presented with progressive dyspnoea.

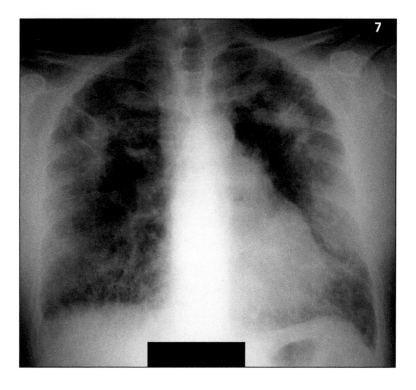

ANSWER 6

Observations (6a)
This frontal chest radiograph demonstrates a well defined pulmonary nodule in the right lower zone. This appears to be a solitary lesion. Arthropathy is noted at the left shoulder joint with associated erosion of the lateral end of the clavicle – this suggests background rheumatoid arthritis. The nodule is therefore likely to be a rheumatoid pulmonary nodule, though other pathology such as a malignant nodule cannot be excluded and follow-up is therefore required. There is no evidence of pulmonary fibrosis.

Diagnosis
Rheumatoid lung.

Differential diagnosis
For lateral end of clavicle erosion:
- Arthropathies – rheumatoid arthritis, gout, scleroderma.
- Hyperparathyroidism.
- Post-traumatic osteolysis (6b).
- Infection – osteomyelitis.
- Neoplastic conditions – myeloma, metastases.
- Hereditary disorders – cleidocranial dysostosis, pyknodysostosis, Holt–Oram syndrome.

Discussion
Rheumatoid lung manifestations can be seen in up to 50% of RA patients. The lung changes are more commonly found in men. CXR features of RA include:
- Interstitial fibrosis that predominantly affects the lower zones.
- Rheumatoid lung nodules – these are usually multiple, and commonly located in the lung periphery or pleurally based. They often cavitate but don't calcify.
- Pleural effusion – usually this is a unilateral exudate. More common in men.

Caplan's syndrome is a condition characterized by pneumoconiosis and RA in coal workers.

Practical tips
- Look for associated bone abnormalities if rheumatoid is suspected, e.g. resorption of the lateral ends of clavicles, erosion of the acromioclavicular, sternoclavicular and shoulder joints.
- Look for effects of drugs used to treat rheumatoid, e.g. steroid use resulting in avascular necrosis (AVN) of the humeral head or vertebral collapse.

Further management
Follow-up of single pulmonary nodules is advised to ensure that the nodule is not a developing primary bronchogenic carcinoma. Fleischner Society guidelines (*Table 1*) suggest dividing patients into high-risk (smokers and other risk factors) and low-risk categories and then organizing subsequent follow-up depending on the size of the nodule.

Further reading
MacMahon H, Austin J, Gamsu G (2005). Guidelines for management of small pulmonary nodules detected on CT scans: a statement from the Fleischner Society. *Radiology* **237**: 395–400.

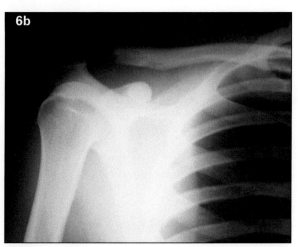

6b Radiograph demonstrates erosion of the lateral edge of the right clavicle following an injury 2 years previously.

Table 1 *Follow-up guidelines for pulmonary nodules*

Nodule size (mm)	Low risk	High risk
<4	No follow-up	CT at 12 months, nil further if unchanged
4–6	CT at 12 months, nil further if unchanged	CT at 6–12 months, then 18–24 months if unchanged
6–8	CT at 6–12 months, then 18–24 months if unchanged	CT at 6 months, then 9–12 months and then 24 months if unchanged
>8	CT at 3, 9 and 24 months +/– PET CT and biopsy	CT at 3, 9 and 24 months +/– PET CT and biopsy

ANSWER 7

Observations (7)
There is widespread abnormal interstitial opacity throughout both lungs with no zonal predominance. This is predominantly of tiny nodules with some reticulation. Poorly defined heart border and hemidiaphragms indicate subpleural involvement. There are large, poorly defined conglomerate masses in both upper zones with surrounding fibrotic changes. These findings are in keeping with progressive massive fibrosis in a patient with underlying pneumoconiosis.

Diagnosis
Progressive massive fibrosis (PMF).

Differential diagnosis
For mass lesion with background pneumoconiosis:
- PMF.
- Bronchogenic carcinoma (increased incidence of adenocarcinoma in scarred lung).
- Granuloma (TB, histoplasmosis).
- Caplan's syndrome (rheumatoid nodules in those with coexisting rheumatoid).
- Any other parenchymal lesion can incidentally co-occur.

Discussion
Pneumoconiosis is a parenchymal lung reaction to chronic inorganic dust exposure. Some typical appearances on chest radiography are:

- Small nodules – silicosis, siderosis, coal worker's pneumoconiosis (CWP).
- Reticulations – asbestosis.
- Reticulonodular opacities – carbon/petroleum products.
- Interstitial pneumonia – cobalt, titanium, nickel, chromium exposure.

Progressive massive fibrosis arises as a consequence of pneumoconiosis and can develop and progress even after dust exposure has ceased. Radiologically, presentation is with large opacities in the mid/upper zones since they usually involve the posterior segment of the upper lobe and superior segment of the lower lobes. Lesions are initially seen in the lung peripheries and extend towards the hila over time. Cavitation and calcification can occur. Cavitation can then lead to secondary infection with *Aspergillus*.

Practical tips
When mass lesions appear in patients with background pneumoconiosis, remember that this may be PMF but that they are also at increased risk of adenocarcinoma.

Further management
CT chest is usually required for further characterization and it is often difficult to definitively differentiate this from bronchogenic carcinoma. In these cases, review within a lung cancer multidisciplinary team setting is required with a view to percutaneous lung biopsy.

CASE 8

History
A 30-year-old male presented with haemoptysis and shoulder pain.

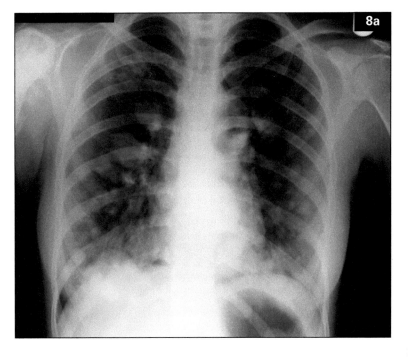

ANSWER 8

Observations (8a)
There are several well defined soft tissue density nodules throughout both lungs with no zonal predominance. The right humerus is seen on the edge of the film and is abnormal in appearance with mottled sclerotic density and apparent periosteal reaction. Further imaging of it is required but the suspicion from this film must be of a sarcoma of the right humerus with associated pulmonary metastases.

Diagnosis
Lung metastases with underlying osteosarcoma.

Differential diagnosis
For multiple lung nodules:
- Neoplastic:
  - Malignant – metastases.
  - Benign – arteriovenous malformation (AVM).

- Infectious:
  - Granulomas – TB, histoplasmosis, coccidioidomycosis, cryptococcus.
  - Abscesses.
  - Septic emboli.

- Noninfectious:
  - Wegener's granulomatosis.
  - Rheumatoid arthritis (RA).

- Infarcts.
- Sarcoid.
- Amyloid.

Discussion
An AP view of the proximal right humerus from this patient is shown (**8b**). It demonstrates a pathological fracture of the right upper diaphysis with a poorly defined underlying lesion involving the metadiaphysis. This has a wide zone of transition with lytic mottled areas and sclerosis. Periosteal reaction is evident and appearances most likely indicate an osteosarcoma.

Metastases to the lung are common and are seen in up to 30% of all patients with malignancy. Common primary tumours are breast, prostate, colon, renal cell carcinoma, melanoma and osteogenic sarcoma. Some clue to the underlying primary can be suspected from the appearances of the metastatic lesion. Squamous cell carcinomas, colon, melanoma, osteosarcoma and cervix metastases are more likely to cavitate. Breast, thyroid, osteosarcoma, testes and ovarian metastases are more likely to calcify. Metastases are commonly multiple and are found in a subpleural location.

Practical tips
- Carefully check that the nodules are truly pulmonary. If no nodules project outside a region of lung covered by ribs, could they be bony? Do nodules extend into the subcutaneous tissues? Figure **8c** shows multiple skin nodules in neurofibromatosis masquerading as pulmonary nodules!

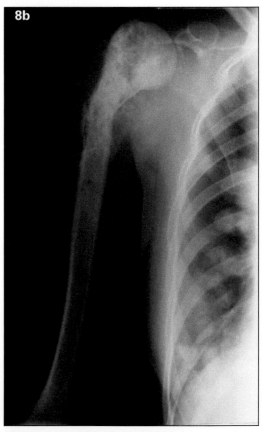

8b AP view of the proximal right humerus from this patient showing a poorly defined lesion in the metadiaphysis of the right humerus with a wide zone of transition, lytic and sclerotic areas. Periosteal reaction is also seen. This is likely to be an osteosarcoma.

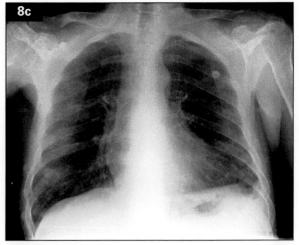

8c Chest radiograph of a patient with neurofibromatosis type 1 with multiple skin nodules.

Answer 8

- Look carefully at the film for a primary malignancy (as in this case) and also metastases elsewhere, such as bone deposits or calcified liver deposits under the right hemidiaphragm.
- Look for cavitation and/or calcification in the nodules to point towards underlying primary/diagnosis.

Further management
- CT chest can identify further nodules and can help to characterize them, i.e. looking for central necrosis, fat, calcification, cavitation.
- Where a primary malignancy cannot be identified then percutaneous biopsy or a surgical video-assisted thorascopic surgery (VATS) procedure can obtain tissue from a nodule for histological characterization.

Further reading
Winer-Muram HT (2006). The solitary pulmonary nodule. *Radiology* **239**: 34–49.

CASE 9

History
A 45-year-old male smoker presented with a cough.

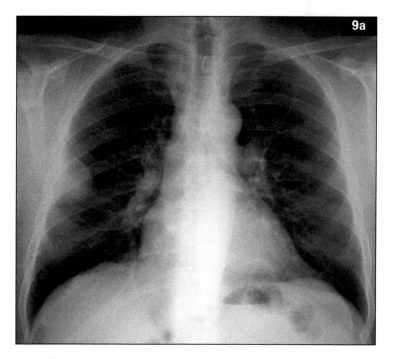

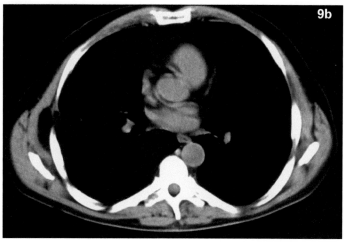

ANSWER 9

Observations (9a, 9b)
PA chest radiograph (**9a**) shows a well defined lesion in the periphery of the right lung forming an obtuse angle with the chest wall. This is consistent with a pleurally based lesion. The single axial image from a CT thorax examination (**9b**) shows a lucent lesion of fat density that extends through the chest wall to a subpleural location.

Diagnosis
Chest wall lipoma.

Differential diagnosis
For pleural lesions:
- Metastasis – lung and breast are the most common primaries, with other adenocarcinomas such as ovary, uterus, pancreas.
- Pleural plaques.
- Loculated pleural effusion.
- Haematoma.
- Lipoma.
- Neurofibroma/schwannoma.
- Rib lesions such as tumour or even healing fracture can be hard to differentiate from pleural lesions. (Figure **9c** is an axial CT image showing a rib-based lesion causing complete destruction of the posterior right 8th rib. The patient had myeloma and appearances are those of a plasmacytoma.)

Discussion
Imaging features on a plain radiograph can usually be used with a good degree of confidence to differentiate pleural lesions from a lung parenchymal lesion.

Important differentiating features that point to a pleural location include:
- Obtuse angle with the chest wall.
- Smooth tapering edges.
- Peripheral location.

Practical tips
- When a pleural soft tissue mass is identified, carefully check the film for supporting evidence of background malignancy.
- An underlying rib fracture points to a subpleural haematoma.
- US can be helpful with the differentiation by determining whether the pleural lesion is fluid or solid.

Further management
No further treatment required for this benign lesion.

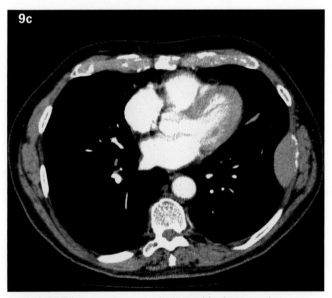

9c Axial CT image shows a rib-based lesion causing complete destruction of the posterior right 8th rib.

CASE 10

History
A 76-year-old male presented with chest pain.

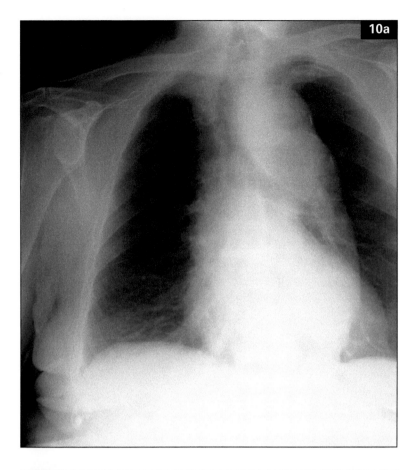

CASE 11

History
A 67-year-old male presented with shortness of breath.

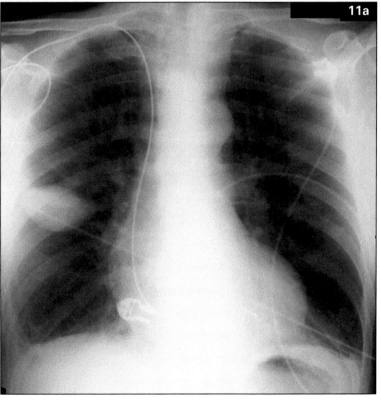

ANSWER 10

Observations (10a)
This AP chest radiograph demonstrates a large mediastinal mass on the left. The arch of the aorta and proximal descending aorta are not seen separate from this mass, which indicates that it arises from the posterior mediastinum. There is curvilinear calcification in the lateral aspect of this mass, which would suggest that the lesion is in fact a dilated aneurysmal thoracic aorta. Comparison with old films would be useful to assess any change.

Diagnosis
Thoracic aortic aneurysm.

Differential diagnosis
Of posterior mediastinal mass:
- Thoracic aortic aneurysm.
- Dilated oesophagus.
- Hernia – hiatus, Bochdalek's.
- Neurogenic tumour – neurofibroma, schwannoma, ganglioneuroma.
- Spinal abscess.
- Extramedullary haematopoiesis.

Of anterior mediastinal mass:
- Thymoma.
- Teratoma.
- Thyroid enlargement with retrosternal extension.
- Lymphoma.

Of middle mediastinal mass:
- Lymph nodes.
- Bronchogenic/duplication cyst.
- Ascending aortic aneurysm.
- Carcinoma of bronchus/trachea.

Discussion
An axial CT image (**10b**) of the chest with IV contrast shows the descending aortic aneurysm. Typical radiological appearances are of a mediastinal mass – the wide tortuous aorta with peripheral curvilinear calcification. Normal CT measurements for the thoracic aorta are <3.5 cm diameter for the ascending aorta and <2.5 cm for the thoracic descending aorta. Surgical repair is considered over 6 cm. In the acute situation, where no old films are available, differentiation from an acute aortic dissection may be necessary. In acute aortic dissection there can be widening of the mediastinum, an irregular fuzzy appearance to the aortic outline and displacement of calcification with additional soft tissue identified lateral to calcification (due to false channel formation).

Characterizing the position of mediastinal masses is useful on plain radiography in order to narrow the differential diagnosis:
- Posterior mediastinum is the space between the posterior aspect of the heart and the thoracic spine, and contains descending aorta, oesophagus, azygous veins and thoracic duct.
- Middle mediastinal space contains heart and great vessels.
- Anterior mediastinal space is from the anterior aspect of the heart to the sternum, and contains thymus and lymph nodes.

Knowing the contents of each space and applying the silhouette sign allows for better identification of what a mediastinal mass may be. For example, in Figure **10c** there is a large, well defined, round mediastinal mass related to the left heart border. The left heart border can be clearly seen, therefore the mass cannot be within the middle mediastinum. Although slightly difficult to assess the region behind the heart, no clear separation can be made between the rounded lesion and the descending aorta, suggesting that the lesion is a posterior mediastinal mass. This is confirmed by the lateral film (**10d**) in the same patient and the lesion was proved to be a neurofibroma.

Practical tips
Lateral films can be very useful in better localizing mediastinal masses.

Further management
If there is clinical concern then CT is usually the next investigation of choice.

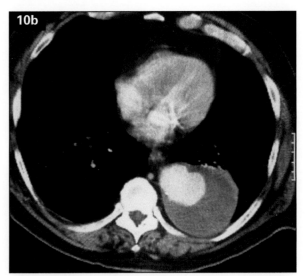

10b Axial CT image of a large descending thoracic aortic aneurysm with marked thrombus.

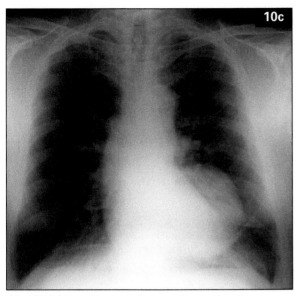 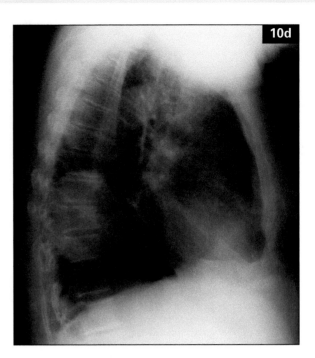

10c, 10d AP and lateral chest radiographs show a posterior mediastinal mass.

ANSWER 11

Observations (11a)
This PA chest radiograph shows a very well defined 5 cm soft tissue density lesion in the right mid zone, in the region of the horizontal fissure. The heart is enlarged with cardiothoracic ratio of 16:26. There is upper zone venous congestion and a slight increase in interstitial opacity. These appearances are in keeping with left heart failure and the right sided opacity could therefore indicate localized pleural fluid in the oblique fissure. Comparison with any recent films or, alternatively, a follow-up film after treatment should confirm resolution of the opacity.

Diagnosis
Pleural pseudotumour.

Differential diagnosis
For solitary lung nodule/mass:
- Neoplastic:
  - Malignant – primary bronchogenic carcinoma, solitary metastasis.
  - Benign – hamartoma, adenoma, arteriovenous malformation (AVM).
- Infectious:
  - Granuloma – TB, histoplasmosis, coccidioidomycosis, cryptococcus.
  - Abscess.
  - Septic embolus.
- Non-infectious:
  - Wegener's granulomatosis.
  - Rheumatoid arthritis (RA).
  - Infarct.
  - Sarcoid.
  - Amyloid.
- Congenital:
  - Bronchogenic cyst.
  - Sequestration.
- Extrapulmonary:
  - Pleural mass/fluid.
  - Rib fracture/lesion.
  - Subcutaneous lesion.
  - External artefact.

Discussion
This is focal accumulation of fluid in the interlobar fissure and is identified on the chest radiograph as having very well defined inferior borders. There are often other features of pleural fluid elsewhere, or features to indicate background pathology such as heart failure that has led to pleural fluid accumulation. The main importance of such a condition is that there is potential to misinterpret it as a focal pulmonary nodule/mass.

(*cont.*)

Answer 11 — Chest Imaging

Practical tips
- Important features in differentiating solitary lesions include:
  - Growth rate – lesions that don't change in size over a period of 2 years can be considered benign. Tumour doubling times (time taken for volume of nodule to increase twofold) have been reported between 1 and 18 months.
  - Margins – irregularity, lobulation and spiculation of the lesion's edge are a good indicator of malignancy. However, 30% of lesions with smooth margins are not benign – usually representing metastases.
  - Presence of fat – this is usually a sure sign of benignity and suggests the diagnosis of a hamartoma. Very occasionally renal cell carcinoma and liposarcoma metastases can also contain fat.
  - Calcification – this is seen in both benign and malignant conditions. Benign lesions usually have calcification with a central nidus, laminated or popcorn appearance. Calcification in malignant lesions usually appears stippled, amorphous or diffuse. Stippled calcification is seen in mucin secreting tumour metastases, e.g. colon, ovary.
  - Cavitation – again this is seen in both benign and malignant lesions. Irregular thick walled cavities are more likely to be malignant than thin, smooth walled ones.
- When an apparent pulmonary opacity has an unusual shape or density, always stop and ask 'could it be in the pleura, chest wall, soft tissue or even external to the patient?' Figure **11b**, for example, shows a very sharply defined calcific density opacity in the right lower zone. It is difficult to imagine what pulmonary pathology this might represent and it is actually a calcified breast fibroadenoma.

Further management
Lateral CXR can be helpful in these cases and if there is still concern then CT chest will usually resolve the issue. (See Case 6, *Table 1* for further management of single pulmonary nodule.)

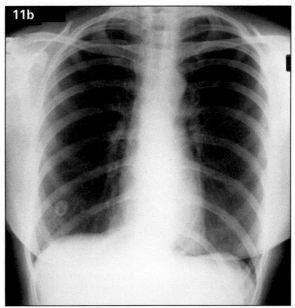

11b Chest radiograph shows a very well defined calcific density in the right lower zone, which actually represents a calcified breast fibroadenoma.

CASE 12

History
A 69-year-old male smoker with ischaemic heart disease, presented with increasing dyspnoea over the last 2 months.

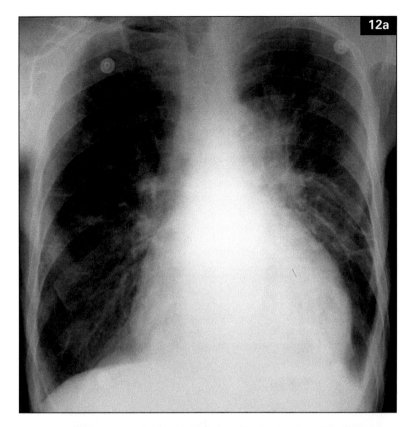

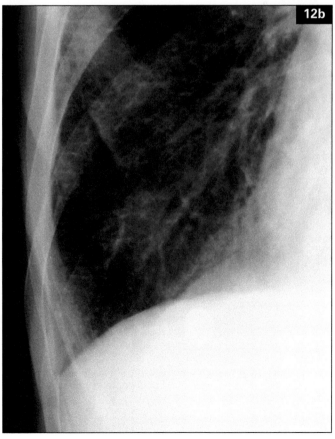

ANSWER 12

Observations (12a, 12b)
The heart looks enlarged but as this is an AP radiograph, it is not possible to be sure. There is a diffuse, bilateral increase in reticular interstitial opacity with Kerley B lines in the right lower zone best seen on the close-up (**12b**). The left hilum is enlarged, and there is a pulmonary nodule in the left upper zone measuring approximately 1.5 cm. A tiny left pleural reaction is also noted.

The most likely explanation is that the patient has a left upper lobe tumour with left hilar adenopathy and lymphangitis carcinomatosa. However, given the history of heart disease and the rather subjective cardiomegaly, it is possible that he could have lung cancer and coexisting left heart failure. A repeat film after treatment for heart failure might help clarify, but he is likely to need staging of the suspected tumour with CT anyway, and this may answer the question.

Diagnosis
Left upper lobe tumour with lymphangitis carcinomatosa.

Differential diagnosis
For tumours causing lymphangitis (anatomically from top down):
- Larynx.
- Thyroid.
- Breast.
- Stomach.
- Pancreas.
- Colon.
- Cervix.

For septal (Kerley B) lines:
- Pulmonary venous hypertension.
- Lymphangitis.

Many other conditions can show septal lines, though the two conditions above rank far above these. Examples include: sarcoid, any chronic fibrosing lung condition, lymphangiectasia, lymphangiomyomatosis, lymphoma and viral pneumonia.

For subpleural nodules:
- Sarcoid.
- Lymphangitis carcinomatosa.
- Silicosis.
- Lymphoma.

Discussion
Certain tumours show a propensity to invade the lung interstitium, both the connective tissue and the lymphatics. Lymphatics become distended by the tumour itself, and also because of congestion resulting from tumour obstruction. Symptoms include dyspnoea and cough.

Plain film signs are of increased reticular/reticulonodular interstitial markings, Kerley A and Kerley B lines. CT shows irregular thickening of the interlobular septae, along the central bronchovascular bundles and subpleural thickening. In addition, there are small peripheral subpleural nodules. Heart failure produces similar appearances on plain film and CT, though the thickening is more likely to be smooth and there will not be the associated lymphadenopathy that is often present in lymphangitis. Like heart failure, lymphangitis usually produces bilateral changes.

Practical tips
- When lymphangitis is diagnosed, look for other signs of malignant spread on available images, i.e. lung metastases, bone deposits.
- CT imaging findings of subpleural nodules and reticulation with interlobular septal thickening are the best diagnostic features. However, if it remains impossible to differentiate interlobular septal thickening of heart failure from lymphangitis on CT scanning, repeat imaging (chest radiograph or perhaps follow-up CT) after treatment for heart failure may resolve the issue.

Further management
Oncological assessment is necessary. If deemed suitable for chemotherapy, a search for the primary tumour is appropriate if not already apparent as in this case. CT scanning of the thorax, abdomen and pelvis is most commonly undertaken.

Further reading
Connolly JE, Erasmus JJ, Patz EF (1999). Thoracic manifestations of breast carcinoma: metastatic disease and complications of treatment. *Clinical Radiology* **54(8)**: 487–494.

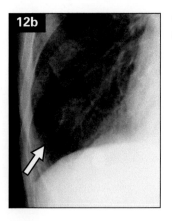

12b Kerley B septal line.

CASE 13

History
A 36-year-old female, otherwise fit and well, presented with acute dyspnoea and left sided chest pain.

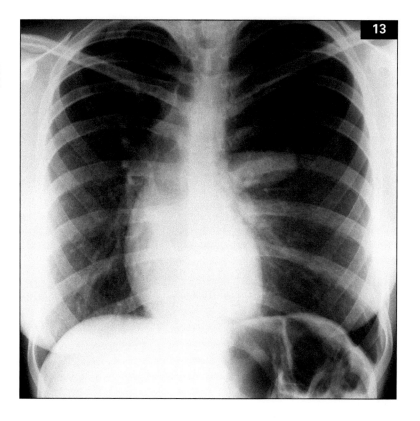

CASE 14

History
A 55-year-old man presented with dysphagia.

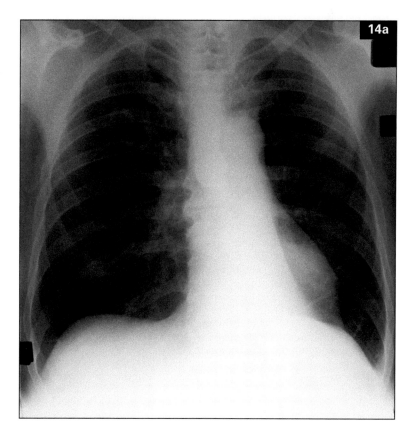

ANSWER 13

Observations (13)
There is a large, well defined, solitary, unilocular thin walled cyst in the medial aspect of the left middle zone. This contains an air-fluid level. A moderate sized left sided pneumothorax is evident with signs of mediastinal and tracheal shift to the right – suggesting that this is a tension pneumothorax. Immediate treatment of this tension pneumothorax is required.

The air-containing mass has presumably ruptured and led to a spontaneous pneumothorax. The fact that this patient is young and otherwise in good health makes most of the causes of large cavitating/cystic masses unlikely. After initial treatment, a search for previous films should be made to see if this is a longstanding benign lesion. Otherwise, further investigation, perhaps with CT, will be required.

Diagnosis
Intrapulmonary bronchogenic cyst.

Differential diagnosis
For solitary cavitating lesion:
- Cavitating neoplasm – squamous cell carcinoma of the lung is the most likely lung tumour to cavitate.
- Lung abscess.
- Cavitating pneumonia.
- Infarct/haematoma.

Discussion
Bronchogenic cysts are usually located in the mediastinum (85%) but can also be intrapulmonary in location (15%). They are more commonly found in the lower lobes and usually in the medial aspect. Typical appearances are of a solitary, unilocular thin walled cyst of uniform density due to thick mucoid fluid content. They can also contain air-fluid levels. Calcification of the wall is rare. They are usually asymptomatic but can be complicated by infection and haemorrhage or can cause compression to adjacent structures, i.e. trachea/airways/oesophagus.

Practical tips
- As always, clinical history is vital in producing a sensible differential diagnosis.
- Tension pneumothorax is an emergency and should be immediately treated or the appropriate clinician should be informed. It arises when air is able to enter the pleural space on inspiration but not escape on expiration. The accumulating air produces increasing mass effect (mediastinum displaced and diaphragm depressed) that compromises ventilation of the other lung and also cardiovascular function.

Further management
Tension pneumothorax is a medical emergency requiring immediate treatment. The increasing pressure must be relieved either with an intercostal chest drain or perhaps even insertion of a cannula into the pleural space in the acute situation.

Further reading
Matzinger M, Matzinger F, Sachs H (1992). Intrapulmonary bronchogenic cyst: spontaneous pneumothorax as the presenting symptom. *American Journal of Radiology* **158**: 987–988.

ANSWER 14

Observations (14a)
This frontal chest radiograph shows a triangular opacity behind the left side of the heart. It obscures the silhouette of the left hemidiaphragm where they meet, and there is depression of the left hilum indicating volume loss. This is the 'sail sign' of left lower lobe collapse.

At least two cavitating pulmonary nodules are present in the right upper lobe and close inspection of the mediastinum reveals residual barium in the upper thoracic oesophagus, terminating abruptly in the mid mediastinum.

The findings suggest that the patient has recently undergone a barium swallow, which has demonstrated a mid-oesophageal tumour. The pulmonary lesions on the right are likely to represent cavitating metastases and the left lower lobe collapse is presumably due to tumour obstruction of the left lower lobe bronchus.

Diagnosis
Oesophageal tumour with left lower lobe collapse and cavitating pulmonary metastases.

Differential diagnosis
Of a veil-like opacity over a hemithorax:
- Left upper lobe collapse.
- Pleural effusion in the supine position.
- Rotated patient position.
- Overlying chest wall abnormality, e.g. gynaecomastia.
- Unilateral airspace opacity.
- Normal, i.e. it is actually the other side that is hypodense!

Of a completely opaque hemithorax:
- Total lung collapse.
- Pneumonectomy – looks like total collapse but there will be evidence of thoracotomy.

Answer 14 — Chest Imaging

- Huge pleural effusion – volume expansion rather than volume loss, i.e. the mediastinum will be displaced away from the side of opacity.

Discussion

The various lobar collapses have their own characteristic appearances but evidence of volume loss is fundamental. Signs to look for include:
- Elevation or 'tenting' of the hemidiaphragm.
- Elevation or depression of the hilum – note that the left is normally higher than right.
- Mediastinal shift in the direction of the collapse.
- Elevation or depression of the horizontal fissure.
- Increased lucency or splayed vessels in the remaining hyperexpanded lobe.

In older adults, an obstructing central tumour must always be excluded. When causing upper lobe collapse, this can sometimes produce the characteristic 'S sign of Golden' (**14b**). The right upper lobe collapses into a triangular upper zone opacity, limited inferiorly by the horizontal fissure. However, the central mass produces an overall 'S' configuration with the fissure. Figures **14c** and **14d** are axial CT images in a patient with subtotal collapse of the right upper lobe with medial collapse of the lobe and significant volume loss as demonstrated by anterior movement of the fissures. A coronal CT reformatted image (**14e**) again shows subtotal collapse of the right upper lobe with volume loss.

(*cont.*)

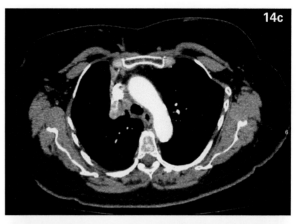

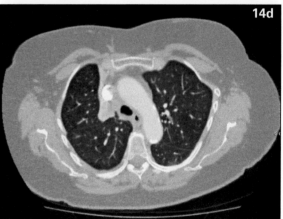

14c, 14d Axial CT images of the upper chest showing collapse of the right upper lobe with anterior and medial collapse. Anterior movement of horizontal and oblique fissures is demonstrated.

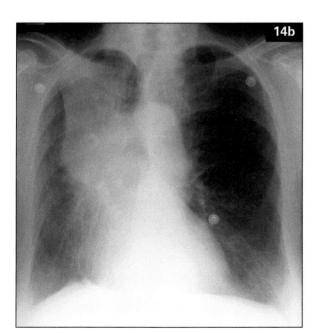

14b Right upper lobe collapse secondary to a central bronchogenic tumour produces an 'S sign of Golden'.

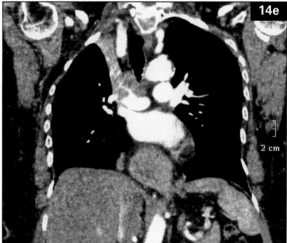

14e Coronal CT reformatted image of the chest showing the medial displacement of the collapsed upper lobe.

Chest Imaging

Answer 14

The left upper lobe has a characteristic appearance when it collapses. Unlike the right upper lobe, there is no horizontal fissure and the whole lobe frequently collapses anteriorly so that no discrete edge is seen. Instead, there is a veil of opacity over the left lung (**14f**). Figure **14g** is a left lateral film that shows how the lobe collapses anteriorly.

The right lower lobe collapses in a similar fashion to the left, but is easier to appreciate because it is not hidden by the heart. Right middle lobe collapse will produce increased opacity in the lower zone too, but unlike lower lobe collapse that obscures the diaphragm silhouette, this obscures the right heart border.

Total lung collapse is illustrated in Figure **14h** (left sided). This causes total opacification of the hemithorax with prominent volume loss on the side of the abnormality – note the grossly displaced mediastinum to the left (this illustration also shows right upper lobe collapse).

Practical tips
- Differentiating collapse and consolidation can sometimes be difficult since they often coexist. Look for signs of volume loss as described above.
- Lateral radiographs are useful in suspected collapse.
- Look for other evidence on the film of a primary bronchogenic tumour, e.g. metastases to lung and bone, previous thoracotomy and radiotherapy change.
- Check the position of endotracheal tube if present – it may have passed too far, occluding a bronchus and causing lung/lobar collapse. (Figure **14h** shows left total lung collapse and right upper lobe collapse due to passage of the endotracheal tube into the bronchus intermedius; the Sengstaken–Blakemore tube *in situ* is unrelated.)

Further management
In the adult patient with no obvious underlying cause, a central or endobronchial tumour needs to be excluded and respiratory referral with a view to bronchoscopy should be made.

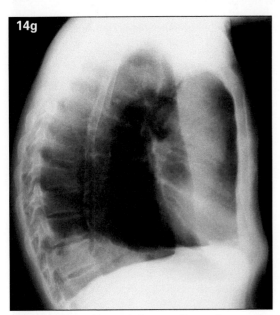

14f, 14g AP and lateral chest radiographs demonstrate left upper lobe collapse, which gives a veiling opacity over the left lung. The left upper lobe collapses anteriorly as shown on the lateral film.

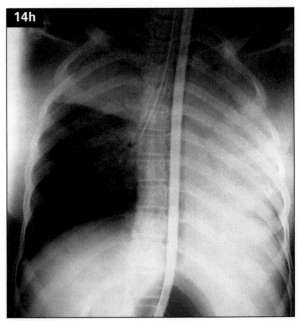

14h Complete collapse of the left lung with right upper lobe collapse.

CASE 15

History
A 68-year-old male presented with slowly progressive dyspnoea.

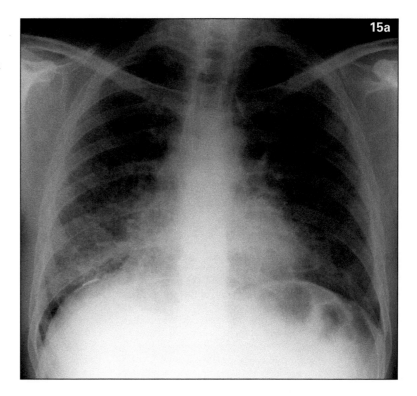

CASE 16

History
A 40-year-old male presented with a long progressive history of dyspnoea and more recent onset cyanosis.

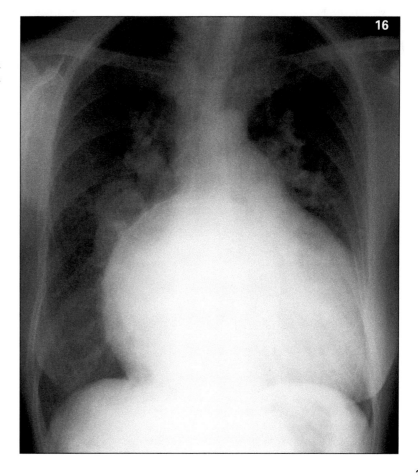

Answer 15

Observations (15a)
This chest radiograph demonstrates bilateral lower zone interstitial reticular opacity with evidence of basal volume loss demonstrated by descent of both hila. The interstitial opacity gives the heart an irregular 'shaggy' border. These appearances are in keeping with basal fibrosis. There is a calcified pleural plaque related to the right hemidiaphragm. The combination of basal fibrosis with pleural disease would suggest asbestos exposure with pulmonary asbestosis and pleural plaques.

Diagnosis
Pulmonary asbestosis.

Discussion
Pulmonary asbestosis is a chronic progressive fibrotic condition secondary to chronic asbestos exposure. Crocidolite (blue) asbestos fibres are most commonly associated with malignant disease and pleural disease. Radiological features are of a fibrosing alveolitis that predominantly affects the bases and is indistinguishable from other causes. Fibrosis can progress to result in progressive massive fibrosis, but this again predominates at the lung bases. Pulmonary asbestosis has a latency period of ~40 years and therefore pleural changes are usually seen prior to lung parenchymal changes.

Other features of asbestos exposure include:
- Pleural effusion – this is the earliest pleural abnormality, with a latency of ~10 years.
- Focal pleural plaques – have a latency of 20–40 years.
- Diffuse pleural thickening.
- Pleural calcification.
- Rounded atelectasis – this is also known as folded lung and arises due to infolding of thickened pleura with associated subsegmental atelectasis. Most commonly seen in the lower lobes, it has the appearance of a rounded subpleural mass abutting thickened pleura, with linear bands extending from the mass into the lung (crow's feet) (15b).
- Malignant mesothelioma – ~90% are related to previous asbestos exposure.
- Lung carcinoma – there is a latency of ~30 years and occurrence is related to the dose of asbestos exposure and to cigarette smoking – which can increase risk by 100-fold.

Practical tips
- Multiple pleural plaques are characteristic for previous asbestos exposure (15c).
- Look for signs of malignancy in patients with asbestos exposure – remember the increased risk of pleural and pulmonary malignancy. Pulmonary masses should be investigated with CT – characteristic findings may permit a confident diagnosis of folded lung in some cases.
- Asbestosis is the 'odd one out' among the inorganic dusts causing pulmonary fibrosis. The other fibrogenic dusts cause *upper zone* fibrosis.

Further management
- Systemic symptoms, e.g. weight loss, should be carefully investigated to exclude mesothelioma or bronchogenic carcinoma, for which these patients are at increased risk.
- In cases where there is still clinical concern about an area of possible folded lung despite imaging, percutaneous biopsy may be required to exclude a malignancy.

Further reading
Akira M, Yamamoto S, Yokoyama K, *et al.* (1990). Asbestosis: high-resolution CT-pathologic correlation. *Radiology* 176: 389–394.

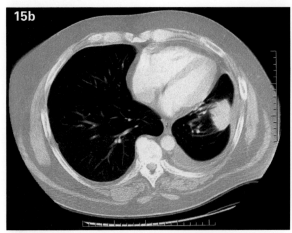

15b CT image of the chest demonstrating a large intraparenchymal lung lesion that is abutting thickened pleura. Vessels appear to be radiating towards the lesion as though pulled towards it.

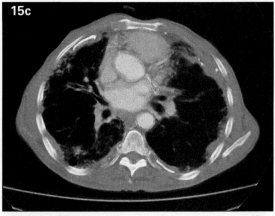

15c Axial CT image shows a right anterior calcified pleural plaque consistent with previous asbestos exposure. There is also subpleural reticulation representing fibrosis and appearances would be of asbestosis.

ANSWER 16

Observations (16)
This frontal chest radiograph shows extreme cardiomegaly. There is marked dilatation of the central and main pulmonary arteries with 'pruning' of peripheral pulmonary arteries. No diffuse lung abnormality is seen.

The findings are indicative of pulmonary hypertension. Given the gross cardiomegaly, a left to right shunt is the most likely cause. However, cyanosis should not occur and its presence suggests the shunt has reversed, that is, the patient has developed Eisenmenger's syndrome.

Diagnosis
Pulmonary arterial hypertension from an undiagnosed ventricular septal defect (VSD) progressing to Eisenmenger's syndrome.

Discussion
Pulmonary arterial hypertension is diagnosed by a sustained mean pressure >20 mmHg (systolic >30 mmHg, diastolic >15 mmHg). Radiological features on a plain chest radiograph that suggest the diagnosis are:
- Increase in size of the main pulmonary artery.
- Reduction in size of peripheral pulmonary arteries known as 'peripheral pruning'.
- Right heart enlargement.
- Calcification of the central pulmonary arteries – a late but characteristic sign.
- Parenchymal mosaic attenuation pattern seen on HRCT.

Primary pulmonary hypertension is idiopathic. The condition can also arise secondary to pulmonary disease or cardiovascular disease, either from an increase in overall pulmonary arterial resistance or from an increase in the overall circulatory volume going through the pulmonary circulation.
- Increased resistance – pulmonary veno-occlusive disease, chronic pulmonary thromboembolism, any chronic ventilatory disorder leading to chronic hypoxia and resulting vasoconstriction in the pulmonary arterial bed.
- Increased flow – left to right shunts, i.e. ASD (atrial septal defect), VSD (ventricular septal defect), PDA (patent ductus arteriosus).

In Eisenmenger's syndrome the pulmonary arterial pressure climbs until it eventually exceeds the pressure in the left heart and the shunt reverses. It is seen in those with pulmonary hypertension from a left to right shunt.

Practical tips
- On a plain chest radiograph, hilar lymphadenopathy can mimic pulmonary arterial hypertension. Clinical history here is vital and CT should be subsequently undertaken in the right clinical setting.
- The diameter of the main pulmonary artery should be less than that of the ascending thoracic aorta. Reversal of this ratio is a sign of pulmonary hypertension.

Further management
Primary pulmonary hypertension has no cure and a dismal prognosis. It is a diagnosis of exclusion so all underlying causes of secondary pulmonary hypertension must be investigated. Cardiology referral with a view to echocardiography would be required initially.

CASE 17

History
A 50-year-old female presented with progressive dyspnoea and intermittent cyanosis of the fingers.

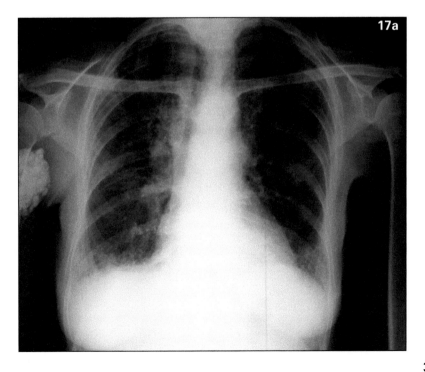

ANSWER 17

Observations (17a)
This frontal chest film shows abnormal reticular interstitial opacity at both lung bases, though there are no features to indicate significant volume loss at the present time. A large area of calcinosis is noted in the soft tissues around the upper right humerus. The combination of findings and clinical history suggests a diagnosis of systemic sclerosis with lower zone pulmonary fibrosis and Raynaud's phenomenon.

Diagnosis
Lower zone pulmonary fibrosis due to systemic sclerosis.

Differential diagnosis
For lower zone pulmonary fibrosis:
- Idiopathic pulmonary fibrosis (IPF) (cryptogenic fibrosing alveolitis – CFA).
- Connective tissue disorders – systemic sclerosis, rheumatoid.
- Asbestosis.
- Drugs – especially certain cytotoxics, e.g. cyclophosphamide, bleomycin, busulphan, etc.

Discussion
This autoimmune disease has also been known as scleroderma, with a subgroup known as CREST syndrome. Current nomenclature is systemic sclerosis with diffuse or limited scleroderma, the latter being the equivalent of CREST syndrome. The condition is three times as common in females and typically presents in the 4th–5th decades. A variety of autoantibodies may be present including ANA and rheumatoid factor. Clinical features are many and varied but include:
- Musculoskeletal – thickened skin, soft tissue calcinosis, Raynaud's, erosive arthritis (see Case 152).
- Lungs – lower zone pulmonary fibrosis, aspiration.
- Oesophagus – hypotonia results in dilatation and dysphagia. Incompetence of the gastro-oesophageal sphincter results in reflux and consequent peptic stricture, aspiration, etc.
- Small bowel – dilatation and slow transit result in bacterial overgrowth and malabsorption. Barium studies show 'hidebound' appearance due to fibrosis pulling the valvulae closer together. Pseudosacculations and pneumatosis in small and large bowel.

The CREST syndrome represents Calcinosis, Raynaud's, oEsophageal dysmotility, Sclerodactyly, Telangiectasia.

Practical tips
- Once lower zone pulmonary fibrosis has been noted on the chest radiograph, examine the film for the following features that may indicate a specific diagnosis:
  - Dilated oesophagus – systemic sclerosis (see Case 152).
  - Erosions of the lateral ends of clavicles – rheumatoid.
  - Pleural plaques – asbestosis.
  - Soft tissue calcification – systemic sclerosis.
  - Signs of malignancy including bony sclerosis from myeloproliferative disorders – cytotoxic induced.
  - Sympathectomy clips – systemic sclerosis (**17b**).
- Remember which disorders cause upper and lower zone fibrosis (refer to the differential diagnosis above, and also that in Case 18 for upper zone fibrosis): sarcoid is the classical upper zone disease, much as IPF is the classical lower zone disease. Thereafter, remember that the upper zones are better aerated and the lower zones better perfused. So, diseases caused by inhaled dust (inorganic or organic, e.g. silicosis and extrinsic allergic alveolitis [EAA] respectively) affect the upper zones, while the lower zones will be affected by blood borne disorders, i.e. drugs and autoimmune conditions. Unfortunately, asbestos is an exception and does not obey this logic.
- As with many fibrotic lung conditions, there is an increased incidence of pulmonary malignancy in systemic sclerosis associated pulmonary fibrosis – check for focal nodules/masses on the chest radiograph. Alternatively, focal airspace opacities may represent aspiration.

Further management
HRCT is the imaging choice in diagnosis and follow-up of interstitial lung disease. CT imaging findings of fibrosis include lung volume reduction, subpleural reticulation, interlobular septal thickening and traction bronchiectasis.

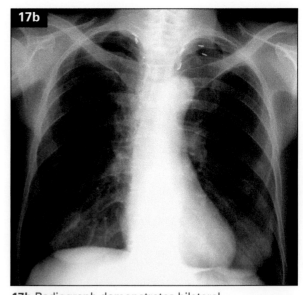

17b Radiograph demonstrates bilateral sympathectomy clips indicating that the patient has undergone treatment for Raynaud's phenomenon.

CASE 18

History
A 33-year-old male presented with back pain and progressive dyspnoea.

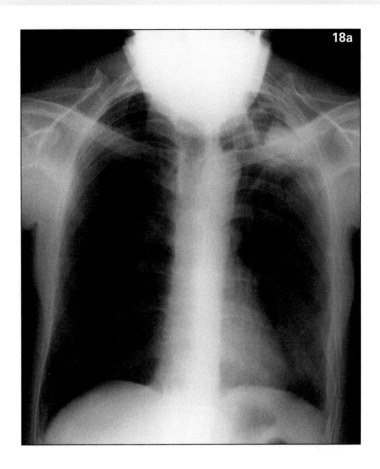

CASE 19

History
A 59-year-old male presented with left arm pain on activity.

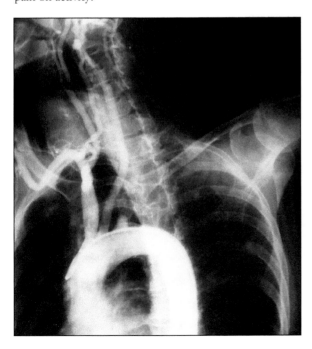
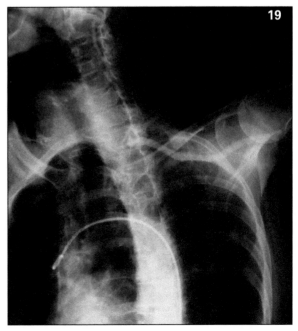

ANSWER 18

Observations (18a)
Plain radiograph of the chest shows changes of upper zone fibrosis with elevation of both hila and upper zone reticular opacities. In addition, there is a cavity in the left upper zone containing a soft tissue density mass with surrounding air crescent. These appearances would be consistent with a mycetoma. The patient also has a marked kyphosis with the head obscuring the lung apices. Moreover, on close inspection, there is a hint of syndesmophyte formation along the right lateral aspect of thoracic spine.

The combination of findings is consistent with upper zone fibrosis associated with ankylosing spondylitis. There is mycetoma formation in the fibrotic cavity in the left upper zone.

Diagnosis
Ankylosing spondylitis.

Differential diagnosis
For upper zone fibrosis (mnemonic – 'STRAD'):
- Sarcoidosis.
- TB.
- Radiation.
- Ankylosing spondylitis.
- Dust inhalation – inorganic (e.g. silica) and organic (i.e. chronic extrinsic allergic alveolitis).

Discussion
Ankylosing spondylitis is an autoimmune disease that most commonly manifests as a seronegative arthropathy, predominantly affecting the axial skeleton (initially sacroiliac joints then thoracic and lumbar spine). It usually presents in the 2nd–4th decade and more frequently affects men (sex ratio of ~5:1). As well as bone involvement, there are respiratory and cardiac manifestations. Respiratory manifestations are seen in ~1% of cases and features include:
- Upper lobe pulmonary fibrosis.
- Reticular/reticulonodular opacities in lung apices.
- Apical bullae and cavitation.
- Paraseptal emphysema.
- Bronchiectasis.

Cardiac features include aortitis involving the ascending aorta with aortic valve insufficiency.

Plain radiographic features of upper zone fibrosis include:
- Elevation of the hila.
- Tenting of the hemidiaphragms.
- Elevation of the horizontal fissure on the right (a good indicator).
- Increased lucency of the lower zone due to hyperexpansion.
- Reticular opacities in the upper zones.

Practical tips
- Clues to help limit the differential diagnosis for upper zone fibrosis include:
  - Kyphosis and 'bamboo spine' indicate ankylosing spondylitis.
  - Egg shell nodal calcification suggests silicosis or sarcoid.
  - Associated calcified granulomata suggest TB.

- Always look for signs of secondary infection/mycetoma in fibrotic cavities (**18b**).
- When pulmonary fibrosis due to ankylosing spondylitis is suspected, look for signs of complications of drug treatment on the film:
  - Avascular necrosis of humeral heads secondary to steroids.
  - Atypical distribution of fibrosis may be secondary to drug treatment.

Further management
Multidisciplinary management is required in this multisystem disease.

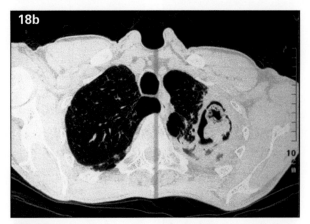

18b CT image in the same patient shows a cavitating lesion in the left upper lobe apical segment containing an Aspergillus fungus ball.

ANSWER 19

Observations (19)
Two spot images from an angiogram investigation at the level of the aortic arch are presented. Both images show the left shoulder joint in an abducted position. The left hand image shows contrast filling of the aortic arch with filling of the brachiocephalic trunk and left common carotid artery. There is filling of the proximal subclavian artery but then there is a complete occlusion with no filling beyond it. The right hand image shows a slightly delayed film with contrast seen in the left vertebral artery (best seen at the level of the C3/4) providing filling of the distal left subclavian artery.

Diagnosis
Subclavian steal syndrome.

Discussion
This is a condition that is usually acquired and caused by atherosclerotic disease. Stenosis of the subclavian artery results in stealing of blood to the arm via retrograde flow in the ipsilateral vertebral artery. Other acquired causes include vasculitis (Takayasu), embolism, aortic dissection, radiation fibrosis and chest trauma. Congenital causes are uncommon. Clinical features include:
- Left arm is more commonly involved than the right.
- Reduced BP by up to 40 mmHg in the affected arm.
- Delayed/weak pulse in the affected arm.
- Subclavian insufficiency – pain, numbness and weakness in the arm that is brought on by exercising the limb. Necrosis of the fingertips.
- Vertebrobasilar insufficiency – syncope can be precipitated by exercising the arm due to the stealing of blood. Headaches, ataxia, vertigo, diplopia, homonymous hemianopia and hemiparesis have all been reported.

Practical tips
Diagnosis can be made noninvasively by US by identifying reversal of Doppler flow in the vertebral artery.

Further management
- CT can be useful to identify/characterize calcified atherosclerotic plaque in the subclavian artery (uncontrasted CT) and also the site/degree of stenosis (arterial phase CT).
- Surgical referral is required for treatment with either balloon angioplasty (+/− stent insertion) or surgical bypass (common carotid to subclavian artery).

Further reading
Chung JW, Park JH, Im JG, *et al*. (1996). Spiral CT angiography of the thoracic aorta. *RadioGraphics* **16**: 811–824.

CASE 20

History
A 44-year-old male having a pre-employment chest radiograph.

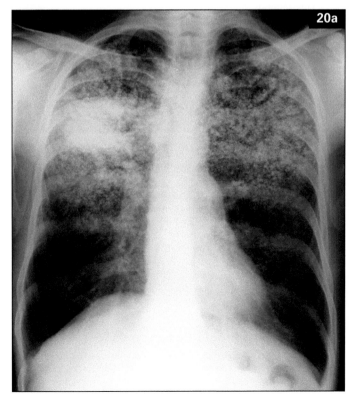

ANSWER 20

Observations (20a)
This chest radiograph shows multiple fine, sand-like, tiny calcified lesions measuring less than 1 mm in diameter, spread throughout both lungs. Both lungs are of normal volume. No other abnormality is seen.

Diagnosis
Alveolar microlithiasis.

Differential diagnosis
With pin-point high-density nodules, the possibilities are fairly limited, as follows:
- Inhaled inorganic dusts such as silicosis. Nodules tend to be a little larger and are predominantly in the middle and upper zones. Coalescence to form larger lesions with cavitation and fibrosis occurs. Egg shell calcification of nodes.
- Other inorganic inhaled dusts such as tin oxide, limestone and marble.

Slightly larger high-density opacities lead to a larger differential in addition to the above:
- Varicella pneumonia – previous infection can appear radiologically with multiple calcified nodules measuring 1–2 mm in size. No lymph node calcification is seen.
- Histoplasmosis – healed infection can also result in multiple tiny calcifications throughout the lungs. Associated with mediastinal lymph node, liver and spleen calcification.
- Metastatic calcinosis – focal calcification within the alveolar septae due to elevated serum calcium and phosphate levels in conditions such as hyperparathyroidism, multiple myeloma, sarcoidosis, milk-alkali syndrome or hypervitaminosis D. There is upper zone predominance and disease can progress to form airspace opacities, consolidative appearances and fibrosis (**20b**).
- Pulmonary haemosiderosis due to mitral valve disease.
- Barium aspiration – hyperdense opacities in the lower zones more common on the right (**20c**).

Discussion
This is a rare condition that affects adults in the 4th–6th decades, resulting in calcification within the alveoli. Usually these patients are asymptomatic, however they can present with dyspnoea on exertion. Radiological appearances can be quite striking with diffuse tiny calcified nodules <1 mm in diameter spread throughout both lungs. The middle and lower zones are preferentially affected. Serum calcium and phosphate are normal. Differentiation from the causes below is usually made by the normal biochemistry, characteristic radiological appearances and the paucity of clinical symptoms relative to the marked radiological changes.

Practical tips
Clinical history is of vital importance when narrowing down a list of differential diagnoses. Alveolar microlithiasis is a good example of where marked radiological changes are associated with a relative lack of symptoms. A simple question to the clinician such as 'how unwell is this patient?' can be most helpful.

Further management
No further management is required in this benign condition.

Further reading
Brown K, Mund DF, Aberle DR, Batra P, *et al.* (1994). Intrathoracic calcifications: radiographic features and differential diagnoses. *RadioGraphics* **14**: 1247–1261.

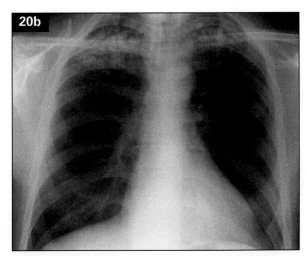

20b Chest radiograph showing bilateral upper zone airspace opacities of metastatic calcinosis.

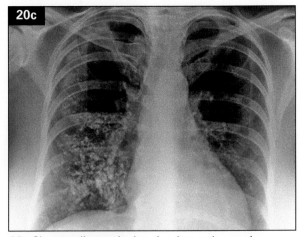

20c Chest radiograph showing hyperdense airspace opacities in the lower zones predominating on the right in a patient who aspirated during a barium swallow examination.

CASE 21

History
A 28-year-old patient presented with deteriorating chronic dyspnoea.

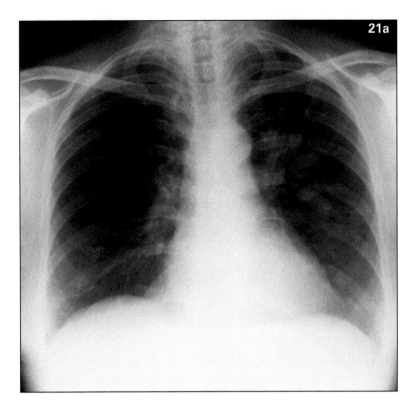

CASE 22

History
A 45-year-old male presented with cardiac arrhythmia and shortness of breath.

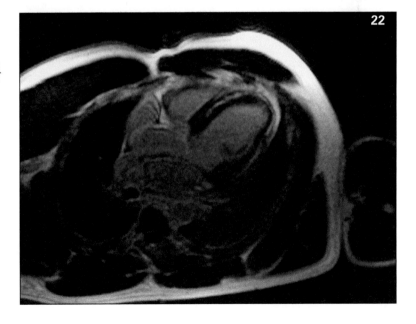

ANSWER 21

Observations (21a)
This frontal chest radiograph shows 'V-shaped' soft tissue opacities around the left hilum that are likely to represent mucous plugs in dilated central bronchi. No segmental collapse is evident. This appearance is described as 'finger in glove' and is a classical appearance of allergic bronchopulmonary aspergillosis.

Diagnosis
Allergic bronchopulmonary aspergillosis (ABPA).

Differential diagnosis
For a 'flitting' pneumonia:
- Eosinophilic pneumonia.
- Aspiration pneumonia.
- ABPA.
- Cryptogenic organizing pneumonia (COP).

Discussion
This is a hypersensitivity condition seen in longstanding asthmatics with sensitivity towards aspergilli. It occurs in 1–2% of asthmatics and more commonly (~10%) in patients with cystic fibrosis. Pulmonary features of the disease are:
- Pulmonary infiltration with eosinophils, which presents as a migratory/flitting pneumonitis of patchy alveolar infiltrates more commonly seen in the upper lobes.
- Cystic bronchiectasis with an upper lobe predominance that is usually central, producing 'ring shadows' on plain radiographs.
- Mucoid impaction in dilated central bronchioles, producing the 'finger in glove' appearance. This can result in segmental/lobar collapse.
- Lobar consolidation.

Axial CT images of a young female patient with ABPA are shown (**21b, 21c**). Figure **21b** shows dilated mucous-filled/plugged upper lobe bronchi, which can be best appreciated on coronal reformats. Figure **21c** demonstrates the typical cystic dilated bronchi with further evidence of mucous-plugging.

Practical tips
Some indication to the underlying cause of bronchiectasis can be made from its distribution and type:
- ABPA – central, cystic/varicose, predominantly in the upper lobes.
- Cystic fibrosis – pan-lobar, affects the upper lobes more than lower lobes (**21d**).
- Post-pertussis infection – cystic, lingula initially affected.
- Hypogammaglobulinaemia – cylindrical. Lower lobe predominance.

Further management
Referral to chest physician is appropriate with further imaging follow-up with HRCT.

Further reading
Williams SM, Jones ET (1997). General case of the day. Allergic (or hypersensitivity) bronchopulmonary aspergillosis (ABPA). *RadioGraphics* **17**: 1597–1600.

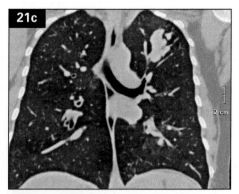

21c Coronal reformat showing the 'finger in glove' mucous-plugging appearance of the bronchi.

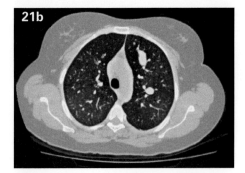

21b Axial CT image showing dilated mucous-filled bronchi in the upper lobes.

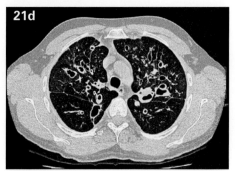

21d Axial CT image showing cystic bronchiectasis in a patient with cystic fibrosis.

ANSWER 22

Observations (22)
This is a single long axis view of the left ventricle at delayed gadolinium enhancement phase. The image shows delayed enhancement of the septal, apical and lateral myocardium with sparing of the endocardium. This pattern of delayed intramyocardial enhancement with a normal endocardium suggests an infiltrative/inflammatory process.

Diagnosis
Cardiac sarcoid.

Discussion
At autopsy cardiac sarcoid is seen in 20–25% of patients with sarcoidosis. However, as few as 5% exhibit any clinical signs. Clinical presentation of sarcoid is with cardiac arrhythmias, cardiomyopathy and heart failure.

Imaging findings of cardiac sarcoid include:
- Cardiac granulomas involving the interventricular septum (hypointensity on T2 weighted images).
- Myocardial enhancement on delayed gadolinium enhancement corresponding to areas of fibrosis, with sparing of the endocardium, allowing for differentiation from the infarcted myocardium of ischaemic heart disease.
- Areas of hypokinesia of the myocardial wall.

Practical tips
Sparing of the endocardium suggests that coronary artery disease is not the underlying diagnosis.

Further management
Look at CXR for respiratory changes of sarcoid.

CASE 23

History
A 50-year-old male patient presented with orthopnoea.

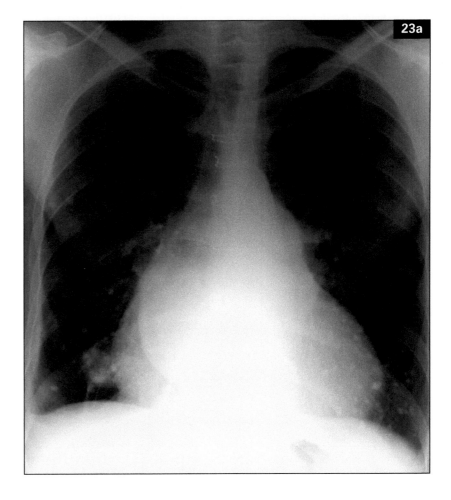

ANSWER 23

Observations (23a)
This chest radiograph shows evidence of previous surgery – there are sternotomy wires and a metallic mitral valve replacement. The heart is enlarged with a cardiothoracic ratio of 21:32. There is a 'double density' seen through the right heart – a sign of left atrial enlargement. Multiple, small (1–5 mm) calcium density nodules are seen in both lungs with mid and lower zone predominance. Upper zone venous diversion and a tiny right pleural effusion suggest pulmonary venous hypertension.

Appearances indicate that the patient has had surgical mitral valve replacement, but there are persisting features of mitral valve disease and signs of left heart failure. He should undergo further assessment of valve and left heart function. The high-density pulmonary nodules indicate pulmonary haemosiderosis, a consequence of elevated pulmonary venous pressure over many years.

Diagnosis
Mitral valve disease.

Discussion
The most common cause of mitral valve disease is rheumatic heart disease, with presentation most commonly seen in middle aged females. It results in left atrial enlargement and pulmonary venous hypertension/heart failure.

Radiographic signs of mitral valve disease are:
- 'Double density' behind the right heart border due to left atrial enlargement.
- Splaying of the carina by the large left atrium.
- Oesophagus displaced to the right.
- Left atrial appendage enlargement. The normal left mediastinal contour has two convexities above the left ventricle – the aortic arch and the main pulmonary artery. Enlargement of the left atrial appendage produces a third 'bump' below the pulmonary artery (**23b**). This is sometimes called the 'third mogul sign' (the term mogul is one used by skiers to describe bumps in the snow!).
- Calcification of thrombus in the left atrium (**23c**).
- Right ventricular hypertrophy.
- Pulmonary venous hypertension, interstitial and pulmonary oedema.
- Pulmonary haemosiderosis – longstanding elevation of pulmonary venous pressure results in oozing of serum into the interstitium. Blood products within this will ultimately be broken down to haemosiderin.

Practical tips
It is difficult to distinguish from plain film whether there is mitral valve stenosis or regurgitation – the radiological consequences and signs are the same and the two can coexist. However, if there is gross left atrial enlargement, there must be a component of stenosis present.

Further management
Cardiac referral with a view to echocardiographic assessment is required. Treatment involves drug therapy for arrhythmias (atrial fibrillation – AF) and to improve cardiac function. Surgical intervention includes percutaneous valve balloon dilatation (high recurrence rates), valvotomy and valve replacement.

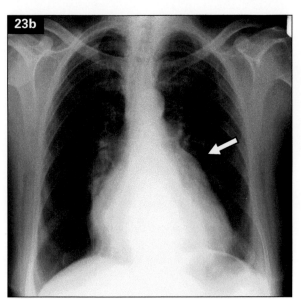

23b Chest radiograph shows enlargement of the left atrial appendage in a patient with mitral stenosis.

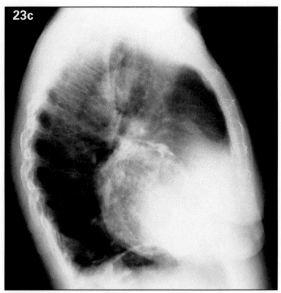

23c Lateral chest radiograph shows curvilinear calcification of the left atrial wall.

Case 24

History
A 70-year-old male was referred for further investigation following initial imaging showing a right lower lobe mass lesion.

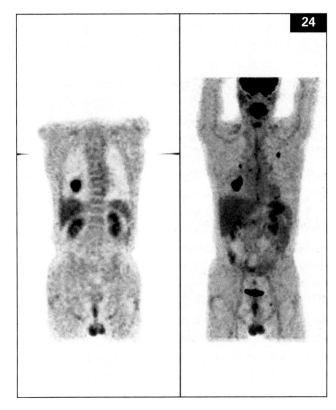

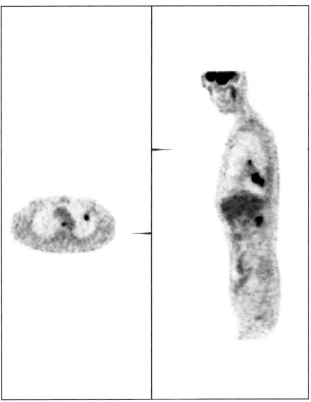

ANSWER 24

Observations (24)
These PET scan images from a PET CT demonstrate a large right lower lobe highly FDG (18 fluoro-2-deoxy-glucose) avid lesion. There is a smaller left upper lobe FDG avid lesion. There is also right hilar uptake as well as uptake in the subcarinal region. Uptake in the region of the oesophagus is also demonstrated. There is no FDG avid lesion in liver or adrenals. No bony lesions are demonstrated.

Diagnosis
Metastatic right lower lobe bronchogenic carcinoma.

Differential diagnosis
The left upper lobe lesion represents either metastases or a synchronous lesion.

Discussion
PET scanning relies on increased uptake of FDG in cell populations with higher metabolic turnover. The main application is oncological imaging; other, less utilized applications include CNS and cardiac imaging. It is essential that PET scans are compared with cross-sectional imaging if no PET CT scan has been performed. Assessing only PET images alone can lead to diagnostic errors, mainly incorrect staging of malignant disease. The CT images (not shown) of this PET/CT scan demonstrated a right sided pleural effusion that turned out to be malignant. Pleural effusions do not demonstrate increased FDG activity.

Among other areas, normal FDG uptake is demonstrated in the brain, heart, salivary glands, liver, spleen as well as upper renal tract and it is also excreted in the urine. Normal bowel uptake is also often demonstrated. Pitfalls include increased FDG uptake in fat (brown fatty tissue); this can simulate malignant nodal disease. In the current study, the increased oesophageal uptake is due to a coexisting reflux oesophagitis.

PET scans can be false negative for small lung metastases or solitary lung nodules. False positive diagnosis on PET scanning also occurs due to infection and inflammation – conditions that are associated with increased glucose turnover.

Practical tips
- In the UK, PET scanning is used mainly as a staging tool. Neurological and cardiac applications are not utilized widely. Among others, PET is used for initial staging and restaging of bronchogenic or oesophageal carcinoma.
- Cancer networks are increasingly utilizing PET prior to planning for curative surgery. A growing application is the assessment of solitary nodules. This is particularly useful in central lesions for which histological confirmation is more challenging and the complication rate is increased.
- A well documented pitfall is a false negative scan for small lung nodules or metastases. Lesions measuring less than 7–8 mm do have a higher false negative rate.
- Lymphoma staging is also widely undertaken. This is very useful for assessment of activity in residual lymphoma masses and also for assessment of early response to chemotherapy. Inflammatory or infected nodal mediastinal masses (histoplasmosis) can also give rise to false positive scans. Correlation with cross-sectional imaging is important in all cases where FDG imaging is undertaken.

Further management
PET CT results should be discussed within a multi-disciplinary team with the purpose of deciding whether the patient would be a candidate for surgical disease clearance.

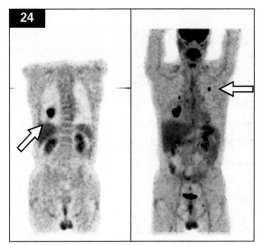

24a Right lower lobe bronchogenic carcinoma (left) and likely metastasis (right).

CASE 25

History
A 45-year-old female, previously resident in the USA, presented for a pre-employment chest radiograph.

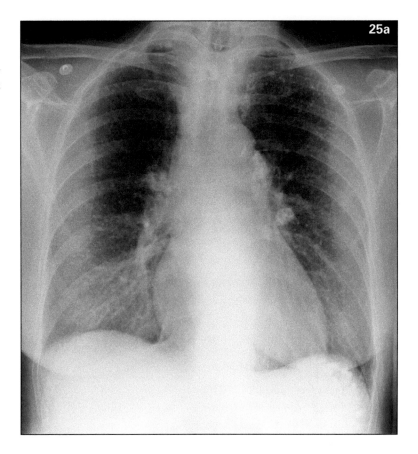

CASE 26

History
A 24-year-old male presented with dysphagia.

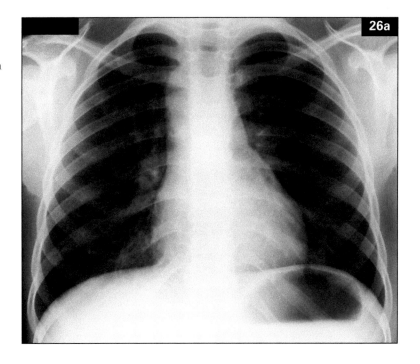

ANSWER 25

Observations (25a)
This frontal chest radiograph demonstrates widespread 1–3 mm diameter miliary nodules seen throughout both lungs with no zonal predominance. The miliary nodules are of calcific density. Popcorn calcification of the left hilar lymph nodes is seen. In addition, there is amorphous calcification seen under the left hemidiaphragm, which is likely to be in the spleen.

Diagnosis
Histoplasmosis.

Differential diagnosis
For increased density miliary opacities:
- Miliary metastases.
- Pneumoconiosis – silicosis, siderosis, baritosis.
- Varicella-zoster (**25b**).
- Haemosiderosis – due to chronic pulmonary venous hypertension, pulmonary haemorrhage, or idiopathic.
- Histoplasmosis.

For popcorn calcification of lymph nodes:
- Sarcoidosis.
- Silicosis.
- Histoplasmosis.
- Coal worker's pneumoconiosis (CWP).
- Lymphoma – post radiotherapy.

For splenic calcification:
- Tuberculosis.
- Histoplasmosis.
- Infarcts secondary to sickle cell disease.
- Hydatid cysts.
- Haematoma.

Discussion
Histoplasma capsulatum is a fungus usually found in temperate climates and most commonly in the northern USA. Infection is by inhalation of air borne fungal spores. These germinate in the alveoli and then spread via the pulmonary lymphatics to the hilar/mediastinal lymph nodes and haematogenously to the spleen. Acute infection usually presents with few nonspecific symptoms, and radiological findings include generalized lymphadenopathy, flitting nonsegmental bronchopneumonia, multiple miliary nodules, popcorn calcification of hilar/mediastinal lymph nodes and splenic calcification. Chronic histoplasmosis is seen in patients with chronic obstructive airways disease and has radiological features of peripheral consolidation and apical fibrosis. Disseminated infection can occur in immunocompromised patients.

Nonpulmonary features of histoplasmosis include pericarditis (5–10%) and rheumatologic syndromes (~6%), e.g. arthralgia, erythema nodosum.

Practical tips
In cases where there are multiple radiological findings, consider the differential diagnosis list for each finding and identify an overlapping diagnosis (easier said than done in a viva situation!).

Further management
Clinical/occupational history and HRCT can be useful to differentiate the possible underlying diagnoses. Respiratory referral with a view to antifungal treatment would be required in the acute infection.

Further reading
Brown K, Mund DF, Aberle DR, *et al*. (1994). Intrathoracic calcifications: radiographic features and differential diagnoses. *RadioGraphics* **14**: 1247–1261.

Wheat LJ, Wass J, Norton J (1984). Cavitary histoplasmosis occurring during two large urban outbreaks. Analysis of clinical, epidemiologic, roentgenographic, and laboratory features. *Medicine* (Baltimore) **63(4)**: 201–209.

Wheat LJ, Connolly-Stringfield PA, Baker RL (1990). Disseminated histoplasmosis in the acquired immune deficiency syndrome: clinical findings, diagnosis and treatment, and review of the literature. *Medicine* (Baltimore) **69(6)**: 361.

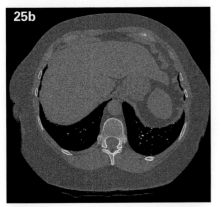

25b Multiple calcified tiny nodules at the left lung base in a patient with old varicella pneumonia.

ANSWER 26

Observations (26a)
This frontal chest radiograph demonstrates a right sided aortic arch. No left sided aortic knuckle is seen. The heart is not enlarged. No focal lung parenchymal abnormality is seen.

Diagnosis
Right sided aortic arch.

Discussion
Diagnosis can be confirmed with arterial phase contrast enhanced CT chest (**26b**). Right sided aortic arch can be associated with several congenital cardiac abnormalities but it can also be seen in patients without cardiac abnormalities. The latter group of patients usually have a right sided aortic arch with an aberrant left subclavian artery (arising as the most distal branch of the aortic arch), which passes behind the oesophagus. This can be seen on a barium swallow examination as a posterior indentation in the barium column of the mid oesophagus. Patients with right sided aortic arch with mirror image branching, such that the left subclavian arises as a branch of the first vessel of the aortic arch, are the group usually associated with cyanotic heart disease. The aorta descends in the right posterior mediastinum (although in a small proportion, <5%, this is on the left).

Practical tips
Right sided aortic arch can give a notch in the posterior aspect of the upper oesophagus on contrast swallow examination.

Further management
No further management is required in this condition.

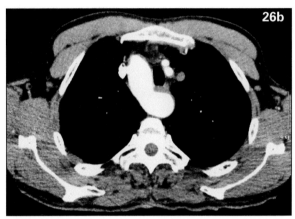

26b Axial CT image demonstrates the right sided aortic arch.

CASE 27

History
A 34-year-old smoker presents with progressively worsening shortness of breath.

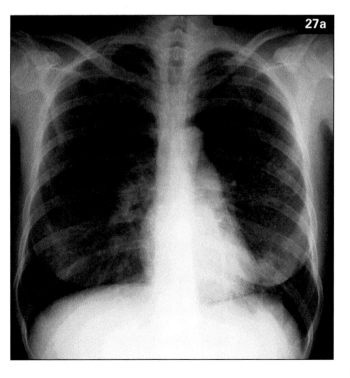

ANSWER 27

Observations (27a)
The chest radiograph shows bilateral thick and thin walled cysts throughout both lungs with preservation of lung volumes. Some small nodules are also seen particularly within the right upper zone. No pleural effusion or pneumothorax is seen. No bony abnormality or soft tissue nodules to suggest neurofibromatosis. In spite of the patient's sex, the widespread distribution and nodularity would make Langerhans cell histiocytosis the most likely diagnosis.

Diagnosis
Langerhans cell histiocytosis.

Differential diagnosis
For cystic lung disease with normal or increased lung volumes:
- Lymphangioleiomyomatosis – affects women in 2nd–6th decades. There are multiple cysts seen throughout the lungs of relatively uniform size (~5 mm) and shape, with no nodule formation. Commonly associated with chylous pleural effusions and recurrent pneumothoraces.
- Neurofibromatosis – predominantly apical cysts.
- Tuberous sclerosis.
- Cystic bronchiectasis.

Discussion
Langerhans cell histiocytosis is a multisystem granulomatous disease, which occurs more commonly in young (3rd–4th decades) adult males, and has an association with cigarette smoking. Pulmonary changes on CXR involve a sequence of changes – initial signs are of nodules that progressively cavitate to result in thick and then thin walled cyst formation. Lung volumes are usually normal or increased in up to 30%. Pneumothoraces are common and can be recurrent. Pleural effusions are rarely associated. HRCT appearances are of centrilobular nodules and complex thin walled cysts that are of variable size and shape and show relative sparing of the apices and costophrenic recesses (27b).

Practical tips
On a CXR, cystic lung disease with normal/increased lung volumes can be differentiated by looking at patient's sex and by identifying other radiological findings:
- Lymphangioleiomyomatosis occurs exclusively in women.
- Neurofibromatosis changes on a CXR include ribbon ribs; soft tissue masses (neurofibromas) seen in posterior mediastinum and skin.
- Tuberous sclerosis is easily identified by the history – being characterized by the triad of mental retardation, seizures and adenoma sebaceum.
- Bronchiectasis produces thicker walled cysts and the thickened airway walls may also be visible along their lengths as 'tramtracking'.

Further management
HRCT can be useful in the follow-up of these patients when looking for potential complications of aspergilloma/mycetoma infection, cavitating nodules and pneumothoraces.

Further reading
Moore AD, Godwin JD, Muller NL, et al. (1989). Pulmonary histiocytosis X: comparison of radiographic and CT findings. *Radiology* 172: 249–254.

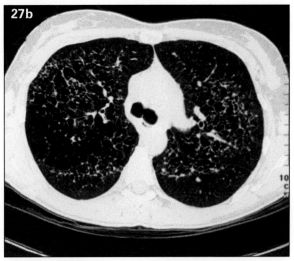

27b Single HRCT image demonstrates multiple central thin walled cysts of varying sizes.

CASE 28

History
A 29-year-old male presented with intermittent pain in both arms. Images **28b** and **28c** were taken just 1 minute apart – what has happened between them?

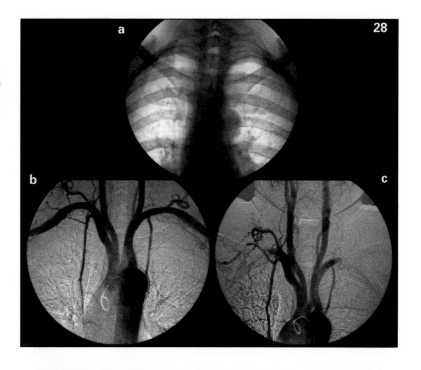

CASE 29

History
A 65-year-old male presented with progressively worsening shortness of breath.

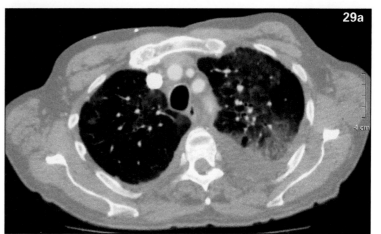

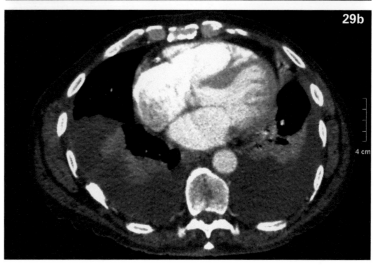

ANSWER 28

Observations (28a, b, c)
Selected images from an arch aortogram. The first image (**28a**) is a pre-contrast image which demonstrates bilateral cervical ribs. The second image (**28b**) shows a pigtail catheter in the arch with contrast injected and normal appearance of the aortic arch and the proximal main branches. The third image (**28c**) shows bilateral occlusion of the subclavian arteries at the level of the thoracic outlet. Given the presence of cervical ribs, it is suspected that the second image was acquired with the arms down, and the third image with the arms elevated.

The patient has thoracic outlet syndrome.

Diagnosis
Thoracic outlet syndrome secondary to bilateral cervical ribs.

Differential diagnosis
Of causes of thoracic outlet syndrome:
- Congenital – cervical rib, fibrous band or abnormal 1st rib.
- Acquired – first rib exostosis or fracture, body habitus.

Discussion
Thoracic outlet syndrome is a clinical syndrome caused by nerve, artery or vein compression in the root of the neck upon elevation of the arms. The vast majority of symptoms arise due to nerve compression and vascular symptoms are found in as few as 2% of symptomatic patients. The subclavian artery and/or vein are transiently occluded with arm movement, but more permanent vascular problems can arise due to the repeated trauma of compression – focal stenosis, poststenotic dilatation and aneurysm formation. The result of this is upper limb ischaemic symptoms with pain, a cold limb and Raynaud's phenomenon. Further complications of poststenotic thrombus formation and subsequent embolism can occur.

Practical tips
Cervical ribs occur in ~3–4% of the population but are only symptomatic in 10% of cases.

Further management
- US is useful as a dynamic test for assessing arterial Doppler signal with the arm in a neutral and elevated position.
- CT/MRI can be useful in identifying the cause of compression if not apparent on plain radiography.

ANSWER 29

Observations (29a, 29b)
Two axial CT images of the chest show features of cardiomegaly, bilateral pleural effusions and patchy 'ground glass' opacity with smooth interlobular septal thickening. This combination of imaging findings would fit with a diagnosis of pulmonary oedema.

Diagnosis
Pulmonary oedema due to heart failure.

Differential diagnosis
For 'ground glass' opacity:
- Pulmonary oedema.
- Infection.
- Haemorrhage.
- Interstitial pneumonias.
- Extrinsic allergic alveolitis.
- Alveolar proteinosis.
- Sarcoidosis.
- Focal areas of 'ground glass' – alveolar cell carcinoma/lymphoma.

For smooth interlobular septal thickening:
- Pulmonary oedema.
- Alveolar proteinosis.
- Pulmonary fibrosis.

For nodular interlobular septal thickening:
- Lymphangitis carcinomatosa.
- Sarcoidosis.

Discussion
Cardiac failure is a diagnosis usually made clinically and confirmed with CXR. The following findings tend to progress in sequence as the condition deteriorates and pulmonary venous pressure increases further:
- Upper zone vascular predominance.
- Interstitial oedema with peripheral reticulations and Kerley B lines.
- Alveolar oedema with a perihilar predominance ('bat's wing' appearance).

The following features provide supplementary evidence to suggest the diagnosis:
- Cardiomegaly with cardiothoracic ratio >50%.
- Pleural effusion.

These same findings are visible on CT. Alveolar fluid often presents as 'ground glass' opacity, which is an increased haziness/attenuation in the lung – and which can be patchy in distribution. 'Ground glass' opacity is a relatively nonspecific imaging finding due to many conditions that cause an overall increase in density within the segment of lung displayed as a pixel on the CT image. There is a long differential diagnosis including any cause of alveolar fluid/consolidation.

Practical tips
A combination of cardiomegaly, pleural effusion and airspace opacity suggests cardiac failure with pulmonary oedema.

Further management
Medical management with CXR radiological follow-up as appropriate.

CASE 30

History
A 65-year-old male was referred for a cardiac MRI to assess cardiac viability.

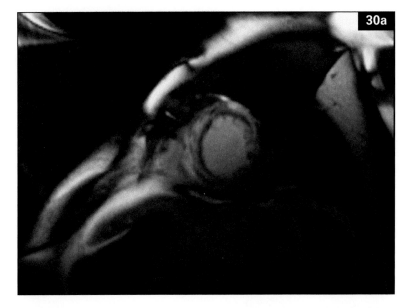

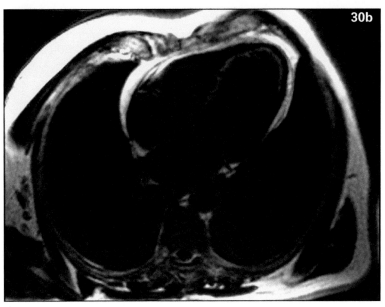

ANSWER 30

Observations (30a, 30b)
The first image (**30a**) is a short axis scan through the left ventricle during the first pass of contrast. There is no contrast enhancement of the thinned left ventricular septal and anterior walls. The visualized posterior, lateral and inferior walls show normal enhancement and are of normal thickness. The second image (**30b**) is a delayed four chamber view showing delayed, prolonged enhancement of the septal, apical and anterolateral wall of the left ventricle. These appearances are of an extensive left ventricular infarct with no evidence that involved areas are viable.

Diagnosis
Left ventricular infarct involving the septal/apical/anterolateral walls.

Discussion
Cardiac MRI has an expanding role and current uses include assessment of:
- Cardiac viability prior to revascularization.
- Cardiac congenital heart defect.
- Cardiac tumours.
- Pericardial disease.
- Cardiomyopathies.

Assessing cardiac viability post myocardial infarction is important since revascularization of live tissue reduces morbidity and mortality. Previously cardiac perfusion was assessed by cardiac nuclear medicine (MIBG – meta-iodobenzylguanidine [scintiscan]) stress testing but there is now an increased role for cardiac MRI.

Short axis cine images are acquired at *first pass* of a bolus injection of gadolinium to determine perfusion. Infarcted myocardium shows no enhancement on first-pass imaging (as demonstrated in this case). In addition, first-pass imaging can show:
- Whether the infarct is transmural or subendocardial.
- Degree of hypo/akinesia.

Delayed enhancement sequences at approximately 5 min show enhancement in infarcted tissue since clearance of contrast from fibrotic tissue is slower than from normal myocardium.

If there is any uncertainty regarding differentiation of ischaemic from infarcted myocardium then cardiac MRI stress testing is performed with *first-pass* images acquired at stress with adenosine and then repeated after 20 min at rest. Areas of hypoenhancement at stress that show recovery at rest represent areas of ischaemia rather than infarction.

Practical tips
Cardiac MRI is a dynamic test that requires assessment of cine images to make a subjective and objective assessment of left ventricular function (ejection fraction).

Further management
Coronary artery atherosclerotic disease is characterized using coronary angiography or coronary artery CT. Patients with ischaemic but viable myocardium may be suitable for revascularization with angioplasty or bypass grafting.

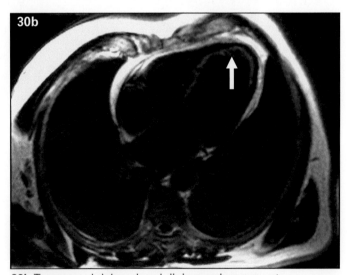

30b Transmural delayed gadolinium enhancement.

CASE 31

History
A 45-year-old female patient presented with chest pain.

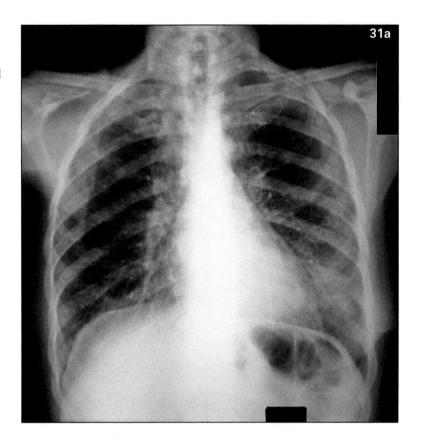

CASE 32

History
A 24-year-old male presented with chest pain after minor trauma.

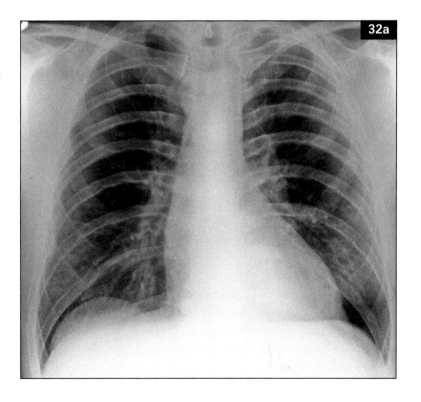

ANSWER 31

Observations (31a)
This chest radiograph shows evidence of a previous right mastectomy. Heart and mediastinal contours are normal. No lung abnormality is seen. There is diffuse sclerosis of all visible bones, most evident in the ribs. Appearances are of diffuse sclerotic metastases from a breast carcinoma primary.

Diagnosis
Mastectomy and sclerotic bone metastases.

Differential diagnosis
For causes of unilateral hypertransradiancy:
- Chest wall abnormality – mastectomy, pectoral muscle atrophy (polio) or absence (Poland's syndrome).
- Pleural abnormality – pneumothorax.
- Lung abnormality – Swyer–James syndrome (consequence of bronchiolitis as a child resulting in a hypoplastic lung with air trapping on expiration), emphysema, bullae, pulmonary embolus (**31b**).

For causes of unilateral hyperdensity:
- Chest wall abnormality – gynaecomastia (unilateral in 40% of cases), breast implant.
- Pleural abnormality – pleural effusion on supine film, pleural thickening.
- Lung abnormality – unilateral pulmonary oedema from lying on one side (**31c**), consolidation, lobar collapse (especially left upper lobe).

Discussion
With breast cancer being such a common malignancy, complications will present frequently on plain radiographs so it is important to note a mastectomy. Another 'tell tale' sign of previous breast cancer is the presence of axillary clips from node sampling.

The mastectomy may first be perceived as a disparity between the overall densities of the two hemithoraces. There are many other causes for this, though sometimes it may not be easy deciding which side is normal.

Practical tips
In any case with a history of breast cancer, the chest radiograph should be scrutinized for features of recurrence. These are classical viva films for exams and also present frequently in everyday practice. Features to look for include:
- Sclerotic/lytic bone metastases (**31d**).
- Lung metastases.
- Lymphangitis carcinomatosa.
- Pleural effusion.
- Axillary lymphadenopathy.
- Right hemidiaphragm elevation secondary to liver metastases.
- Pulmonary pneumonitis/fibrosis from radiotherapy.

Further management
- In cases where clinical history and examination do not reveal an obvious cause for the relative differences in chest lucency – CT chest would be appropriate.
- Isotope bone scan may identify distant bone metastases.

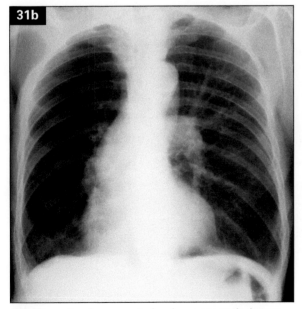

31b There is a large central pulmonary embolus on the right with marked reduction in vascular markings on this side.

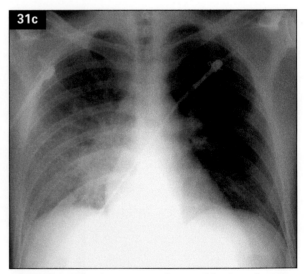

31c Unilateral pulmonary oedema with pleural effusion and airspace opacity on the right.

31d Multiple poorly defined lytic lesions are seen throughout the ribs bilaterally.

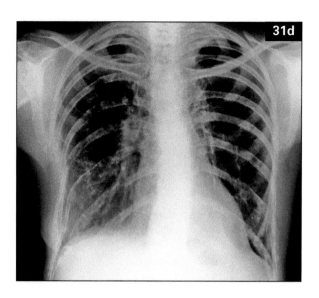

ANSWER 32

Observations (32a)
The chest radiograph shows no focal lung abnormality and no rib fracture or pneumothorax from the recent trauma. However, there is bilateral inferior rib notching involving the 3rd–8th ribs. The aortic knuckle is not well seen but there is no other mediastinal contour abnormality. The heart is not enlarged. There is no evidence of previous cardiac surgery. No other specific bony or soft tissue abnormalities are seen.

The most likely diagnosis is coarctation of the aorta – the patient's blood pressure should be checked in both arms and compared with that in the legs for confirmatory evidence.

Diagnosis
Inferior rib notching due to coarctation of the aorta.

Differential diagnosis
For inferior rib notching:
- Arterial:
  - Coarctation of the aorta.
  - Subclavian obstruction after Blalock–Taussig shunt for tetralogy of Fallot.

- Venous: SVC obstruction.
- Arteriovenous malformations (AVM).
- Neurogenic, neurofibromatosis.

For superior rib notching:
- Rheumatoid arthritis, scleroderma and systemic lupus erythematosus (SLE).
- Hyperparathyroidism.
- Neurofibromatosis.
- Marfan's syndrome.
- Restrictive lung disease.

Discussion
The most common cause of inferior rib notching is coarctation of the aorta. This can be of two types:
- Preductal – the hypoplastic narrowed segment is long. These patients present in infancy and early childhood with congestive cardiac failure. Prognosis is worse than for those who present with the postductal type.
- Postductal – this usually consists of a short narrowed segment, immediately distal to the site of the ligamentum arteriosum (**32b**). Presentation is usually in later childhood, and is with hypertension, differential blood pressures in the upper and lower limbs and/or a heart murmur.

(*cont.*)

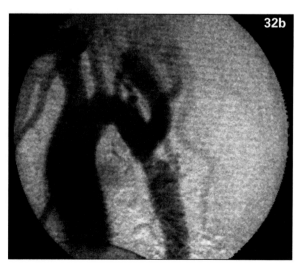

32b Single angiographic image shows postductal stenosis of the descending thoracic aorta, with poststenotic dilatation.

Answer 32 — Chest Imaging

On chest radiographs, the focal narrowing of the aorta is classically made more evident because of pre- and poststenotic dilatation producing a classic 'figure of 3' sign. Obscuration of the arch, as in this case, is also recognized. Rib notching on the inferior surface of the 3rd–8th ribs can usually be seen in untreated patients by 8 years. Rib notching occurs due to dilatation of the posterior intercostal arteries, which act as collateral vessels. Since the 1st and 2nd posterior intercostal arteries arise from the costocervical trunk of subclavian artery rather than descending aorta, they do not form a collateral path and hence do not cause rib erosion.

Coarctation of the aorta is associated with several other congenital anomalies such as bicuspid aortic valve, patent ductus arteriosus (PDA), ventricular septal defect (VSD), tricuspid atresia and transposition of the great vessels. There is also an association with Turner's syndrome.

Practical tips
- When suspected from plain films and clinical findings, MR or CT angiography has now largely replaced conventional angiography as the next investigation of choice (**32c**).
- When inferior rib notching is noted check:
  - The aortic contour for the 'figure of 3' sign.
  - Is there evidence of previous repair, e.g. thoracotomy scar?
  - The heart for evidence of left ventricular hypertrophy, i.e. elevation of the apex.
  - Are there features to indicate neurofibromatosis, e.g. cutaneous soft tissue nodules?
- When rib notching is unilateral, suspect an aberrant subclavian artery origin on the unaffected side.

Further management
Surgical treatment for coarctation of the aorta involves resection and end to end anastomosis, prosthetic patch graft, subclavian flap aortoplasty or balloon angioplasty.

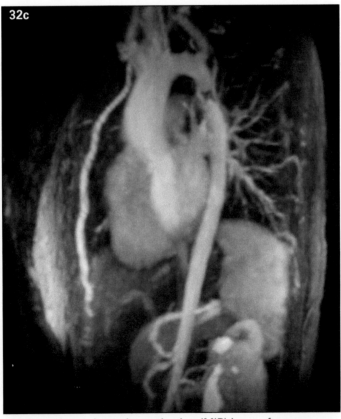

32c A maximum intensity projection (MIP) image from an MRA examination of the thoracic aorta.

CASE 33

History
A 38-year-old man was being investigated for transient neurological episodes.

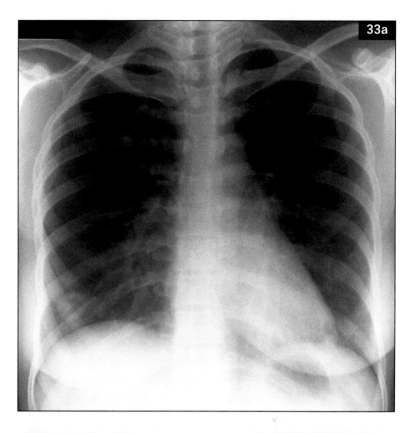

CASE 34

History
A 52-year-old woman with oesophageal cancer presented complaining of chest pain.

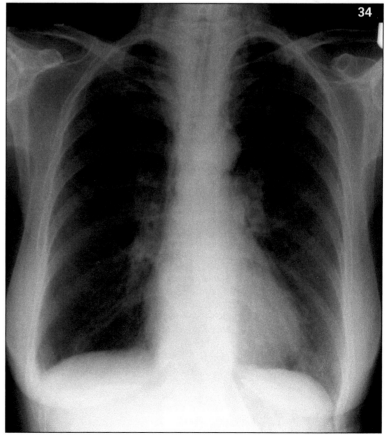

ANSWER 33

Observations (33a)
There are some increased tubular soft tissue density opacities in the right lower zone, suggestive of abnormal vessels, leading to a faint pulmonary nodule. There is a further nodular opacity in the right upper zone, again with the suspicion of vessels running to it from the right hilum. The left lung is clear and the mediastinal outline normal.

Given the clinical details, pulmonary arteriovenous malformations giving rise to paradoxical emboli and TIAs must be presumed. Contrast enhanced CT would confirm.

Diagnosis
Pulmonary arteriovenous malformation (AVM).

Differential diagnosis
Single or multiple pulmonary nodules from other causes.

Discussion
Pulmonary AVMs are abnormal vascular communications between pulmonary arteries and veins (95%) or systemic arteries and pulmonary veins. Most commonly, they are of the simple type, with a single artery feeding a focal aneurysmal segment and a single draining vein. Complex lesions have more than one artery and/or vein. Figure **33b** is a single angiographic image that demonstrates the large feeding vessel to a solitary AVM.

Multiple pulmonary AVMs may be associated with Osler–Weber–Rendu syndrome. They are usually asymptomatic until the 3rd–4th decade when they can present with local effects – haemoptysis, dyspnoea on exertion and cyanosis with clubbing (due to right to left shunt); or with distal effects – cerebrovascular accident (CVA) or brain abscess due to paradoxical emboli. Lesions enlarge with age.

Practical tips
The 'finger in glove' appearance from mucoid impaction of central airways in allergic bronchopulmonary aspergillosis can look similar in some ways to the vessels supplying an AVM. However, there is a nodule at the end of these vessels in AVM.

Further management
Angiographic assessment and treatment with embolization or balloon occlusion is now the preferred management.

Further reading
Coley SC, Jackson JE (1998). Pulmonary arteriovenous malformations. *Clinical Radiology* **53**(6): 396–404.

Pick A, Deschamps C, Stanson AW (1999). Pulmonary arteriovenous fistula: presentation, diagnosis, and treatment. *World Journal of Surgery* **23**(11): 1118–1122.

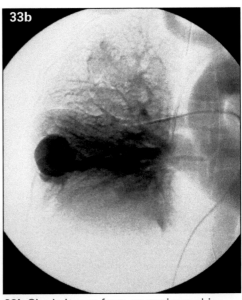

33b Single image from an angiographic investigation demonstrating a large feeding vessel to the pulmonary AVM.

ANSWER 34

Observations (34)
This chest radiograph shows a normal sized heart and clear lungs. There is, however, evidence of air within the mediastinum – best seen around the left heart border and aortic arch. Below the medial left diaphragm, a stent is just about visible across the gastro-oesophageal junction.

It is likely that there has been oesophageal perforation from the stented oesophageal tumour.

Diagnosis
Pneumomediastinum from perforation of stented oesophageal cancer.

Differential diagnosis
For causes of pneumomediastinum:
- Alveolar rupture in acute asthma.
- Oesophageal rupture due to malignancy, trauma, violent vomiting (Boerhaave's syndrome – usually associated with a left sided pleural effusion).
- Extension from peritoneum – pneumoperitoneum.
- Iatrogenic – following oesophageal balloon dilatation/stenting, bronchoscopy, mediastinoscopy, positive pressure ventilation.

Discussion
Pneumomediastinum is an uncommon condition that is usually asymptomatic but can present with neck or chest pain. In itself it rarely leads to any complications but it can be a useful diagnostic sign for an underlying medical condition that does need treatment. Although a rare condition in adults, it is seen in children and most commonly in neonates.

Radiological features include:
- Thin line following the mediastinal contours, as in this case. This line represents the pleura, lifted away from the mediastinal soft tissue by air.
- Streaky air lucencies in the mediastinum.
- 'Continuous diaphragm' sign where lucency is seen behind the heart, connecting the two domes of the diaphragm.

Practical tips
- Assess the ribs for any sign of trauma.
- Assess the lung fields for a lesion that might have warranted bronchoscopic/surgical investigation.
- Look for air under the diaphragm to indicate pneumoperitoneum.
- Look for an effusion to suggest oesophageal injury, or oesophageal stent, as in this case.

Further management
Chest CT after the patient has drunk some water-soluble contrast, or a water-soluble contrast swallow, can confirm an oesophageal tear and leak and help to identify the site.

Further reading
Gerazounis M, Athanassiadi K, Kalantzi N, Moustardas M (2003). Spontaneous pneumomediastinum: a rare benign entity. *Journal of Thoracic and Cardiovascular Surgery* **126**(3): 774–776.

CASE 35

History
A 50-year-old male presented to A&E with recurrent acute-on-chronic dyspnoea.

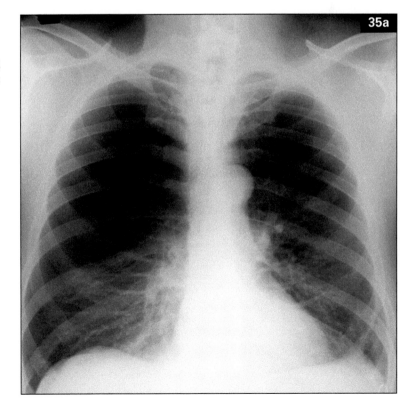

ANSWER 35

Observations (35a)
There is a large area of increased lucency in the right mid and upper zone with no visible lung markings. There is no visible lung edge, however, to suggest this is a pneumothorax. Moreover, there is crowding of vessels in the lower zone. The appearances are likely to indicate a large upper lobe bulla. There are no focal pulmonary opacities to indicate superadded infection. Comparison with any available old films should help confirm this interpretation. A general reduction in density in the left upper zone suggests that similar pathology is developing here too.

Diagnosis
Large right sided bulla.

Discussion
A bulla is a large dilated airspace within the lung with a wall less than 1 mm thick. They are usually produced by alveolar destruction in emphysema. Impaired ventilation of the rest of the lung can result in dyspnoea, as well as that due to the background chronic lung disease.

Confusion can arise when the absence of lung markings leads to the erroneous diagnosis of pneumothorax. This can have dire consequences if an intercostal chest drain is then mistakenly placed in the bulla! An expiratory film makes a pneumothorax easier to detect (because it enhances the contrast differential between pleural air and lung parenchyma) but probably won't help resolve diagnostic confusion with a bulla. Patients with chronic lung disease may well have previous films that show a bulla to be longstanding.

Practical tips
A pneumothorax leads to two findings: a visible lung edge and hypodensity with absent lung markings lateral to this (**35b**). A bulla has absent lung markings but not the discrete lung edge. Conversely, skin folds (seen most frequently in babies and the elderly) can produce a pseudo lung edge but there will be lung markings lateral to it (**35c**).

Further management
If diagnostic uncertainty continues after expert review of the films, then occasionally CT of the thorax may be needed to differentiate bullae from pneumothorax.

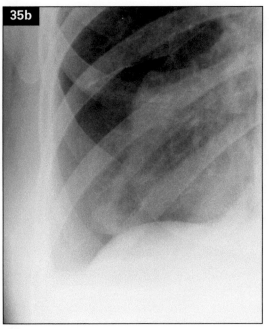

35b Image demonstrates a small pneumothorax with no lung markings lateral to the lung edge.

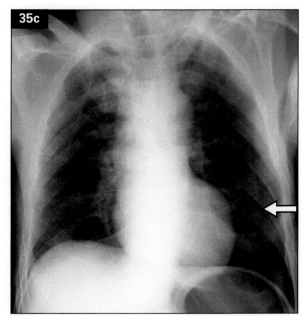

35c Chest radiograph demonstrates a skin fold giving an apparent lung edge but lung markings are visible lateral to it.

CASE 36

History
A 15-year-old male with diabetes presented with recurrent chest infections.

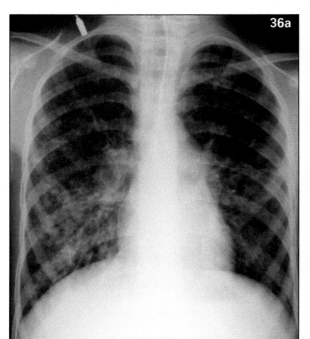
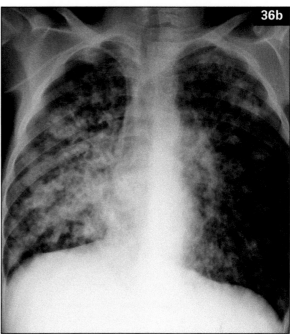

36a, 36b Sequential chest radiographs taken 4 months apart.

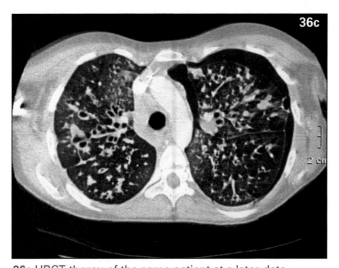

36c HRCT thorax of the same patient at a later date.

ANSWER 36

Observations (36a, 36b, 36c)
This frontal chest radiograph (36a) demonstrates widespread, fairly symmetrical lung parenchymal abnormality that is central in distribution and characterized by bronchial wall thickening and cystic bronchiectatic change. Some larger soft tissue density nodules are seen in the lower zones, which likely represent mucous plugs. Bilateral lobulated hilar enlargement is seen with the right sided lymphadenopathy being more evident. Appearances are of cystic fibrosis.

Chest radiograph (36b) from the same patient taken at a later date demonstrates more advanced disease with more mucous plugging and hyperinflated lungs secondary to air trapping. Peribronchial cuffing and thickened nontapering bronchi are evident. A right subclavian central line is noted, presumably for the administration of IV antibiotics.

A CT image (36c) of the chest on lung windows shows typical features of CF with cylindrical bronchiectasis and a central distribution, peribronchial cuffing, mucous plugging and focal atelectasis. It also shows the most common complication of a pneumothorax on the left side.

Diagnosis
Cystic fibrosis (CF).

Discussion
Cystic fibrosis is an autosomal recessive multisystem condition that is characterized by exocrine gland dysfunction due to mucous plugging arising secondary to a fault in cell chloride transport. The condition affects whites with a geographical distribution affecting Europeans and Ashkenazi Jews. Diagnosis is usually made in children, with the majority being diagnosed within the first year of life with the clinical presentation of meconium ileus and respiratory symptoms. Pulmonary complications are the predominant cause of death and survival is limited to ~30–40 years.

Radiological features of CF on a chest radiograph are:
- Cystic/cylindrical bronchiectasis.
- Peribronchial cuffing/thickening.
- Mucous plugging with secondary atelectasis due to obstruction.
- Hilar lymphadenopathy.
- Allergic bronchopulmonary aspergillosis (ABPA).

Respiratory complications of CF include pneumothorax, haemoptysis and cor pulmonale. Chronic pulmonary infection can lead to hypertrophic pulmonary osteoarthropathy (HPOA).

Cystic fibrosis is a multisystem disease: as well as causing meconium ileus (in children) and meconium ileus equivalent (in adults), it can also cause pancreatic insufficiency, biliary cirrhosis, portal hypertension, malabsorption due to gallbladder disease, cholelithiasis and clubbing (36d).

Practical tips
- Typical presentation is of widespread pulmonary disease in a young patient.
- Tunnelled central lines in patients are used for long term drug treatment with antibiotics or chemotherapy. Again this is a clue to the underlying diagnosis.
- Look for complications of CF – pneumothoraces and secondary infections.
- Though not a common site, HPOA can occur in the humerus and may thus be visible on the edge of the film.

Further management
Follow-up in these patients is best performed with HRCT, which can answer the important questions when lung transplant is considered – is there coexistent *Aspergillus* infection? Are there complicating features, e.g. pneumothoraces?

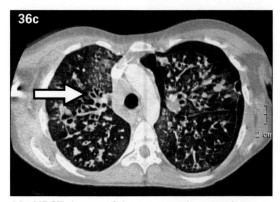

36c HRCT thorax of the same patient at a later date.

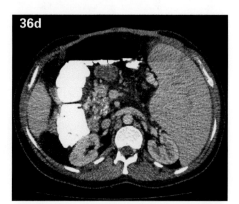

36d Single axial CT image demonstrates significant splenomegaly due to portal hypertension and pancreatic calcification secondary to recurrent bouts of acute pancreatitis.

CASE 37

History
A 34-year-old IV drug user presented with cough and severe shortness of breath. He is noted to be significantly hypoxic on presentation. This series of chest radiographs were taken at presentation, day 3 and day 7.

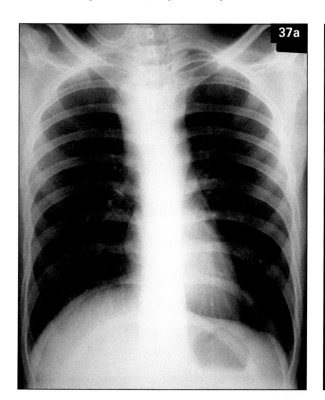
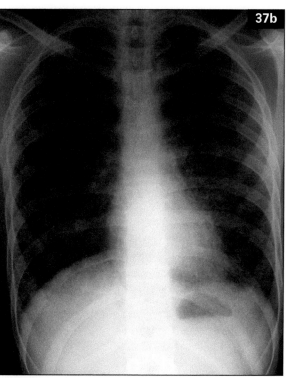
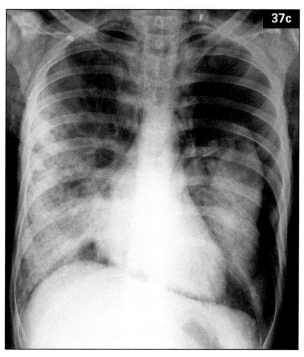

ANSWER 37

Observations (37a, 37b, 37c)
The first chest film taken at presentation (**37a**) shows no obvious radiological abnormality. The next radiograph from 3 days later (**37b**) shows bilateral mid and lower zone reticular/granular interstitial infiltrate with no evidence of volume loss. The third film from 7 days after presentation (**37c**) shows bilateral consolidative change affecting both lungs. There is a pneumothorax on the left with subtotal collapse of the left lung. Surgical emphysema is noted.

It is notable that the patient was initially very symptomatic with a relatively normal chest film and then showed rapid pulmonary changes over several days. The history of IV drug abuse raises the possibility of background HIV infection and the sequence of radiological appearances is typical for *Pneumocystis carinii* pneumonia.

Diagnosis
Pneumocystis carinii pneumonia (PCP).

Discussion
P. carinii pneumonia is the most common cause of interstitial pneumonia in immunocompromised patients. Radiological findings can be very variable but the typical pattern of development is as follows:

- Normal chest radiograph is seen in up to 40% of patients, especially early on in the infection.
- Bilateral diffuse perihilar airspace/granular/reticular opacities is the typical appearance.
- Progression to diffuse airspace consolidation with air bronchograms.
- Pleural effusions are seen in ~20% of cases.
- Response to treatment occurs over a period of ~1 week.
- Atypical features (seen in ~5%) include upper lobe thin and thick walled cysts, lung nodules, mediastinal and hilar lymphadenopathy.
- Treatment with aerosolized pentamidine alone results in the disease affecting upper lobes.

Complications of PCP are common, e.g. pneumothorax and superimposed TB/fungal infections.

Appearances on CT include a patchy mosaic/'ground glass' pattern with subsegmental sparing and coexistent thin walled cysts and pneumatoceles. Appearance of nodules on CT imaging is suggestive of a second disease process being involved – metastases, lymphoma, septic emboli or Kaposi's sarcoma.

Bilateral gallium uptake is seen prior to radiological changes being evident.

Practical tips
A strong index of suspicion for PCP should be maintained when an immunocompromised patient presents with dyspnoea. As in this case, symptoms can be out of proportion to the initial radiographic changes.

Further management
Diagnosis is confirmed with sputum cytology or bronchoscopy and lavage. Treatment is with IV co-trimoxazole.

Further reading
Kuhlman JE, Kavuru M, Fishman EK, Siegelman SS (1990). *Pneumocystis carinii* pneumonia: spectrum of parenchymal CT findings. *Radiology* **175**: 711–714.

Chapter 2

ABDOMINAL IMAGING

PLAIN ABDOMINAL RADIOGRAPHS

As always, a systematic approach is required to be able to extract the most information from a radiograph. The order suggested is a guide and should be adapted to your own preferences and adjusted for each individual case.

General assessment

Rapidly assess the quality of the film, ensuring that there is adequate coverage – are the hernial orifices covered in the patient who appears to have small bowel obstruction? In addition, make a quick assessment of the film to exclude two important diagnoses that are surgical emergencies and will require immediate management:
- Perforation.
- Toxic megacolon.

Lines

Identify any lines that are present, e.g. postsurgical drains, NG tubes, urinary catheters and peritoneal dialysis catheters. The presence of peritoneal dialysis catheters or postsurgical drains may offer a simple explanation for free intraperitoneal gas.

Gas pattern

Differentiating small from large bowel is very difficult in young children and one can usually only say whether a problem is in the proximal or distal bowel. In adults, features used to distinguish the two include position in the abdomen; diameter (large bowel <5 cm, small bowel <3 cm); valvulae conniventes traverse the whole width of small bowel but this is not so with the colonic haustrations; solid faeces only seen in colon.

The range of 'normal' bowel gas patterns is rather wide, but from experience, one should quickly know whether the amount and distribution of bowel gas are very abnormal. Unusually shaped collections of gas (e.g. triangular) should raise suspicion of gas outside the GI tract and lead you to examine the area very closely. Check carefully for gas in areas of the abdomen where it is not normally seen, e.g. over the liver (either as pockets of gas or within the biliary tree) or in the retroperitoneum. Don't forget to check for bowel loops extending below the inguinal ligament indicative of hernia.

Exclude bowel dilatation and wall thickening. If there is dilatation, decide whether it is small or large bowel and then try to establish the 'cut-off' point. Later cases illustrate specific features to check for when one suspects small or large bowel obstruction.

Soft tissue organs

Check the size and outline of the liver, spleen and kidneys. Also check the psoas outlines which may be obscured by retroperitoneal pathology.

Calcification

Look at the rest of the film for calcified densities such as gallstones (only 5–10% visible on plain radiographs) and renal tract calculi (80–85% visible on plain radiographs). Common incidental calcific opacities include mesenteric nodes, phleboliths, vascular calcification and uterine fibroids. Calcification within the solid organs may be more significant however. Unusual calcified opacities may allow for a specific diagnosis such as a pelvic dermoid.

Bones

Assess the bones of the vertebral column and pelvis for incidental pathology or findings that might be relevant to intra-abdominal disease such as sacroiliac joint changes associated with inflammatory bowel disease.

Periphery of the film

Conclude by looking at peripheral structures. For example, pathology at the lung bases that might mimic abdominal pathology, incidental lesions in the abdominal wall.

ABDOMINAL CT

The first question to ask yourself when looking at an abdominal CT is what type of contrast has the patient been given, i.e. oral/IV/both and during what phase has imaging been carried out. The typical phase for abdominal

Abdominal Imaging

imaging is portal–venous (60–70 seconds delay) but other phases, e.g. pre-contrast, arterial, delayed, are useful in characterizing specific lesions.

Axial images will commonly be presented and you can proceed in one of two ways – either assess all structures on each axial image then proceed to the next image, or, alternatively, assess each organ in turn over a series of slices before moving on to the next organ. In reality, a combination of the two is often used but the latter ensures nothing is missed.

As well as searching for focal lesions within the organs, other features to check include the following:

- Liver:
  - Overall attenuation (e.g. reduced in fatty change) and enhancement homogeneity.
  - Size and contour (e.g. irregular contour in cirrhosis).
  - Patency of normal vascular structures.
  - State of intrahepatic bile ducts.
- Gallbladder – check for stones, the density of bile, wall thickening and pericholecystic fluid. Carefully assess the extrahepatic bile ducts.
- Pancreas – check for calcification; the state of the pancreatic duct, peripancreatic collections and inflammatory changes.
- Spleen – check size and adjacent varices.
- Kidneys – is the attenuation of the kidneys correct for that phase of scan? Is there collecting system dilatation? Check the adrenals above.

Then systematically evaluate the non-solid organs:

- Aorta – as well as overall size, check for dissection and patency of main branches. Check major venous patency at the same time, excluding deep vein thrombus.
- Bladder, ovaries/uterus.
- Lymphadenopathy.
- Intra-abdominal fat – peritoneal soft tissue deposits are easily overlooked unless the abdominal fat is carefully scrutinized.
- Colon, ileum and stomach.
- Free gas/fluid.
- Bones and lung bases.

CASE 38

History
A 53-year-old male presented with a history of gradually progressive dysphagia.

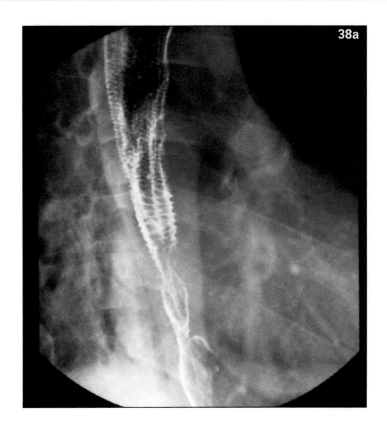

CASE 39

History
A 78-year-old female presented with rectal bleeding.

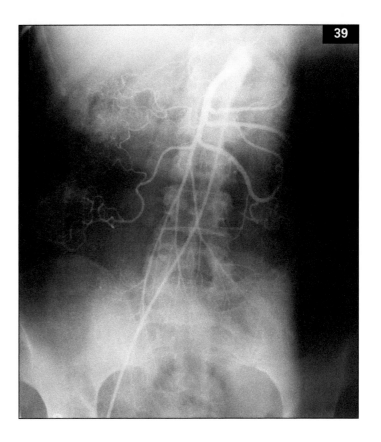

ANSWER 38

Observations (38a)
Single AP image from a double contrast barium swallow examination shows a short, smoothly tapered narrowing in the lower oesophagus just superior to the gastro-oesophageal junction and a small hiatus hernia. The oesophagus proximal to this has delicate transverse mucosal folds, the so-called feline oesophagus. This appearance is associated with gastro-oesophageal reflux and leads to the conclusion that the short stricture is a peptic stricture.

Diagnosis
Peptic stricture feline oesophagus.

Differential diagnosis
For oesophageal strictures:
- Lower oesophagus:
  - Peptic stricture secondary to gastro-oesophageal reflux.
  - Scleroderma – affected patients have an incompetent lower oesophageal sphincter and reduced peristalsis resulting in marked gastro-oesophageal reflux.
  - NG intubation – prevents closure of the lower oesophageal sphincter.
  - Zollinger–Ellison syndrome.

- Upper and mid oesophagus:
  - Barrett oesophagus – acquired condition characterized by columnar metaplasia secondary to chronic gastro-oesophageal reflux/oesophagitis. Premalignant condition with an increased risk of adenocarcinoma of the oesophagus.
  - Caustic ingestion – usually long, smooth narrowing forms 1–3 months post ingestion.
  - Mediastinal radiotherapy – usually long, smooth narrowing forms 4–8 months post radiotherapy.
  - Skin diseases – epidermolysis bullosa, pemphigoid, erythema multiforme.

Other less common causes of strictures include Crohn's disease, *Candida* oesophagitis and Behçet's disease.

Discussion
Peptic strictures have this typical appearance of short (1–4 cm), smooth, tapered, concentric narrowing in the lower oesophagus. Associated radiological findings include intramural pseudodiverticulosis (**38b**) and feline oesophagus (so called because this is the normal appearance in cats). Longitudinal scarring can cause fixed transverse folds but these can be differentiated from feline oesophagus since they are only seen in the region of the stricture and do not extend more than half way across the oesophagus, giving a 'step ladder' appearance.

Practical tips
Previous CXRs can be useful in identifying a cause for a stricture – look for a tumour that might have been irradiated or features of aspiration pneumonia/hiatus hernia.

Further management
Gastroenterology referral with a view to direct visualization and confirmation of diagnosis with endoscopy.

Further reading
Luedtke P, Levine MS, Rubesin SE, *et al.* (2003). Radiologic diagnosis of benign esophageal strictures: a pattern approach. *RadioGraphics* **23**: 897–909.

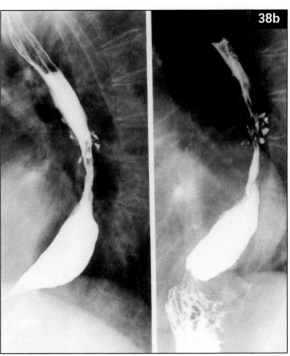

38b Contrast barium swallow shows flask shaped outpouchings with a narrow neck of intramural pseudodiverticulosis.

ANSWER 39

Observations (39)
Single image from a mesenteric angiogram examination shows an abnormal cluster of vessels and contrast 'blush' in the caecum.

Diagnosis
Angiodysplasia.

Differential diagnosis
Of lower GI haemorrhage:
- Diverticular disease.
- Colonic carcinoma.
- Colonic angiodysplasia.
- Inflammatory colitis.
- Mesenteric varices.

Discussion
Angiodysplasia is the most common cause of occult bleeding in the large bowel, predominantly affecting the elderly population. The condition is characterized by vascular ectasia of the colonic circulation, most commonly affecting the caecum and ascending colon. The condition leads to chronic low-grade blood loss but can also lead to episodes of severe lower GI bleeding. There is an association with valvular heart disease, specifically aortic stenosis.

Diagnosis can be made with selective mesenteric angiography or CT angiography. Both are able to identify bleeding when the rate is as little as 1 ml/min. Three levels of abnormality are identified:
- In early disease, a densely contrast filled dilated vein is seen within the bowel wall.
- As the disease progresses, a vascular tuft can be seen at the lesion site.
- Further progression shows an early filling vein during the arterial phase of scanning.

Mesenteric angiography has the advantage of proceeding directly to treatment with embolization.

Practical tips
CT is excellent at identifying the bleeding point when there is active GI bleeding. Always perform a pre-contrast scan prior to the arterial phase scan so that high-contrast intraluminal blood can be differentiated from high-contrast bowel food content/debris.

Further management
Surgical resection is the definitive treatment when endoscopic treatments have not controlled bleeding.

CASE 40

History
A 35-year-old farmer presented with mild ache in the right upper abdomen for several months.

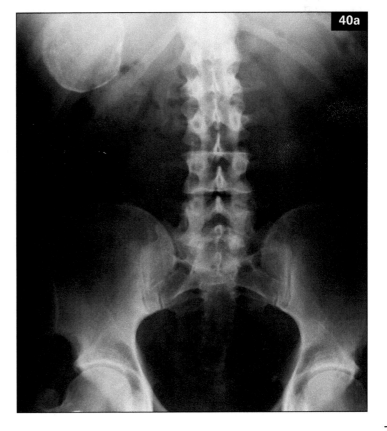

ANSWER 40

Observations (40a)
There is a large, well defined lesion in the right upper quadrant, which has thin, curvilinear calcification of its wall. This is projected over the liver and is probably intrahepatic, though a calcified gallbladder cannot be excluded from this film. This is a solitary lesion with no other abnormality seen. Given the appearances and patient's young age and occupation, a hydatid cyst of the liver is most likely. Further imaging with CT would help confirm the location of the lesion and the likely diagnosis. Serological tests for hydatid disease should also be undertaken.

Diagnosis
Hydatid disease.

Differential diagnosis
Of calcified liver lesion:
- Metastasis – especially colorectal cancer.
- Primary liver tumour.
- Infection – hydatid, TB.

Discussion
Hydatid disease is acquired through infection by the parasitic tapeworm *Echinococcus granulosus*. Dogs are the definite host with the human acting as an accidental host following accidental ingestion of eggs from canine faeces. The liver is the most commonly involved organ and presentation is with abdominal pain, jaundice, biliary colic with eosinophilia in 20–50%.

In the liver, infection results in the formation of a cyst, which is more commonly found in the right lobe; the size of the cyst ranges up to 50 cm but is ~5 cm on average and multiple in 20% of cases. The cyst is composed of three layers – the outer pericyst, middle laminated ectocyst and the inner endocyst.

Radiological features are:
- Variable appearance ranging from a simple unilocular cyst to a complex heterogeneous cystic mass.
- Daughter cysts are characteristic but are a rare finding. Their presence is noted by a 'racemose' appearance. Initially daughter cysts are well defined and round and are seen at the periphery of the mother cysts. They progress to form large, irregular shaped cysts filling the mother cyst.
- Can also contain debris (hydatid sand), internal septations and wall calcification.
- Calcification is seen in 20–30% of hydatid cysts and is usually curvilinear or ring like. Dense calcification is seen as the cyst starts to heal.
- On CT, the appearance is of a cyst with a high attenuation wall on unenhanced CT even without calcification.
- MRI appearance is of a cyst with a low signal rim.
- On CT/MRI, the wall and septae enhance with contrast, which can aid in the differentiation between hydatid cyst and a simple liver cyst.

Complications are of cyst rupture (50–90% of cases) and infection.

The lungs are the second most common site of involvement in adults and the most common in children. There is a predilection for the lower lobes and disease is more commonly seen on the right. Cysts are multiple in 20% and bilateral in 20% of cases. Figure **40b** shows several left sided, well defined round intrapulmonary lesions. Calcification is rare. When air infiltrates between the layers of the cyst wall it can give the appearance of a 'meniscus' sign, 'onion peel' sign and finally the 'water lily' sign, when there is complete separation of the endocyst from the pericyst. Rupture of the cyst can result in surrounding consolidation.

Practical tips
- Benign liver cysts are common, but all cysts should be closely inspected for atypical features, e.g. hyperattenuating wall or wall calcification suggestive of abscess/hydatid; poorly defined edges, which may suggest the lesion is in fact a metastasis.
- Cystic lesions involving liver and lungs should suggest infective/malignant underlying diagnosis until proven otherwise.

Further management
Management can be either medical (two benzimidazoles are commonly used, albendazole and mebendazole) or surgical (cystectomy or partial organ resection).

Further reading
Pedrosa I, Saíz A, Arrazola J, *et al.* (2000). Hydatid disease: radiologic and pathologic features and complications. *RadioGraphics* **20**: 795–817.

Polat P, Kantarci M, Alper F, *et al.* (2003). Hydatid disease from head to toe. *RadioGraphics* **23**: 475–494.

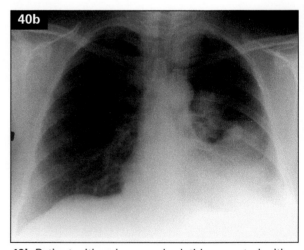

40b Patient with pulmonary hydatid presented with several large, well defined nodules in the left lung with no calcification.

Abdominal Imaging Case 41

CASE 41

History
A 67-year-old, overweight female patient, with no past medical history, presented with vague abdominal pain, nausea and vomiting.

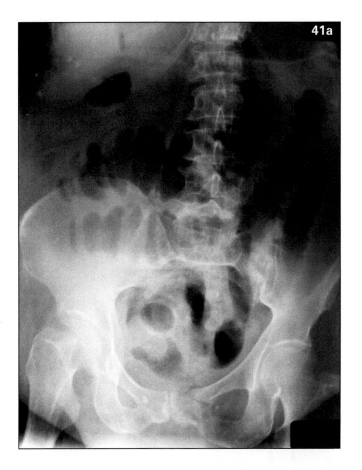

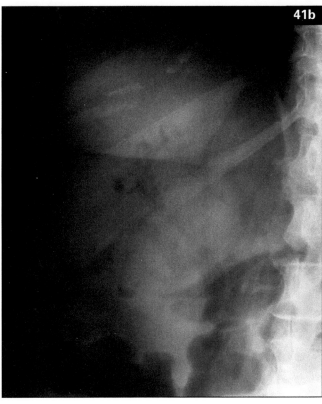

ANSWER 41

Observations (41a, 41b)
AP abdominal radiograph shows distended loops of gas-filled small bowel but absent colonic gas. Together with the clinical history, appearances are consistent with small bowel obstruction. There is no evidence of free gas on these films but on the second image there is an abnormal collection of air over the central liver that has a somewhat linear/branching configuration. This is consistent with air in the biliary tree. In the right side of pelvis, there is a round opacity showing peripheral calcification – this is likely to indicate an obstructing gallstone.

Diagnosis
Gallstone ileus.

Discussion
Gallstone ileus is relatively rare, accounting for 1–2% of all mechanical obstructions (though more in the elderly). The most common scenario is of a stone eroding through from gallbladder to duodenum – the cholecystoduodenal fistula leads to pneumobilia and the stone then impacts in the small bowel. The fistula can also be from the common duct, and can extend to the colon or stomach instead of the small bowel.

Occasionally, the diagnosis can be made on plain films with Rigler's triad of small bowel obstruction, pneumobilia and ectopic gallstones. Often, however, the gallstone is not seen on plain film since the stones frequently have a predominant composition of cholesterol with little calcification. An axial CT scan of the abdomen (**41c**) confirmed a gallstone ileus with a 5 cm diameter laminated gallstone found in the distal ileum. The bowel was collapsed distal to the site of stone impaction. At laparotomy, the stone was milked back to the jejunum and removed.

Practical tips
- Always check for air in the biliary tree on the small bowel obstruction abdominal film.
- Tiny locules of air in the biliary tree tend to be centrally located in the liver (**41d**) compared with portal vein gas, which is seen in the periphery.
- Biliary tree gas can also be seen as a normal finding in patients who have had a previous sphincterotomy or following a recent ERCP (endoscopic retrograde cholangiopancreatography).

Further management
Mechanical small bowel obstruction is a surgical emergency.

Further reading
Gurleyik G, Gurleyik E (2001). Gallstone ileus: demographic and clinical criteria supporting preoperative diagnosis. *Ulus Travma Derg* **7(1)**: 32–34.

Pangan JC, Estrada R, Rosales R (1984). Cholecystoduodenocolic fistula with recurrent gallstone ileus. *Archives of Surgery* **119**: 1201–1203.

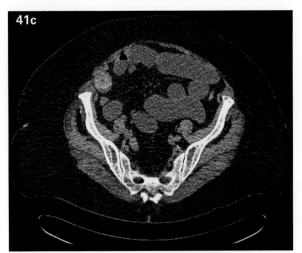

41c Axial CT image shows a calcified gallstone within the lumen of the distal ileum with dilated loops of small bowel seen proximally.

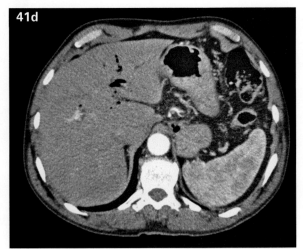

41d Axial CT image shows central locules of gas within the biliary tree.

CASE 42

History
A 68-year-old male is admitted with hepatic encephalopathy.

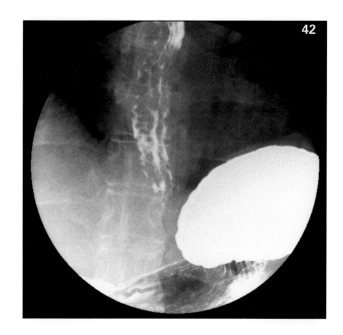

CASE 43

History
An asymptomatic 22-year-old male presented with deteriorating renal function.

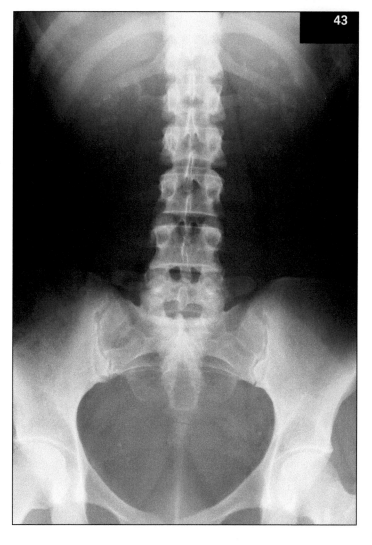

ANSWER 42

Observations (42)
Image from a double contrast barium meal examination shows multiple serpiginous filling defects in the lower oesophagus. Normal appearances of the gastric fundus are observed. Appearances are consistent with oesophageal varices and the distribution suggests that these are 'uphill'.

Diagnosis
Oesophageal varices.

Differential diagnosis
For oesophageal varices:
- Varicoid carcinoma of oesophagus.

For gastric varices (i.e. causes of thickened gastric folds):
- Hypertrophic gastritis.
- Ménétrier's disease.
- Lymphoma.
- Splenic vein thrombosis.

Discussion
Oesophageal varices have a very typical appearance on contrast swallow examination of dilated, smooth, serpiginous filling defects. Varices collapse in the erect position and are best imaged with the patient prone. There are two types:
- Uphill varices (found in the lower oesophagus); these are characterized by collateral blood flow from the portal vein via the azygous vein to the superior vena cava (SVC). These arise due to liver cirrhosis and due to IVC/hepatic vein/splenic vein thrombosis or obstruction.
- Downhill varices (found in the mid and upper oesophagus); these are characterized by collateral blood flow from the SVC via the azygous vein into the IVC, and arise due to SVC obstruction from conditions such as lung tumour, lymphoma and retrosternal goitre.

Gastric varices are seen in combination with oesophageal varices in patients with portal hypertension. When seen in the absence of oesophageal varices, splenic vein thrombosis should be suspected. Again, appearances are of smooth, serpiginous or grape-like filling defects; most commonly seen in the gastric fundus.

Practical tips
- Best images are obtained with the patient in a prone position.
- Further investigation with an ultrasound of the abdomen should be advised to look for cirrhosis and portal hypertension.

Further management
Treatment is aimed at controlling portal hypertension with medical and surgical (transjugular intrahepatic portosystemic shunt – TIPS) means. Treatment of bleeding varices and preemptive treatment of nonbleeding varices is achieved with endoscopic banding and sclerotherapy.

ANSWER 43

Observations (43)
This plain abdominal radiograph shows multiple small foci of calcification over both renal areas in the region of the renal medulla rather than renal cortex. No stones are seen elsewhere along the course of the renal tracts.

Diagnosis
Renal medullary nephrocalcinosis.

Discussion
Medullary nephrocalcinosis represents calcification in the distal convoluted tubules, i.e. in the renal pyramids. There are many causes and the underlying pathology can rarely be determined on a plain radiograph – clinical history is far more important here.

The causes are:
- Renal tubular acidosis (RTA).
- Endocrine causes – hyperparathyroidism, hyperthyroidism, Cushing's.
- Medullary sponge kidney.
- Idiopathic hypercalcuria.
- Renal papillary necrosis.
- Hypervitaminosis D.
- Milk-alkali syndrome.
- Malignancy – bone metastases, multiple myeloma, paraneoplastic syndrome.
- Primary hyperoxaluria.

Practical tips
- The most common causes of symmetrical medullary nephrocalcinosis are hyperparathyroidism and RTA.
- The most common cause of asymmetrical medullary nephrocalcinosis is medullary sponge kidney.

Further management
Underlying cause must be identified – particularly treatable causes.

Further reading
Dyer RB, Chen MY, Zagoria RJ (1998). Abnormal calcifications in the urinary tract. *RadioGraphics* **18**: 1405–1424.

CASE 44

History
A 34-year-old male presented with nausea and vomiting.

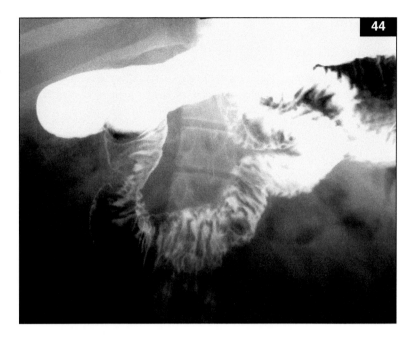

CASE 45

History
A 68-year-old male presented with postprandial bloating.

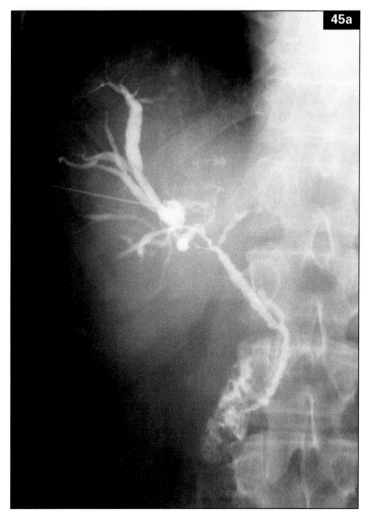

ANSWER 44

Observations (44)
This is a single AP image from a double contrast small bowel barium examination. There is focal, eccentric narrowing of the second part of the duodenum, with predominant notching of the lateral wall. Appearances of the duodenum superior and inferior to this are completely normal.

Diagnosis
Annular pancreas.

Differential diagnosis
For annular pancreas:
- Sphincter of Oddi oedema (secondary to impacted stone or pancreatitis)/carcinoma – usually produces an eccentric lesion but this is predominantly medially located.
- Duodenal adenocarcinoma – usually presents with an annular concentric lesion with shouldering and ulceration. There is an association with Gardner's syndrome and coeliac disease.

Discussion
Annular pancreas is a disorder characterized by failure of rotation of the ventral bud of the pancreas resulting in pancreatic tissue encircling the duodenum. The second part of the duodenum is involved in 85% of cases. Usually patients are asymptomatic, but the condition can present at any age, with 48% of cases presenting in adulthood. There is an association with other congenital abnormalities when the condition presents in childhood – tracheo-oesophageal atresia, duodenal atresia, imperforate anus, Down's syndrome.

Clinical presentation can be with:
- Polyhydramnios – *in utero*.
- Persistent vomiting, 'double bubble' – in neonates.
- Nausea, vomiting and abdominal pain – in adults.

The condition is complicated by an increased incidence of acute and chronic pancreatitis and periampullary peptic ulcer.

Practical tips
Carefully examine the film for gallstones or small bowel features of coeliac disease (small bowel dilatation, flocculation of contrast, featureless smooth small bowel lumen/folds, jejunization of ileal loops and poor peristalsis) to suggest another diagnosis.

Further management
- CT will confirm pancreatic tissue encircling the duodenum.
- ERCP (endoscopic retrograde cholangiopancreatography) or MRCP (magnetic resonance cholangiopancreatography) shows a normally located main pancreatic duct in the body of the pancreas, and a small duct in the head of the pancreas encircling the duodenum.

Further reading
Rizzo RJ, Szucs RA, Turner MA (1995). Congenital abnormalities of the pancreas and biliary tree in adults. *RadioGraphics* **15(1):** 49–68.

ANSWER 45

Observations (45a)
Single image from a percutaneous cholangiogram is shown. The percutaneous needle is seen with the tip in a proximal intrahepatic biliary duct. There is clear abnormality of the common duct, which has several strictures with duct dilatation and beading. No filling defects are seen to indicate gallstones. Contrast is seen in the duodenum with no obstructing lesion seen at the level of the sphincter of Oddi.

Diagnosis
Primary sclerosing cholangitis (PSC).

Differential diagnosis
For PSC:
- Sclerosing cholangiocarcinoma.
- Acute ascending cholangitis.
- Bile duct carcinoma – this can rarely involve the biliary system in a diffuse manner producing multiple tumour strictures.

Discussion
Primary sclerosing cholangitis is a progressive fibrosing inflammatory condition affecting both intrahepatic and extrahepatic bile ducts. The condition is strongly associated with inflammatory bowel disease (ulcerative colitis [UC] found in 70%, Crohn's in 15%). Other associations include retroperitoneal and mediastinal fibrosis, chronic active hepatitis, Riedel's thyroiditis, pancreatitis and Sjögren's syndrome. Presentation is with progressive fatigue, pruritus and jaundice. Biochemical changes are found with elevated serum bilirubin and alkaline phosphatase.
- Imaging features on cholangiography (MRCP/ERCP): there are multifocal strictures affecting intra- and extrahepatic bile ducts with skip lesions. The classic pattern is of a 'beaded' appearance with alternating segments of stenosis and dilatation (45b).
- Imaging features on CT: ducts have the appearance of strictures, dilatation, beading and pruning.
- Imaging on US: usually normal but may show duct wall thickening.

Complications of PSC include:
- Gallstones.
- Biliary cirrhosis.
- Portal hypertension.
- Cholangiocarcinoma.

Practical tips
MRCP is now the noninvasive diagnostic investigation of choice.

Further management
The only curative treatment for this condition is liver transplantation. Medical palliative care involves treatment of the symptoms of cirrhosis, portal hypertension, chronic cholestasis (pruritus and malabsorption) and ductal complications such as strictures and ascending cholangitis. A multidisciplinary approach is therefore adopted requiring hepatologists, transplant surgeons and interventional radiologists.

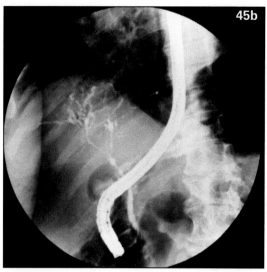

45b Single image from an ERCP examination showing multiple strictures with poststenotic dilatation giving a beaded appearance.

CASE 46

History
A 67-year-old male presented with abdominal pain and vomiting.

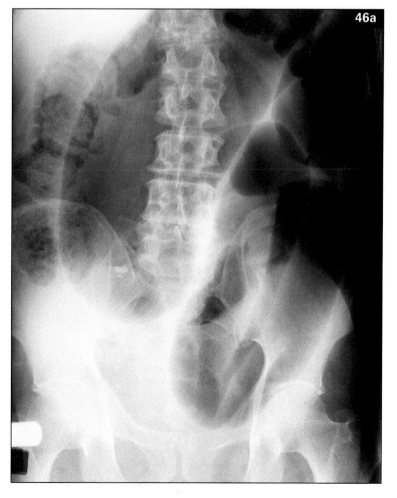

ANSWER 46

Observations (46a)
This plain abdominal radiograph shows a large, ahaustral gas-filled viscus arising from the left side of the pelvis and extending into the upper abdomen. The loop is projected over the left side of pelvis and descending colon with its apex under the left hemidiaphragm. The medial walls of the loop form a summation line. There are several dilated loops of descending colon evident with absence of gas in the rectum. The features are typical of sigmoid volvulus and there is no free intraperitoneal gas seen to indicate perforation.

Diagnosis
Sigmoid volvulus.

Differential diagnosis
For large bowel obstruction:
- Colonic malignancy.
- Inflammatory strictures: Crohn's, ischaemia, diverticulitis.
- Volvulus.
- Infectious processes: TB, amoebiasis.
- Extrinsic lesions: abscess, bladder/prostate/uterine tumour, endometriosis.

Discussion
Volvulus account for ~10% of large bowel obstructions in the UK, the most common type being sigmoid volvulus. This occurs more commonly in the elderly. The twisting of the sigmoid colon on its mesenteric axis is usually a chronic problem with superimposed acute episodes, and represents a closed loop obstruction. Radiologically, the features are of large bowel obstruction with a markedly dilated loop of colon seen arising from the left iliac fossa. The volvulus is characterized by an ahaustral inverted U-shaped loop of colon. The medial walls produce a summation line and together with the lines of the lateral walls create the classic 'coffee bean' appearance. Several radiological features have been documented as typical, though the most specific are:
- Apex of the loop under the left hemidiaphragm.
- Inferior convergence of the loop in the left side of the pelvis – the main axis of the loop therefore extends from left iliac fossa towards right upper quadrant.
- 'Left flank overlap' sign – loop overlaps descending colon.
- Medial wall summation line.

Other features described include 'liver overlap' and 'pelvic overlap' signs (where the loop overlaps liver and left iliac bone, respectively); apex of loop above T10; an air to fluid ratio >2:1.

Diagnostic confusion can be resolved with a barium enema examination. This demonstrates a smooth, tapered beak-like end of the barium column termed the 'bird's beak' sign. Treatment involves the placing of a rectal flatus tube.

Practical tips
Caecal volvulus (**46b**) can sometimes be a confusing differential. It represents twisting just above the ileocaecal valve and can usually be differentiated from sigmoid volvulus by several features:
- Caecal volvulus usually occurs in a younger age group: 30–50 years.
- Dilated obstructed caecum often dilates to fill the left upper quadrant (although in many cases vertical rotation occurs with caecum still filling the right iliac fossa). The main axis will be opposite that of sigmoid volvulus however, extending from the right iliac fossa towards the left upper quadrant.
- Some haustral markings are still evident, unlike sigmoid volvulus.
- There may well be small bowel dilatation but the rest of the colon will be undilated, unlike sigmoid volvulus.

Further management
Urgent surgical referral with a view to insertion of a flatus tube to decompress the bowel.

Further reading
Burrell HC, Baker DM, Wardrop P, Evans AJ (1994). Significant plain film findings in sigmoid volvulus. *Clinical Radiology* **49**: 317–319.

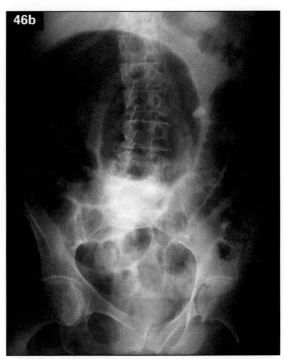

46b Caecal volvulus with a dilated caecum extending up into the right upper quadrant. Small bowel is dilated secondary to this obstruction but large bowel is collapsed helping to differentiate caecal from sigmoid volvulus.

Abdominal Imaging — Cases 47, 48

CASE 47

History
A 35-year-old female presented with abdominal pain and vomiting.

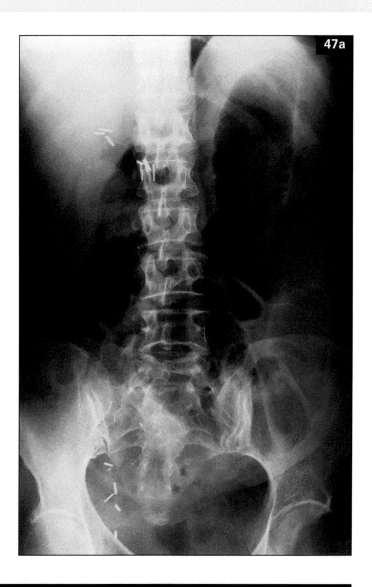

CASE 48

History
A 38-year-old woman underwent contrast enhanced CT for further evaluation of a lesion noted on ultrasound.

(see page 88 for case answer)

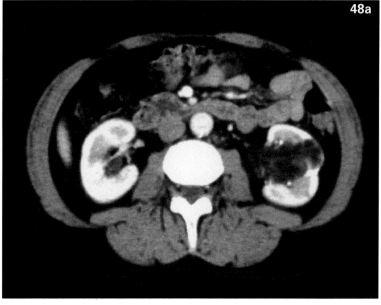

ANSWER 47

Observations (47a)
Multiple dilated loops of gas-filled small bowel that measure more than 3 cm in diameter are seen within the central abdomen. No gas is seen within the large bowel and appearances are consistent with small bowel obstruction. Surgical clips are noted in the right side of pelvis along with cholecystectomy clips in the right upper quadrant. Adhesions are therefore the most likely cause of the obstruction.

Diagnosis
Small bowel obstruction from adhesions.

Differential diagnosis
For small bowel obstruction:
- Adhesions – account for up to 60% of small bowel obstructions.
- Hernia.
- Gallstone ileus.
- Small bowel or caecal malignancy.
- Intussusception.
- Malrotation and volvulus.

Discussion
Small bowel obstruction can have a varied presentation on plain abdominal radiography. The classical appearance is of central abdominal small bowel loops dilated to >3 cm in diameter with a paucity of gas in the large bowel. Other appearances can be of:
- 'String of beads' sign due to small air-fluid levels in fluid-filled obstructed loops of small bowel (**47b**).
- Absence of gas in the small bowel due to complete obstruction and complete fluid filling of loops (**47c**).

Small bowel can be differentiated from large bowel using the following features:
- Presence of valvulae conniventes which extend across the width of the bowel. Colonic haustra do not traverse the whole lumen.
- Dilated bowel located in the central abdomen rather than the periphery (**47d**).
- Diameter of loops is <5 cm.
- Absence of solid faeces.

Practical tips
Always check the film to try to identify the underlying cause of the obstruction:
- Check hernial orifices at the groin – there should be no bowel gas extending below the position of the inguinal ligament (a line from pubic tubercle to anterior-superior iliac spine) (**47e, 47f, 47g, 47h**).
- Look for evidence of previous surgery, as in this case.
- Look for air in the biliary tree and radio-opaque gallstones outside the territory of the gallbladder as indicators of gallstone ileus.
- Examine bones for metastatic lesions, which can point to malignancy.
- Always remember to check for free gas secondary to perforation!

Further management
CT is the investigation of choice for small bowel obstruction and it can identify both the site and cause of obstruction and also the complications. Mechanical small bowel obstruction is a surgical emergency.

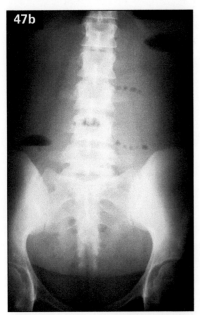

47b Plain abdominal radiograph demonstrating the 'string of beads' sign.

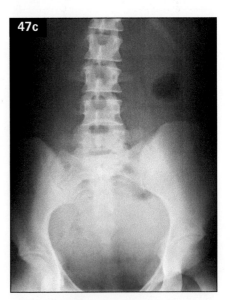

47c Plain abdominal radiograph demonstrating complete absence of small bowel gas due to fluid filling.

Answer 47 — Abdominal Imaging

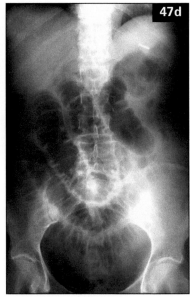

47d Classic distribution of dilated small bowel: dilated loops are centrally located within the abdomen.

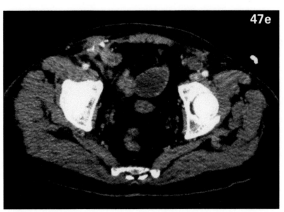

47e Axial CT image shows that there has been a previous attempted hernia repair with a mesh noted *in situ*. There has, however, been a recurrence with dilated bowel going into the hernia and completely collapsed bowel emerging from it. This shows that this is the level of obstruction.

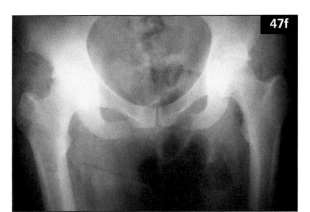

47f Pelvis radiograph shows loops of small bowel below the inguinal ligament.

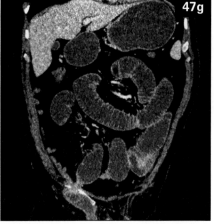

47g Coronal CT reformatted image in the same patient demonstrates a right sided inguinal hernia.

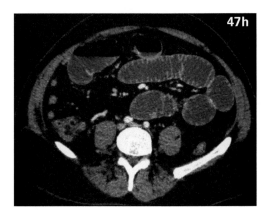

47h Axial CT image of a patient with small bowel obstruction.

ANSWER 48

Observations (48a)
A large central mass lesion is demonstrated in the left kidney. This is slightly heterogeneous but has a predominantly fatty density. Appearances are consistent with left renal angiomyolipoma.

Diagnosis
Angiomyolipoma.

Discussion
Angiomyolipoma is a benign lesion containing fat, blood vessels and smooth muscle. They tend to present in two groups of patients:
- Women in their 4th–7th decades where lesions arise spontaneously and tend to be *solitary and unilateral*.
- Young patients with tuberous sclerosis where *multiple and bilateral* lesions are seen in up to 75% of patients (48b).

They are also seen rarely in autosomal dominant polycystic kidney disease (ADPKD) and neurofibromatosis.
- Appearance on US: typical appearance is of a well defined echobright lesion due to a high fat content (48c). There can be a variable degree of reduced echogenicity depending on the amount of smooth muscle and/or haemorrhage.
- Appearance on CT: again, appearance is of a well defined fat-containing lesion with some areas of higher attenuation tissue. Identification of fat (HU <–20) within a renal lesion is highly specific for an angiomyolipoma.
- Appearances on MRI: a fat suppression sequence can be very useful in confirming intralesional fat content.

The main complication of these lesions is haemorrhage and the risk is related to size. Lesions greater than 4 cm in diameter have a risk of spontaneous bleeding of approximately 50%.

Practical tips
Identification of fat in a renal lesion is very specific for angiomyolipoma.

Further management
Small lesions (<4 cm) are usually asymptomatic but lesions >4 cm are almost always symptomatic with pain and a risk of haemorrhage. Lesion resection or nephrectomy should be considered in these patients. Transcatheter arterial embolization is an alternative.

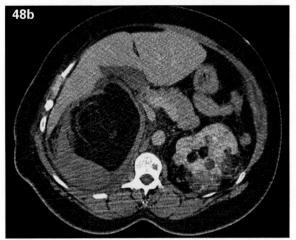

48b Single axial CT image demonstrating multiple low-attenuation lesions in both kidneys in a patient with tuberous sclerosis.

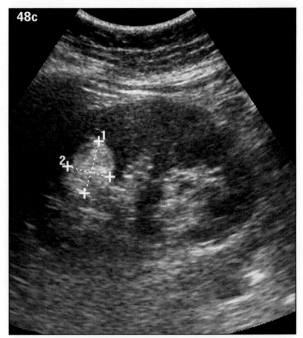

48c US appearances of angiomyolipomas, which appear as well defined hyperechoic lesions.

CASE 49

History
A 30-year-old male presented with abdominal swelling over several months.

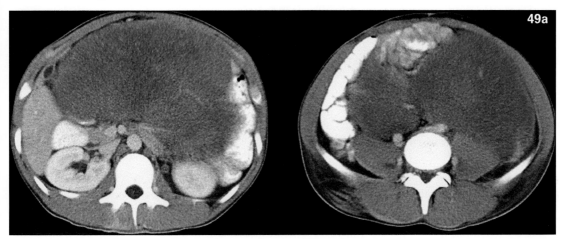

49a Selected images from a recent contrast enhanced CT study.

49b A barium enema done on the same patient 3 years previously.

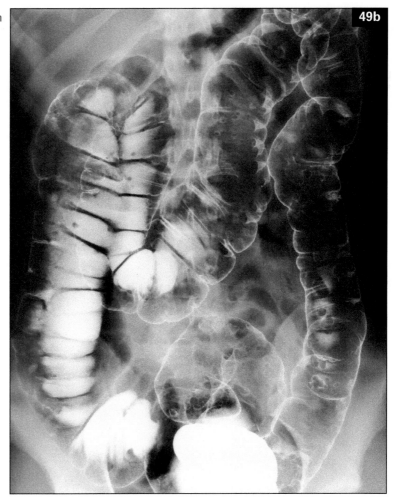

ANSWER 49

Observations (49a, 49b)
The two CT images (**49a**) demonstrate a large, well defined soft tissue mass in the central abdomen. This displaces adjacent bowel loops and most likely originates in the mesentery.

The single image (**49b**) from a double contrast barium enema examination shows multiple small, well defined mucosal filling defects throughout the colon consistent with widespread colonic polyposis. Multiple polyps throughout the colon suggest an underlying genetic condition.

Diagnosis
Familial adenomatous polyposis (FAP) with mesenteric desmoid tumour.

Discussion
Familial adenomatous polyposis is an autosomal dominant disease (chromosome 5) characterized by multiple colonic adenomatous polyps that inevitably progress to colorectal cancer within 20 years of diagnosis. Treatment involves prophylactic total colectomy in early adult life and genetic screening of family members from the second decade with a view to prophylactic surgery. All patients have colonic polyps but small bowel and gastric adenomas are also found (periampullary cancer is the most common cause of death once colectomy has been performed).

Other associated features include:
- Desmoid tumours.
- Mesenteric fibrosis.
- Gastric hamartomas.
- Hypertrophy of retinal pigment epithelium.

Gardner and Turcot syndromes are variants of FAP. Gardner syndrome also includes:
- Osteomas of the skull and mandible.
- Dental abnormalities – dentigerous cysts, odontoma, hypercementoma, supernumerary teeth.
- Soft tissue tumours such as fibroma, lipoma, leiomyoma, neurofibroma.
- Epidermal cysts.
- Association with thyroid cancer.

Turcot syndrome is FAP with associated CNS malignancy such as medulloblastoma.

Other polyposis conditions are:
- Peutz–Jeghers – autosomal dominant (AD) hamartomatous polyposis condition with features of mucocutaneous pigmentation (usually brown pigmented freckling on the mucous membranes of lips and gums) and multiple polyps found predominantly in the stomach and small bowel, with a few also seen in the large bowel. Hamartomas have no malignant potential but the condition is associated with an increased risk of upper GI tract malignancies. Complications of the condition include:
  - Malabsorption.
  - Transient intussusception.
  - Carcinoma of the GI tract.
  - Carcinoma of breast, pancreas, ovary, endometrium and testes.

- Cowden's syndrome – AD condition characterized by multiple hamartomatous polyps, breast and thyroid malignancy and skin lesions.
- Cronkhite–Canada syndrome – hamartomatous colonic polyps are associated with alopecia, skin pigmentation and nail atrophy.

Practical tips
- Images should be carefully inspected for a coexistent colonic tumour as well as extracolonic malignancies.
- Intussusception in adults indicates an underlying bowel pathology, whereas in children it can be idiopathic.

Further management
Surgical referral is required for prophylactic colectomy, as is referral for genetic screening of relatives.

Further reading
Galiatsatos P, Foulkes WD (2006). Familial adenomatous polyposis. *American Journal of Gastroenterology* **101**(2): 385–398.

49b Multiple polyps.

CASE 50

History
A 43-year-old male presented with abnormal liver function tests.

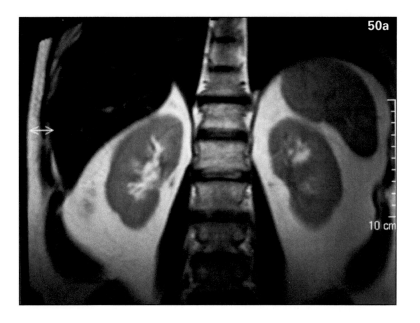

CASE 51

History
A 19-year-old male presented with multiple episodes of renal colic.

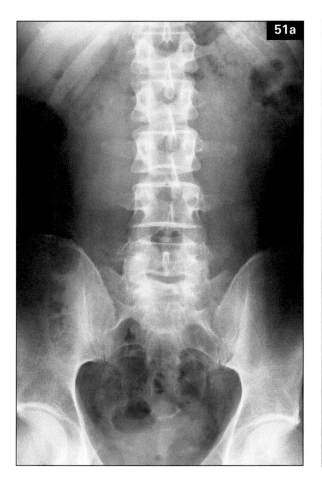
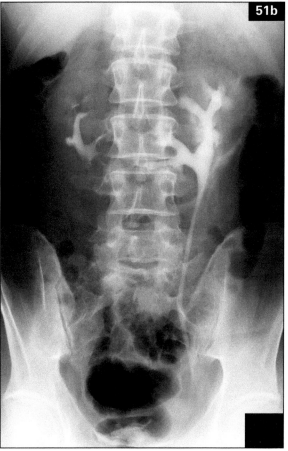

ANSWER 50

Observations (50a)
This single T1 weighted coronal image shows a striking reduction in signal intensity throughout the liver parenchyma. This is likely to indicate iron overload. It is notable that the spleen retains normal signal intensity so the liver abnormality is most likely due to haemochromatosis.

Diagnosis
Haemochromatosis.

Discussion
Primary haemochromatosis is an autosomal recessive condition characterized by increased absorption and deposition of iron within several organs including liver, pancreas, heart and pituitary gland. Patients are usually asymptomatic until the 2nd decade, then they present with a varied clinical picture due to iron deposition in:
- Skin – hyperpigmentation.
- Liver – cirrhosis, hepatomegaly.
- Pancreas – diabetes.
- Heart – arrhythmias, dilated cardiomyopathy.
- Musculoskeletal – arthralgia.
- Pituitary – pituitary failure with signs of impotence, testicular atrophy, hair loss.

Radiologically, imaging of the abdomen shows marked abnormality of the liver. Accumulation of iron results in the liver being of diffusely reduced signal on MRI. The degree of iron deposition has been shown to correlate with the MRI appearances. Unenhanced CT of the liver demonstrates increased attenuation (>75 HU). Follow-up in these patients is important due to the hepatic complications of cirrhosis and the increased risk of hepatocellular carcinoma.

Arthropathy of haemochromatosis is similar to that of calcium pyrophosphate deposition disease. Chondrocalcinosis is a feature. Typically, appearances are of squaring of the metacarpal heads due to flattening and peripheral small, hook-like spurs (**50b**). Osteopenia is also common.

Practical tips
Multiple transfusions for chronic haematological disorders can lead to iron overload, i.e. transfusion siderosis. MRI will show hypointensity in the liver *and* spleen in this condition. This helps differentiate it from haemochromatosis where the spleen shows normal signal on MRI.

Further management
In the course of follow-up, ultrasound monitoring may be useful due to the high risk of developing cirrhosis and hepatocellular carcinoma.

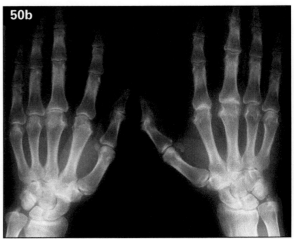

50b Radiograph of both hands shows flattening of the 2nd and 3rd metacarpal heads with loss of joint space, giving a squared appearance. Early spur formation is seen on the lateral aspect of the 2nd metacarpal of left hand.

ANSWER 51

Observations (51a, 51b)
Images are control and delayed prone abdominal radiographs from an IVU series. The control film shows medially located appearance of both kidneys and although the superior poles of both are identifiable, inferior poles are not. The delayed IVU image (**51b**) shows medial location of the pelvicalyceal systems, which are anteriorly orientated. No filling defects are identified.

Diagnosis
Horseshoe kidney.

Discussion
This is the most common fusion abnormality of the kidneys. It is more commonly found in male patients and has an incidence of 1 in 300. The kidneys are joined at their lower poles in 90% of cases, by a parenchymal/fibrous isthmus band (**51c**). The long axis of the kidneys is medially orientated with anterior rotation, such that the renal pelvises are anteriorly located. The condition is complicated by urinary stasis with renal stone formation, infection and reflux. Vesicoureteric reflux and hydronephrosis secondary to ureteropelvic junction obstruction are common. There is a reported increase in

Answer 51

the incidence of renal adenocarcinoma, transitional cell carcinoma and Wilms' tumour. In addition the kidney is more susceptible to injury following abdominal trauma.

Horseshoe kidney is associated with:
- Genitourinary abnormalities: hypospadia, cryptorchidism, ureteral duplication, bicornuate uterus.
- Cardiovascular abnormalities.
- Skeletal abnormalities.
- CNS abnormalities.
- Trisomy 18.
- Turner's syndrome.

Practical tips
- On an IVU, check for filling defects, which could represent a renal calculus or transitional cell carcinoma.
- On US, look for a renal cell carcinoma.
- On plain radiography, look for signs of bony metastases anal stones.

Further management
Follow-up may be considered due to increased incidence of renal malignancy.

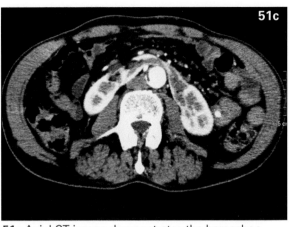

51c Axial CT image demonstrates the horseshoe kidney with a narrow isthmus of tissue extending anterior to the aorta and IVC.

CASE 52

History
A 64-year-old male with weight loss.

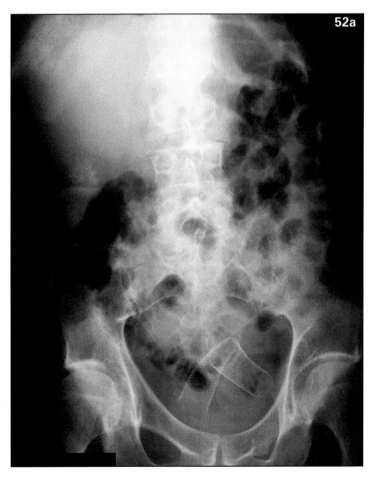

ANSWER 52

Observations (52a)
Single AP radiograph of the abdomen shows a metallic stent within the central pelvis, which presumably lies in the rectum or distal sigmoid colon. It is likely that this stent has been inserted to relieve symptoms from a colorectal tumour. The rest of the bowel gas pattern is unremarkable with no evidence of obstruction.

There are, however, amorphous, poorly marginated areas of calcification seen in the region of the liver and these likely represent calcified liver metastases. Ultrasound or CT should be undertaken, and a contrast enhanced CT (**52b**) of this patient does confirm the presence of calcified liver metastases.

Diagnosis
Stented rectal tumour with calcified liver metastases.

Differential diagnosis
For calcified liver metastases:
- Mucinous adenocarcinomas – colon, rectum, ovarian, breast and stomach.
- Osteosarcoma.
- Endocrine pancreatic carcinoma.
- Medullary carcinoma of thyroid.
- Lung cancer.

Discussion
Colorectal carcinoma is the third most common cancer diagnosed in the developed world. Rectum and sigmoid are the most common sites of lesions. Where surgical resection is not possible or appropriate, stents can provide symptomatic relief and prevent obstruction.

The liver is the most common site for metastatic spread after regional lymph nodes.

Practical tips
- As with all radiographs that show evidence of likely primary malignancy, once this has been noted, look carefully for metastatic disease elsewhere on the film.
- Classically, colorectal cancers metastasize to the liver due to the venous drainage of bowel via the portal venous system. However, the venous drainage of the rectum interfaces with the systemic venous drainage at the anal canal and thus pulmonary metastases are said to be more likely in rectal cancer than other colonic tumours. In reality, pulmonary metastases are not an uncommon finding in colon or rectal cancer.

Further management
TNM (tumour–node–metastases) staging must be accomplished as for most tumours. Tumour staging of rectal cancer is done with MRI (**52c**) (along with local nodal staging). The primary reason for MRI is to assess proximity of tumour to the mesorectal fascia – this is the plane along which the surgeon dissects in a total mesorectal excision (TME) procedure. This boundary is thus referred to as the circumferential resection margin (CRM). If local tumour spread extends close to it, the surgical margin may well be contaminated with tumour with the attendant risk of local recurrence. Identifying patients where the CRM is threatened in this way means they can be selected for preoperative radiotherapy or chemotherapy to reduce this risk. Distal nodal disease and metastases can be assessed with CT or MRI but if the chest is also to be imaged to exclude pulmonary metastases, CT is required for this component at least.

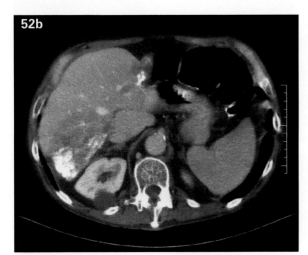

52b Axial CT image confirms calcified liver metastases.

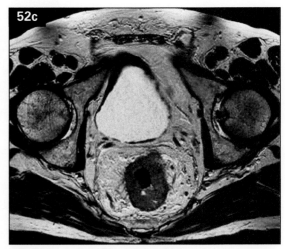

52c Thin section T2 weighted image shows a circumferential rectal tumour with wall breach at the left anterolateral wall (12–2 o'clock) consistent with this being a T3 tumour.

CASE 53

History
A 35-year-old female presented with abdominal pain and per rectal bleeding for 3 months.

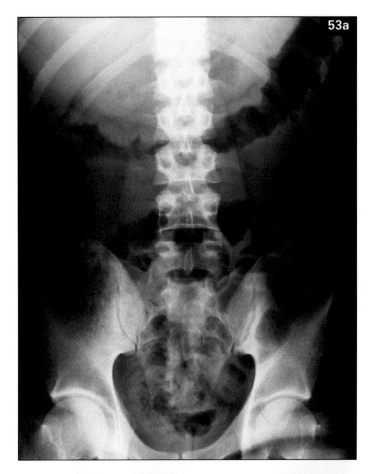

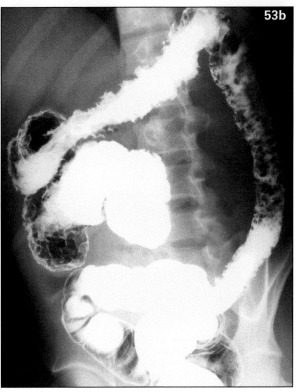

ANSWER 53

Observations (53a, 53b)
Plain abdominal film of adult patient shows marked wall thickening of the transverse colon with thumb-printing. The sigmoid loops show no such abnormalities and the rectum contains faeces. The double contrast barium enema film confirms extensive mucosal ulceration and a somewhat cobblestone appearance that extends from caecum to the descending colon. The colon distal to this is normal. The appearances are in keeping with colitis, and sparing of the more distal colon makes Crohn's disease more likely than ulcerative colitis. It is notable that the sacroiliac joints are normal.

Diagnosis
Crohn's disease.

Differential diagnosis
For terminal ileal disease:
- TB – usually has more severe involvement of the caecum (**53c**). There is often evidence of pulmonary TB.
- Radiation ileitis.
- Yersinia.

For thumb-printing:
- Inflammatory colitis – Crohn's, ulcerative colitis (UC).
- Ischaemic colitis.
- Infectious colitis/pseudomembranous colitis.
- Diverticulitis.
- Other causes: endometriosis, amyloidosis, hereditary angioneurotic oedema, lymphoma.

Discussion
Crohn's disease is a chronic, inflammatory, granulomatous disease that can affect any part of the bowel from oesophagus to rectum. Small bowel is most commonly involved and the terminal ileum is involved in over 95% of cases (**53d**). Presentation is usually in the 2nd–4th decades with symptoms of abdominal pain, diarrhoea, per rectal bleeding, weight loss and features of malabsorption.

Radiological features are:
- Aphthous ulcers – shallow ulcers with surrounding oedema.
- Fissures, sinuses and fistulae – Crohn's is the third most common cause of fistulae after idiopathic causes and diverticulitis. The fistulae can be between loops

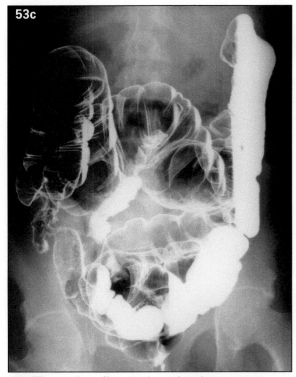

53c TB can also affect the bowel and appearances can mimic those of Crohn's disease. Caecal involvement with features of stricturing and ulceration is more common than terminal ileal involvement.

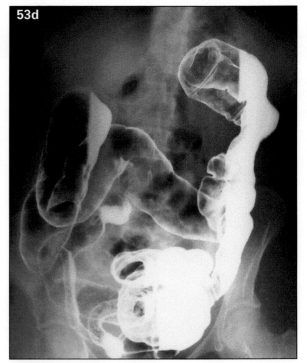

53d Decubitus film from a barium enema series shows marked narrowing of the terminal ileum in a patient with Crohn's disease.

Answer 53 — Abdominal Imaging

of bowel, between inflamed bowel loops and other abdominal viscera, e.g. colovesical or from bowel to the skin.
- Cobblestone mucosa – longitudinal and transverse ulcers separated by oedematous mucosa.
- Thickening of small bowel folds.
- Separation of small bowel loops due to inflammation and oedema of wall.
- Mucosal granularity with <1 mm rounded mucosal lesions.
- Pseudopolyps – inflammatory or hyperplastic mucosa.
- Strictures – often multiple.
- Skip lesions with discontinuous disease are seen in >90% of cases.

CT imaging features (**53e**) are demonstrated in this case of a young male patient who has had a previous terminal ileal resection for Crohn's disease. There is now recurrence of disease in the neoterminal ileum with features of:
- Thickening of the bowel wall.
- Marked stranding of the surrounding fat due to inflammation.
- Engorged and dilated mesenteric vessels referred to as the 'comb sign' due to the similarity in appearance to the teeth of a comb.
- Skip lesions with two involved segments shown on this single axial image.

MR imaging (small bowel enterography) features are demonstrated in Figures **53f–53i**. The fat suppressed coronal/axial images (**53f**, **53g**) show bowel wall thickening in the proximal ileum.

(*cont.*)

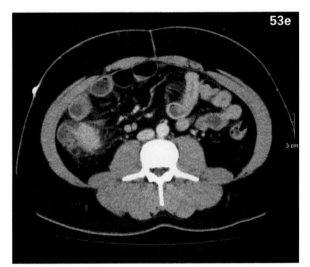

53e CT image shows recurrence of disease in the neoterminal ileum post surgical resection. There is small bowel wall thickening and oedema with inflammatory change in the surrounding tissues.

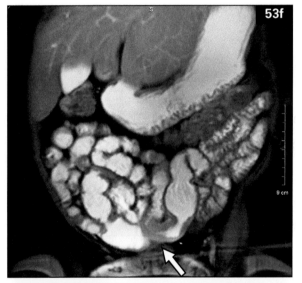

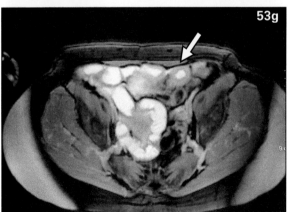

53f (coronal), **53g** (axial) fat suppressed images showing bowel wall thickening of a loop of proximal ileum. Dynamic images are obtained and viewed in cine mode to see how this focus of bowel contracts.

Answer 53

The pre- and post-contrast T1 weighted coronal images (**53h, 53i**) show enhancement of an involved loop of small bowel in the central lower abdomen.

Treatment is both medical and surgical, with a high rate of recurrence even after resection (almost 40%), particularly in the neoterminal ileum following distal ileal resections.

Practical tips
- Terminal ileal involvement, skip lesions and multiple strictures are the best signs for Crohn's disease. When assessing colonic disease, remember that UC almost always involves the rectum and has a continuous distribution without skip lesions. However, if a UC patient has had steroid enemas, the rectum may look normal.
- Always look for signs of complications of Crohn's, i.e. adenocarcinoma (risk increased up to 20-fold), lymphoma, toxic megacolon, perforation, abscess, fistulae.
- Always look for signs of extraintestinal manifestations of disease on the film. Check for sacroiliac joint disease, gallstones, hypertrophic osteoarthropathy.
- Always look for signs of drug treatment of disease on the film. Check femoral heads for evidence of avascular necrosis from steroid treatment.

Further management
- Initial diagnosis in suspected cases is often confirmed with a small bowel barium study (follow through or enteroclysis). Sometimes a more acute presentation with abdominal pains may lead to the diagnosis first being suggested by CT. Capsule endoscopy is a newer investigation that may also first identify disease. Once the diagnosis is made, follow-up imaging with MRI is ideal as this incurs no radiation risk in what are frequently young patients. CT imaging remains equally useful, however, when complications such as abscess formation are suspected.
- Treatment includes medical and surgical disciplines.

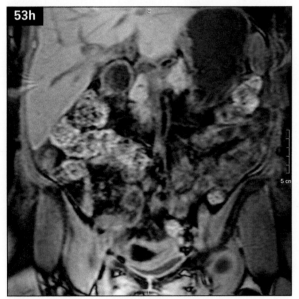 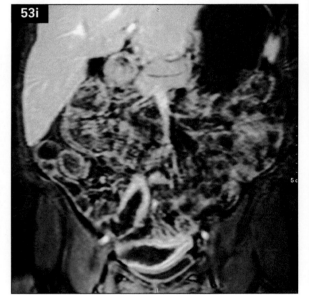

53h (pre-contrast), **53i** (post-contrast) coronal images of the colon showing enhancement in the thickened small bowel loops in the lower abdomen.

CASE 54

History
A 54-year-old male presented with dyspepsia.

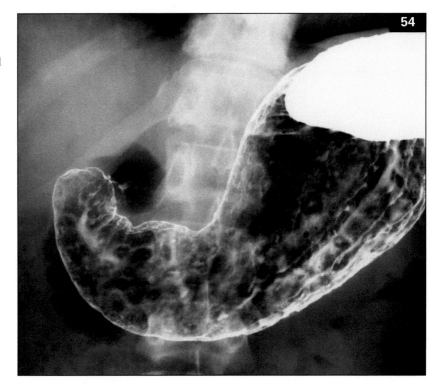

CASE 55

History
A 29-year-old male presented with progressive dysphagia.

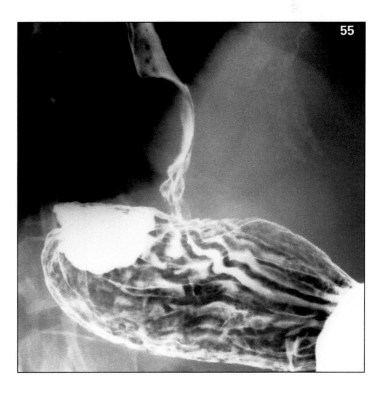

ANSWER 54

Observations (54)
Single image from a double contrast barium meal examination shows multiple, small dense foci of contrast within the antrum and body of the stomach. These are surrounded by a lucent halo representing oedema. There is some irregular thickening of the gastric folds, with the target lesions appearing to be orientated along these.

Diagnosis
Erosive gastritis.

Differential diagnosis
For aphthous ulceration:
- Erosive gastritis.
- Crohn's disease.
- Barium precipitate artefacts.

For gastric fold thickening:
- Erosive gastritis.
- Zollinger–Ellison syndrome.
- Crohn's disease.
- Malignancy – lymphoma, carcinoma.
- Benign reactive lymphoid hyperplasia.
- Ménétrier's disease.

Discussion
Gastritis often has this aphthoid appearance with varioliform ulcers, consisting of a tiny dense focus of barium surrounded by a radiolucent halo of oedema giving a 'target lesion' appearance. Lesions are usually multiple. The antrum is preferentially affected with spread towards the fundus, lesions appearing to be longitudinally orientated along the rugal folds.

Causes:
- In 50% of cases, no causative abnormality is identified.
- Peptic disease.
- Drugs – aspirin, NSAIDs, steroids.
- Alcohol.
- Infection – herpes simplex, cytomegalovirus (CMV), *Candida*.
- Crohn's disease – usually there are signs of Crohn's disease in other locations, most commonly the terminal ileum.

Practical tips
On the contrast examination look for features in the oesophagus of an infective cause for the gastric appearances or for oesophageal varices pointing to alcohol as an underlying cause.

Further management
Gastroenterology referral with a view to endoscopy.

ANSWER 55

Observations (55)
Single image from a barium swallow examination shows a lesion in the lower oesophagus, just superior to the gastro-oesophageal junction. The lesion is well defined with a smooth edge, indenting the oesophageal lumen. No ulceration or infiltration is seen. Appearances suggest a benign intramural mass, most likely a leiomyoma.

Diagnosis
Leiomyoma of the oesophagus.

Differential diagnosis
For smooth oesophageal mass lesion:
- Neurofibroma.
- Lipoma.
- Haematoma, e.g. from instrumentation.
- Duplication cyst – can simulate an intramural mass.

Discussion
This is the most common benign tumour of the oesophagus. It is usually found in young adults, being slightly more common in males. Growth is slow and presentation is with dysphagia, odynophagia and possibly haematemesis.

Radiological features are:
- Well defined, large, smooth intramural mass extending into the oesophageal lumen.
- Forms an obtuse angle with the adjacent mucosa – good sign of a benign lesion.
- Usually found in the mid and lower oesophagus.
- Calcification is sometimes seen and is virtually diagnostic since it is the only oesophageal tumour to calcify.
- Ulceration is rare.
- May be multiple in ~3%.
- Uniform contrast enhancement on CT.

Practical tips
Smooth, well defined, slow growing oesophageal lesions are likely to be benign.

Further management
Gastroenterology referral with a view to direct visualization with endoscopy.

CASE 56

History
A 24-year-old male patient presented with dysuria.

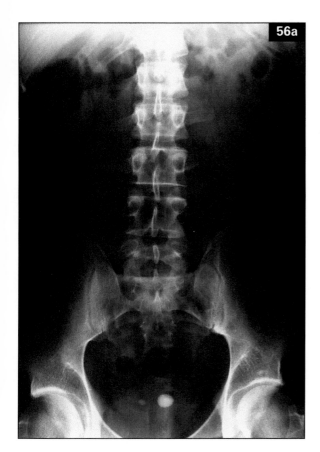
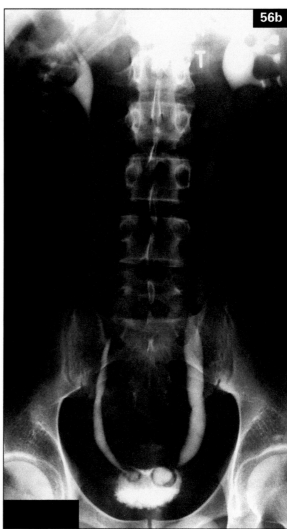

ANSWER 56

Observations (56a, 56b)
The AP postmicturition image (**56b**) from an IVU series shows bilateral dilatation of the distal ureter with a 'cobra head' appearance. There is a surrounding thick halo of lucency within the bladder, representing oedema. These appearances are of bilateral ureteroceles. The control film (**56a**) demonstrates bilateral calculi in the pelvis that lie within these ureteroceles.

Diagnosis
Bilateral ureteroceles.

Differential diagnosis
For radiolucent bladder filling defects on IVU:
- Ureterocele.
- Bladder tumour.
- Radiolucent calculus.
- Sloughed renal papilla.
- Gas secondary to fistula, cystitis, idiopathic causes and trauma.
- Island prostate – enlarged central zone can appear as a central bladder lucency.

Discussion
A simple or orthotopic ureterocele is a congenital prolapse of the distal ureter and its orifice into the bladder. It is usually an incidental finding in adults and is bilateral in a third of cases. Figure **56c** shows how a ureterocele can produce a less specific type of filling defect when the bladder is full and Figure **56d** shows the typical ultrasound appearance. The main complication is of obstruction, which can cause collecting system dilatation and renal failure. There is also an increased risk of stone formation and it is therefore imperative to check the control film in every patient – as in this case!

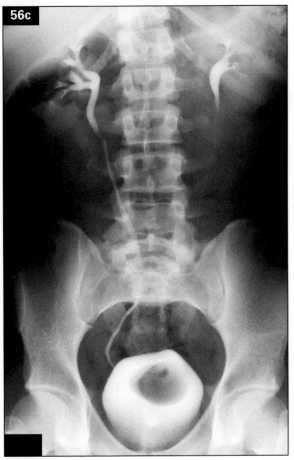

56c IVU film in a patient with a full bladder showing a radiolucent filling defect.

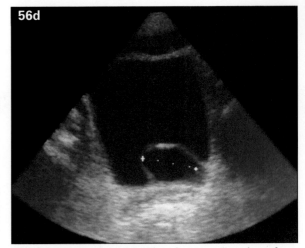

56d US image of the bladder shows protrusion of the distal ureter into the bladder, indicating that these are orthotopic ureteroceles and not pseudoureteroceles.

Answer 56

Pseudoureteroceles can have a similar appearance and are caused by obstruction of a normal ureter. Differentiation between the two types can be made using ultrasound or oblique films, which show no protrusion of the ureter into the bladder lumen with pseudoureteroceles.

Causes of pseudoureteroceles include:
- Oedema of the distal ureter secondary to impacted stone, infection, radiotherapy.
- Bladder tumour (**56e**).

Practical tips
Always remember to check the control film of an IVU.

Further management
While a small asymptomatic ureterocele may not require treatment, recurrent urinary tract infection (UTI), calculi, pain and obstructive uropathy are indications for surgical intervention.

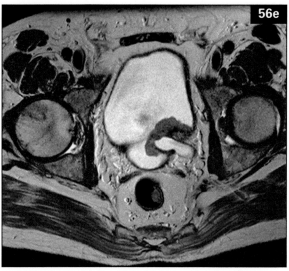

56e Single axial T2 weighted image of the pelvis shows a pseudoureterocele secondary to a large bladder tumour.

CASE 57

History
A 36-year-old male presented with progressive dysphagia.

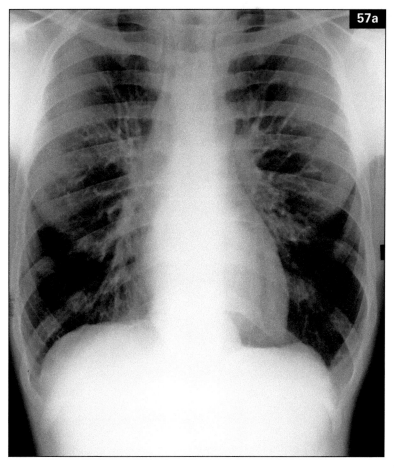

ANSWER 57

Observations (57a)
This frontal chest radiograph of an adult patient shows an added convex soft tissue density along the right mediastinal border and behind the heart. There is no normal gastric air bubble beneath the left hemidiaphragm. The findings suggest dilatation of the oesophagus secondary to chronic distal obstruction, most likely due to achalasia. A barium swallow would confirm.

Diagnosis
Achalasia.

Differential diagnosis
- Secondary achalasia due to a stricture at the gastro-oesophageal junction. There will be normal peristalsis however.
- Chagas' disease is essentially the same as achalasia but the neurenteric plexus damage is due to *Trypanosoma cruzi* infection.

Discussion
Achalasia is a motility disorder that is idiopathic in aetiology, characterized by degeneration of Auerbach's plexus. This results in a failure of relaxation of the caudal oesophagus at the gastro-oesophageal sphincter. Presentation is with progressive dysphagia. Investigation is with a contrast swallow examination (57b), which may show features of:
- 'Vigorous achalasia' – multiple tertiary contractions in the distal oesophagus can be the earliest sign.
- 'Bird's beak' deformity – symmetrical stenotic segment of oesophagus at the gastro-oesophageal junction. Imaging the patient erect allows best demonstration with contrast forcing its way through the gastro-oesophageal sphincter when the hydrostatic pressure of the barium column in the oesophagus is sufficiently high.
- Mega-oesophagus – dilatation of the oesophagus that can involve its entire length.
- Relaxation of the lower oesophageal sphincter can be induced with amyl nitrate inhalation.

Achalasia is complicated by an increased risk of developing an oesophageal squamous cell carcinoma.

Practical tips
- Check lungs for pulmonary changes of previous aspiration.
- Check for evidence of pulmonary metastases from secondary oesophageal malignancy (or indeed if the dilated oesophagus is due to a primary malignancy rather than achalasia).

Further management
- The condition is further investigated with pressure measurements (manometry) and endoscopy.
- Treatment is most commonly by pneumatic dilatation of the gastro-oesophageal sphincter. Surgical myotomy is considered where there is disease recurrence.

57b Two images from a barium swallow examination show a dilated oesophagus containing food debris, which narrows down to form the classical 'bird's beak' appearance at the gastro-oesophageal junction.

CASE 58

History
An 18-year-old male presented with headaches.

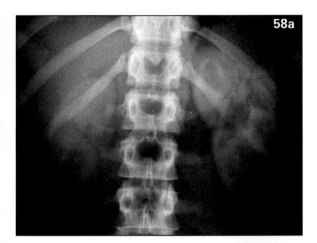

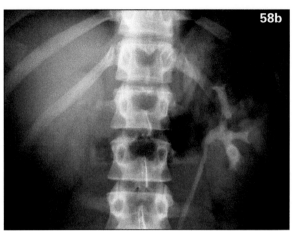

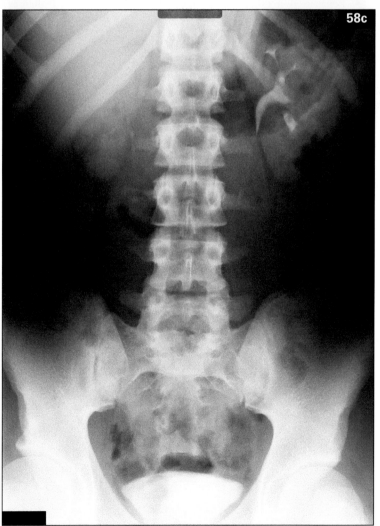

58a, 58b, 58c IVU films taken at 0, 5 and 10 minutes following contrast injection.

Answer 58

Observations (58a, 58b, 58c)
Three images from an IVU series are provided but no control film (which would normally be assessed prior to interpretation of the post-contrast films). Images show unilateral increasingly dense and persistent nephrogram on the right. The right kidney shows uniform smooth reduction in size when compared to the left. There is delayed excretion of contrast by the right kidney on the 10 minute film (**58c**). These appearances suggest unilateral right renal artery stenosis. The young age of the patient makes fibromuscular dysplasia more likely than atherosclerosis as the underlying pathology.

Diagnosis
Renal artery stenosis.

Differential diagnosis
For persistent dense nephrogram:
- Unilateral:
  - Obstruction – acute obstruction is the most common cause of this sign.
  - Renal artery stenosis/ischaemia.
  - Renal vein thrombosis.
  - Acute bacterial pyelonephritis.
  - Acute papillary necrosis.

- Bilateral:
  - Hypotension/shock.
  - Acute tubular necrosis.
  - Acute glomerulonephritis.
  - Causes of unilateral change involving both kidneys.

Discussion
There are two main causes of renal artery stenosis:
- Atherosclerosis (80–90%) – usually in the proximal 2 cm of the renal artery; affects older population >50 years; more common in men; bilateral in one-third.
- Fibromuscular dysplasia (10–20%) – usually in the mid and distal renal artery; affects young adults and children; more common in women; bilateral in two-thirds.

Less common causes include vasculitis, arterial dissection and thromboembolic disease.

Hypertension in neurofibromatosis is a consequence of phaeochromocytoma and/or renal artery stenosis, with a smooth stenosis seen in proximal renal artery.

In this patient, a renal angiogram was performed and showed a smooth narrow stenosis in the mid portion of the right renal artery (**58d**) and this would be in keeping with the underlying diagnosis of fibromuscular dysplasia of the renal artery.

The consequence of renal artery stenosis is systemic hypertension as a result of overactivity of the renin–angiotensin system. Treatment is aimed at medically controlling hypertension and with renal artery angioplasty.

Practical tips
- If there is bilateral delayed persistent nephrogram with absent or decreased excretion, then the patient needs to be immediately checked to ensure that contrast anaphylactic shock has not occurred.
- Magnetic resonance or CT angiography is the preferred investigation for this condition in the modern era.

Further management
Attempted renal artery angiography and angioplasty are usually advised.

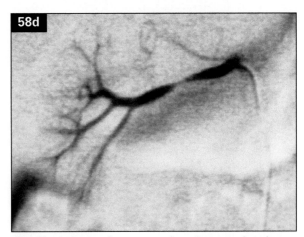

58d Single image from a renal angiogram showing a stenosis in the mid portion of the right renal artery.

CASE 59

History
A 37-year-old female presented with acute abdominal pain.

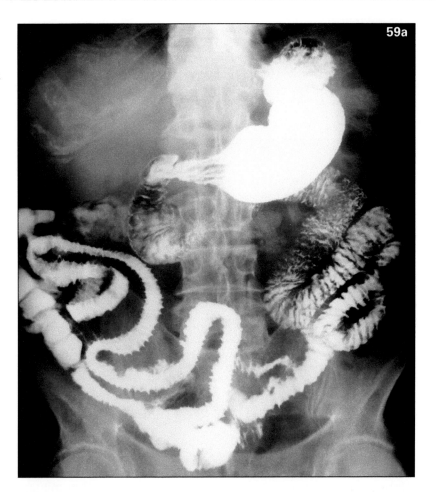

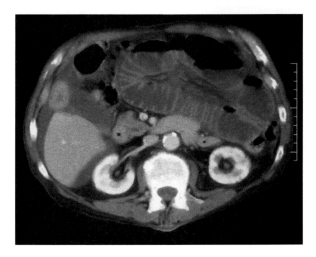

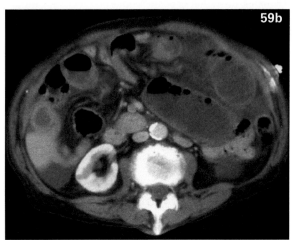

ANSWER 59

Observations (59a, 59b)
Single image from a barium follow-through examination shows smooth thickened small bowel folds. Selected axial images from an IV contrast enhanced CT scan of the abdomen again demonstrates smooth thickening of bowel folds in dilated loops of fluid-filled small bowel. In addition, there is thrombus seen in the mid superior mesenteric vein.

Diagnosis
Small bowel ischaemia secondary to superior mesenteric vein (SMV) thrombosis.

Differential diagnosis
For smooth thickened folds:
- Haemorrhage.
- Ischaemia:
  - Acute – embolus, Henoch–Schönlein purpura (HSP).
  - Chronic – vasculitis, thromboangiitis obliterans, radiotherapy.
- Oedema:
  - Hypoproteinaemia– cirrhosis, nephrotic syndrome, protein-losing enteropathy.
  - Angioneurotic oedema.
- Lymphatic obstruction – lymphoma, mesenteric fibrosis, intestinal lymphangiectasia.

Discussion
Small bowel/mesenteric ischaemia can present very acutely with symptoms of acute abdominal pain, vomiting, diarrhoea and rectal bleeding. This is usually due to arterial thrombus, dissection or acute venous obstruction. Chronic ischaemia usually due to chronic arterial thrombus has a more indolent symptomatology with longstanding grumbling abdominal cramps, postprandial pain, weight loss and malabsorption. Other causes of ischaemia include vasculitis, bowel obstruction, radiotherapy and acute abdominal inflammation, e.g. pancreatitis, appendicitis.

Radiological features of acute small bowel ischaemia include:
- Bowel wall thickening/oedema.
- Enhancement pattern of the bowel wall can be increased or decreased (**59c**).
- Stranding of the surrounding fat.
- Pneumatosis intestinalis, which is a late sign and indicative of necrotic bowel.
- Free intra-abdominal gas due to perforation of necrosed bowel.
- Portal venous gas is seen in premorbid patients.

In chronic ischaemia, there can be additional complications of strictures (which tend to be long, smooth and symmetrical), ulceration and atrophic valvulae conniventes. The splenic flexure and the proximal descending colon are most commonly affected due to the transition from superior to inferior mesenteric arterial supply at this point.

Practical tips
- Look carefully for linear gas shadows within the bowel wall indicative of intramural gas.
- Portal vein gas is usually seen in the periphery of the liver as well as centrally, in contrast to biliary gas, which is usually only central. This is a premorbid sign in adults.

Further management
Investigation with CT can both diagnose and identify the complications of ischaemia.

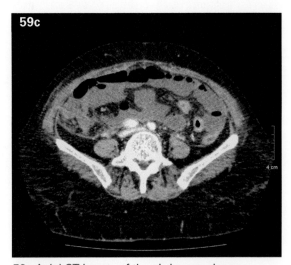

59c Axial CT image of the abdomen shows dilated fluid-filled loops of non-enhancing ischaemic small bowel.

CASE 60

History
A 23-year-old male presented with a history of renal tract calculi.

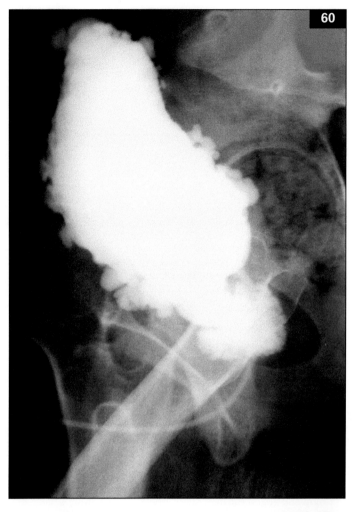

CASE 61

History
A 57-year-old male presented with lower abdominal pain.

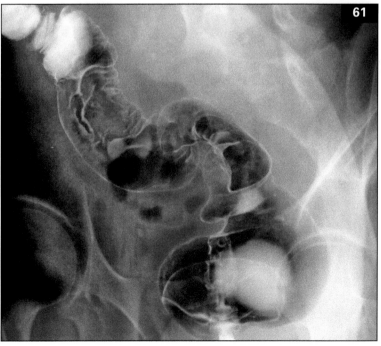

ANSWER 60

Observations (60)
Single oblique radiograph of the pelvis from an IVU shows a small, shrunken, spastic trabeculated bladder with multiple diverticula, with a superiorly pointed dome. This is the so-called 'pine tree' appearance of a neurogenic bladder.

Diagnosis
Neurogenic bladder.

Differential diagnosis
For small bladder:
- Infection – schistosomiasis/TB.
- Iatrogenic – postsurgery/radiotherapy.
- Neurogenic.
- Transitional cell carcinoma (TCC) – asymmetric bladder contraction with thick wall and filling defects.
- Extrinsic compression – usually gives a pear shaped bladder appearance.

Discussion
Bladder innervation is by the parasympathetic nerves S2–S4. Injury to these nerves causes denervation of the detrusor muscle, giving this appearance of a shrunken, heavily trabeculated bladder, with an irregular thickened wall and multiple diverticula. Causes include:
- Congenital anomalies – myelomeningocele, spina bifida.
- Spinal trauma.
- Diabetes mellitus.
- Infection – syphilis, herpes.
- Spinal neoplasm.

Practical tips
Inspect IVU films carefully to look for a spinal abnormality, which can help to determine the underlying cause of the bladder abnormality.

Further management
In the absence of an easily identifiable cause, lumbosacral spine MRI can be useful.

ANSWER 61

Observations (61)
Single image from a barium enema examination demonstrates a well defined, smooth, eccentric filling defect in the distal sigmoid colon. This appears to be extraluminal in origin and lies on the mesenteric aspect of the bowel. A similar lesion is seen in the pouch of Douglas. Multiple lesions centred in an intraperitoneal location suggest the diagnosis of intraperitoneal metastases.

Diagnosis
Colonic metastases.

Discussion
Tumours spread to the mesentery via four routes:
- Direct invasion along the mesenteric vessels and fat – seen with gastric, pancreatic, colonic and biliary cancers; 40% of patients with adenocarcinoma of the pancreas have tumour extending along the mesenteric root at diagnosis.
- Extension via mesenteric lymphatics – colonic, ovarian, breast, lung, carcinoid and melanoma cancers can spread to mesenteric lymph nodes, though lymphoma is more common.
- Haematogenous spread – commonly from melanoma, breast and lung primaries, metastases involve the antimesenteric border of the bowel via small arteries. They can act as the lead point for intussusception. Up to 7.5% of melanoma patients show small bowel involvement.
- Intraperitoneal seeding – breast, ovarian, pancreatic and gastric tumours are the most common primaries responsible for intraperitoneal 'drop' seeding. These lesions involve the mesenteric borders. Appearances are of a focal mass or diffuse stellate appearance on CT, but on double contrast barium imaging, appearances are of a focal extrinsic indentation of the bowel. This involves the pouch of Douglas (50%) and commonly the superior/anterior border of the sigmoid. The distal ileum and medial border of the caecum are also often involved.

Practical tips
The most common underlying cause for intraperitoneal malignant disease is ovarian cancer.

Further management
Clinical review of patient to try and localize a likely primary tumour. CT scanning will confirm peritoneal disease and may well reveal the primary tumour.

Further reading
Sheth S, Horton KM, Garland MR, Fishman EK (2003). Mesenteric neoplasms: CT appearances of primary and secondary tumors and differential diagnosis. *RadioGraphics* 23: 457–473.

CASE 62

History
A 46-year-old female, recently emigrated to the UK from Africa, presented with symptoms of urinary frequency and urgency.

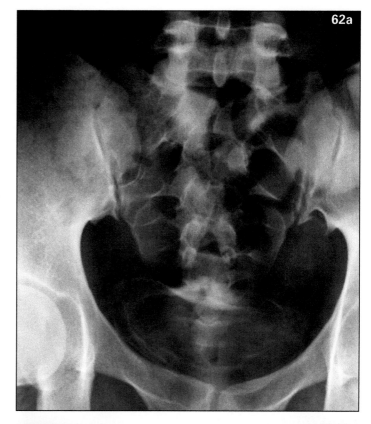

CASE 63

History
A 45-year-old diabetic presented with pyrexia and abdominal pain.

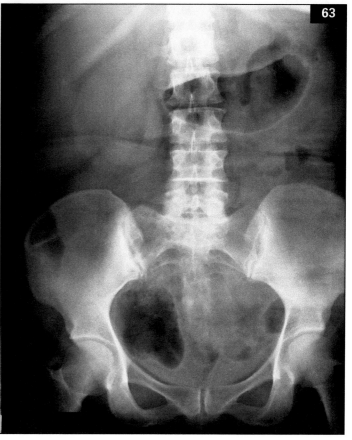

Answer 62

Observations (62a)
This single coned view of the pelvis shows curvilinear wall calcification of a relatively normal capacity bladder. No calcification of the lower ureters is seen. No discontinuity in the calcification is seen.

The history of residence in Africa raises the possibilities of bladder TB and schistosomiasis. The absence of gross bladder contraction makes the latter more likely, but it would also be helpful to review a full length abdominal film to look for upper tract calcification. Transitional cell tumour must also be excluded.

Diagnosis
Schistosomiasis.

Differential diagnosis
For calcified bladder wall:
- Cancer – primarily transitional cell carcinoma (TCC) but also other rarer bladder tumours.
- Radiotherapy.
- Infection – TB and schistosomiasis.

Discussion
Schistosomiasis is one of the most common parasitic infections, affecting 8% of the global population. *Schistosoma haematobium* is the female parasite which affects the genitourinary system. Unlike TB, which tends to affect the kidneys first and then spreads caudally, schistosomiasis has a reverse involvement and usually is confined to bladder and lower ureters. (Another case of bladder schistosomiasis [62b] is shown – note the absence of upper tract calcification that one might see in TB.)

Classically, the patient presents with urinary frequency, urgency and dysuria. Imaging findings are of:
- Calcification of the bladder – which results in reduced bladder filling capacity and increased postmicturition residual volume.
- Calcification of the lower ureters.
- Lower ureteric strictures.
- Ureteritis cystica.

Complications of disease affecting the genitourinary system include:
- Cystitis.
- Vesicoureteric reflux and subsequent pyelonephritis.
- Increased risk of squamous cell carcinoma of the bladder.

Other systems can be affected:
- Liver – oval migration results in portal hypertension and subsequent oesophageal varices.
- Respiratory system – diffuse granulomatous lung lesions.

Practical tips
- Schistosomiasis involves bladder and lower ureters and results in a calcified, nonshrunken bladder. TB involves the kidneys and spreads via the ureters to involve the bladder. It is very unusual to have isolated bladder involvement with TB and the degree of bladder contraction is more marked than in schistosomiasis.
- Discontinuity of calcification in the bladder wall should arouse suspicion of bladder cancer.

Further management
Follow-up in these patients is required since the latency for development of squamous cell carcinoma of the bladder can be up to 30–35 years.

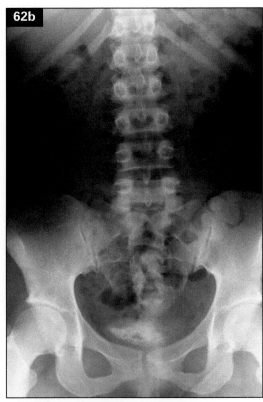

62b Calcification of the bladder is seen in schistosomiasis with absence of upper tract calcification to help differentiate from TB.

ANSWER 63

Observations (63)
Supine abdominal radiograph demonstrates gas within the left pelvicalyceal system and upper ureter. No intra-parenchymal renal gas is seen. No gas is seen in the right renal tract or in the bladder.

Diagnosis
Emphysematous pyelitis.

Differential diagnosis
Of cause of gas in the urinary tract:
- Emphysematous pyelonephritis/pyelitis/cystitis.
- Gas forming perinephric abscess.
- Trauma.
- Iatrogenic – urinary diversion procedures.
- Urinary tract fistula to bowel due to inflammation, e.g. Crohn's, diverticulitis or spreading malignancy.

Discussion
Emphysematous pyelitis is a condition in which infective organisms produce gas, which is confined within the renal pelvicalyceal system. In emphysematous pyelonephritis, gas also forms within the renal parenchyma – a life-threatening condition that requires prompt diagnosis and treatment. There is an increased incidence of these conditions in patients with diabetes mellitus and women are three times more commonly affected than men. *Escherichia coli* is the causative organism in 70% of cases with *Klebsiella*, *Proteus*, *Candida* and *Pseudomonas* organisms also being found. In emphysematous pyelonephritis, small gas bubbles are initially seen on plain radiographs involving the renal parenchyma; this progresses to give a diffuse mottling in more advanced disease and then progresses to produce a crescent of perinephric gas when there is extension into the perirenal fat.

Practical tips
CT is the best imaging modality for assessing extent and location of gas.

Further management
Depends on cause but obviously infective causes require prompt, appropriate antibiotic treatment.

Further reading
Joseph RC, Amendola MA, Artze ME, *et al.* (1996). Genitourinary tract gas: imaging evaluation. *RadioGraphics* 16: 295–308.

CASE 64

History
A 39-year-old female presented with early satiety and epigastric pain.

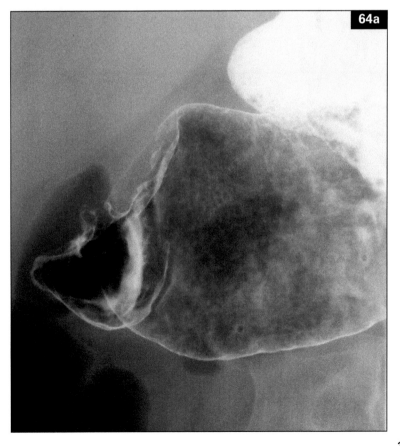

ANSWER 64

Observations (64a)
Single image from a double contrast barium meal examination shows a well defined smooth walled ovoid mass lesion in the gastric antrum. A central smooth ulcer is present and no calcification is seen.

Diagnosis
Leiomyoma of the stomach.

Differential diagnosis
For target lesions:
- Neurofibroma.
- Lipoma (**64b**).
- Ectopic pancreatic rest.
- Metastases – commonly breast, lung, renal and malignant melanoma.
- Haemangioma.

Discussion
This is the second most common benign gastric tumour after gastric polyps. Like oesophageal leiomyoma, these are slow growing lesions and are usually asymptomatic until they increase in size, when there may be epigastric pain and bleeding. The gastric antrum and pylorus are the most common sites affected. The majority of these lesions extend intraluminally (60%) and form well defined ovoid defects. They are more likely to ulcerate than oesophageal leiomyoma with ulceration seen in up to 50%. Calcification is rare.

Complications include:
- Bleeding.
- Obstruction.
- Intussusception – tumour can act as a lead point.
- Malignant degeneration – seen in up to 15–20% of cases.

Practical tips
Smooth, well defined, slow growing gastric lesions are likely to be benign.

Further management
Although radiological appearances suggest this to be a benign lesion, referral for endoscopy +/– biopsy should be made.

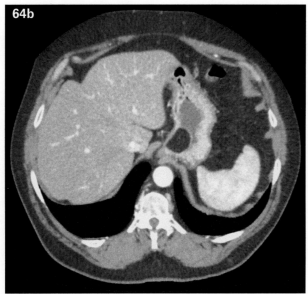

64b Axial CT image demonstrating a well defined, smooth, rounded lesion in the stomach, which has clearly the same attenuation as intra-/extra-abominal fat. This has appearances of a gastric lipoma.

CASE 65

History
A 45-year-old female presented with per rectal bleeding.

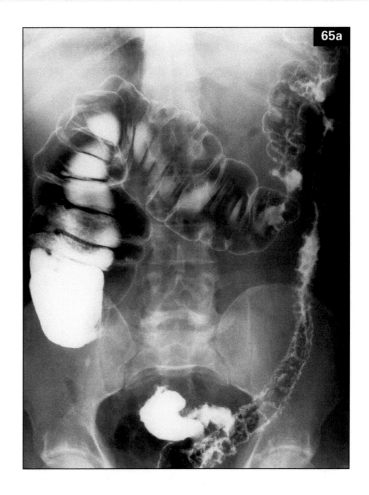

CASE 66

History
A 42-year-old smoker with a family history of bowel cancer.

(see page 118 for case answer)

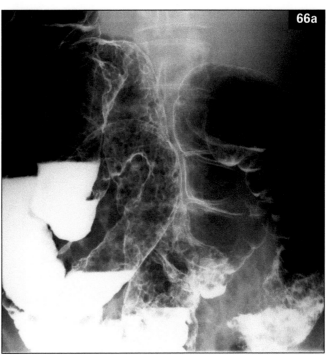

ANSWER 65

Observations (65a)
Single image from a double contrast barium enema examination shows abnormality of the colon that extends from the rectum to the mid transverse colon. There are features of luminal narrowing with mucosal irregularity, granularity and shallow ulceration. The disease process appears continuous along the affected segments with no further lesions seen. Normal appearances of the ileocaecal region. Normal sacroiliac joints. The appearances are in keeping with a colitis, most likely ulcerative colitis.

Diagnosis
Ulcerative colitis (UC).

Discussion
Ulcerative colitis is an idiopathic inflammatory bowel disease with involvement predominantly of the mucosa and submucosa of the large bowel. There are two peaks of presentation – 3rd–5th decades and 7th–8th decades. The most common presentation is with bloody diarrhoea and abdominal pain.

The rectum is almost always involved (96% of cases) with continuous, concentric and symmetric involvement of the colon more proximally. The terminal ileum is involved in 10–25% due to backwash ileitis. In acute inflammation there are findings of:

- Thickening of bowel wall (**65b**).
- Significant bowel wall thickening can lead to the classical 'thumb-printing' appearance.
- Widening of the presacral space.
- Fine mucosal granularity.
- Superficial ulceration.
- Pseudopolyps – islands of oedematous mucosa.
- Collar button ulcers (**65c**).

Appearances in the chronic stage:
- Colon becomes rigid with luminal narrowing due to chronic inflammation, and loss of haustrations – 'leadpipe' colon.
- Coarse granular mucosa.
- Inflammatory polyps.
- Backwash ileitis.

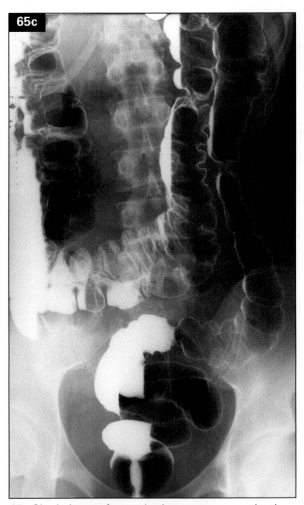

65b Single axial CT image shows continuous thickening of the colonic wall involving sigmoid colon. The surrounding fat is 'dirty' (increased attenuation) due to inflammatory change. Appearances are of an acute active colitis though the appearances here are not specific for an underlying cause.

65c Single image from a barium enema examination shows multiple shallow barium-filled ulcers in the left sided colon.

Answer 65

The condition is complicated by:
- Perforation from toxic megacolon in 5–10% – the most common cause of death (**65d**).
- Colonic adenocarcinoma – this complicates up to 5% of UC patients with risk highest when there is pancolitis or onset at a young age(<15 years) and increases with chronicity of disease. The rectosigmoid is the most common location for neoplastic transformation.
- Colonic strictures – usually a single, short, smooth stricture is found, most commonly in the rectum/sigmoid.

In addition, as with Crohn's disease, there are a variety of extracolonic complications which include iritis, pyoderma gangrenosum, chronic active hepatitis, sclerosing cholangitis and seronegative arthritis (Figure **65e** demonstrates sacroiliitis with early sclerosis of both sacroiliac joints).

Practical tips
- Differentiation of Crohn's from UC is often possible from the imaging findings:
  - Crohn's characteristically has multiple, eccentric, transmural, skip lesions; preferential involvement of terminal ileum. Fistulae and deep ulcers are common features.
  - UC characteristically has a continuous, concentric, symmetric involvement that extends proximally from the rectum and only occasionally involves the terminal ileum. Fistulae, fissures and deep ulceration are not features.
  - Remember that although the rectum is always involved in UC, it may appear spared if steroid enemas have been used.

- Look for intestinal complications of UC including malignancy, toxic megacolon, pneumatosis intestinalis and perforation.
- Look for extraintestinal complications of UC such as sacroiliitis.
- Look for complications of treatment, e.g. steroids causing avascular necrosis (AVN) or osteoporosis.

Further management
A combined medical/surgical approach to disease management should be taken.

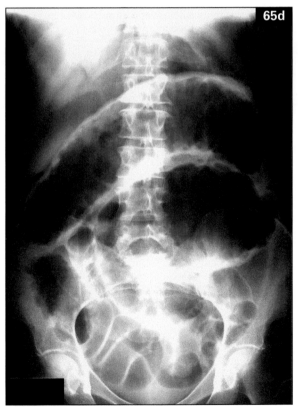

65d Abdominal radiograph with features of toxic megacolon and perforation.

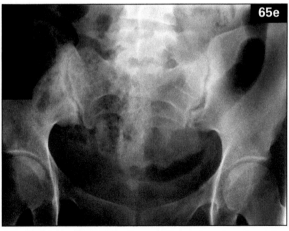

65e Pelvic radiograph shows bilateral early sclerosis of both sacroiliac joints.

ANSWER 66

Observations (66a)
Single image from a double contrast barium examination is shown. There are multiple submucosal lesions seen scattered throughout the colon with no regional predominance. Close inspection shows that these are due to gas-filled cysts in the bowel wall. No free intra-abdominal gas is seen to suggest perforation. No linear gas collections are seen. No portal vein gas is seen.

Diagnosis
Pneumatosis cystoides intestinalis.

Discussion
Pneumatosis cystoides intestinalis is usually a benign condition of middle aged people who tend to be asymptomatic but can present with symptoms of vague abdominal pain, diarrhoea and mucous discharge. Radiological findings are of multiple small 1–5 mm gas-filled cysts in a subserosal/submucosal distribution. They are more commonly found on the mesenteric rather than antimesenteric side of the colon. The cysts can rupture leading to pneumoperitoneum but with no symptoms of peritonitis. This cystic pneumatosis is usually a benign, innocuous condition and is associated with chronic obstructive pulmonary disease, perhaps due to air tracking from ruptured alveoli and along the mesentery via the retroperitoneum. There is also an association with mucosal disruption elsewhere in the GI tract, e.g. peptic ulcer disease.

Practical tips
Air in the bowel wall due to infarction typically appears more linear (66b) and may be associated with portal vein gas in premorbid cases.

Further management
Pneumatosis of the colon is usually not clinically significant – the importance here is to treat the patient, not the x-ray.

Further reading
Pear BL (1998). Pneumatosis intestinalis: a review. *Radiology* **207**: 13–19.

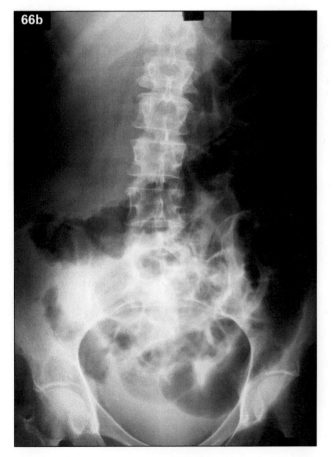

66b Abdominal radiograph shows linear gas opacity within the wall of the transverse colon in a patient with ulcerative colitis.

CASE 67

History
A 56-year-old male with lung cancer.

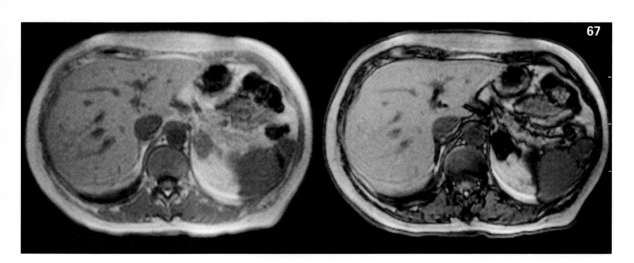

CASE 68

History
A 46-year-old male presented with recurrent urinary tract infections.

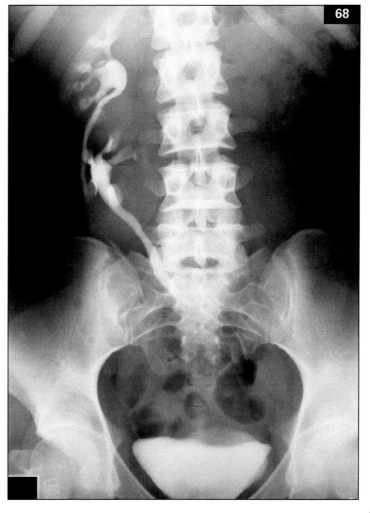

ANSWER 67

Observations (67)
Selected 'in and out of phase' T1 weighted axial images of the abdomen are provided, the out of phase image lying to the right. There is enlargement of the left adrenal gland which appears of intermediate signal intensity on T1 in phase and shows signal 'drop out' on the T1 out of phase image. Appearances on this chemical shift MRI are consistent with fatty content and indicative of a benign adenoma.

Diagnosis
Adrenal adenoma.

Discussion
Adrenal lesions are found in ~9% of the general population. Adrenal adenomas are the most common adrenal lesion. Imaging features can be used to differentiate benign adenomas from primary malignant (carcinoma, phaeochromocytoma) or metastatic adrenal lesions.

Imaging features for differentiation of an adenoma from metastasis are:
- Adenomas are mostly <2.5 cm in size; lesions >4 cm in size are more likely to be metastases or adrenal carcinomas.
- Lesions showing no growth over 6 months are usually benign.
- On unenhanced CT – adenomas often contain intracellular fat, lowering the overall density on CT. When <10 Hounsfield units (HU), this is highly specific for adenoma (96% specificity). Some adenomas contain less fat and so a lesion with HU >10 may represent adenoma or malignant lesion.
- On IV contrast enhanced CT – both adenomas and metastases enhance, but adenomas washout more rapidly. After a plain scan, acquire postcontrast scans at 60 s (early) and 10 min (delayed).

$$\% \text{ washout} = \left(\frac{\text{early} - \text{delayed}}{\text{early} - \text{unenhanced}}\right) \times 100$$

Washout >60% has sensitivity and specificity ~90% for the diagnosis of adenoma.

- On chemical shift MRI – signal drop out on the out of phase imaging is seen with adenomas. Lesions without significant intracellular fat (e.g. metastases) don't show any signal difference on in/out of phase imaging. The sensitivity and specificity are similar to, if not better than, those of contrast enhanced CT.
- PET may be useful when CT and MRI fail to characterize an adrenal mass. Malignant lesions show increased uptake of FDG (18 fluoro-2-deoxyglucose) (>liver activity) while benign lesions do not (<liver activity).

Practical tips
An incidental enlarged adrenal picked up on US/CT/MRI should be further investigated with a chest radiograph to look for a lung neoplasm.

Further management
Adrenal adenoma should be followed up after 6 months. Lesions that grow by over 1 cm in this time or those that measure over 4 cm should be considered for surgery. Hormonally active lesions may also be considered for surgery.

Further reading
Mayo-Smith WW, Boland GW, Noto RB, Lee MJ (2001). State-of-the-art adrenal imaging. *RadioGraphics* **21**: 995–1012.

ANSWER 68

Observations (68)
Single image from an IVU study is provided without a control film. It shows renal ectopia with both kidneys being located on the right side. This is crossed fused renal ectopia. There is no associated hydronephrosis.

Diagnosis
Crossed fused renal ectopia.

Discussion
Crossed renal ectopia involves a kidney being located on the opposite side of the midline from its ureteral orifice. It is more common for the left kidney to have migrated to the right, with the crossed kidney lying inferior to the normal kidney. Usually the kidneys are fused and are associated with aberrant renal arteries.

It is associated with:
- Renal calculi.
- Infection.
- Reflux.
- Megaureter.
- Cryptorchidism.
- Urethral valves.
- Multicystic dysplasia.

Practical tips
Try to identify complications of the condition such as renal scarring from recurrent infections, or hydronephrosis due to obstruction from stones/urethral valves.

Further management
No active management is required.

CASE 69

History
A 25-year-old female presented with fatigue and steatorrhoea for 12 months.

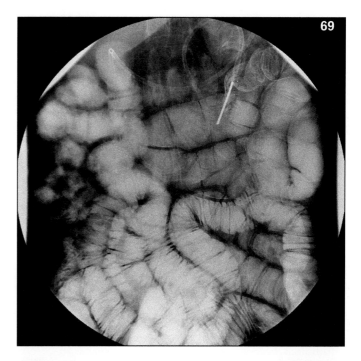

CASE 70

History
A 26-year-old male was involved in a road traffic accident.

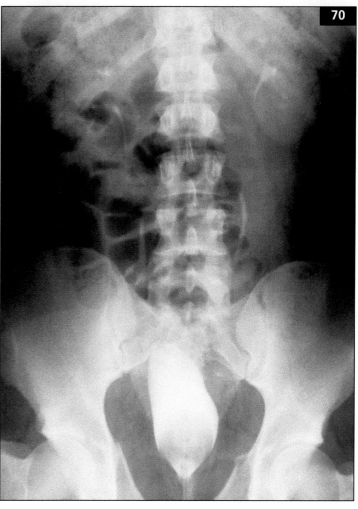

ANSWER 69

Observations (69)
Single image from a small bowel enema examination is shown. The tip of the small bowel enema catheter is seen in the proximal duodenum. The examination demonstrates a reversal of fold pattern with an increased number of folds seen in the ileum and a reduction in the number of small bowel folds seen in the proximal jejunum. These features suggest malabsorption in the proximal small bowel such as coeliac disease.

Diagnosis
Coeliac disease.

Discussion
Coeliac disease is a gluten-sensitive enteropathy characterized histologically by villous atrophy. The duodenum and jejunum are affected more than the ileum because some proximal gluten digestion means that less reaches the distal small bowel. It classically presents with steatorrhoea and diarrhoea, but more commonly presents in less specific ways such as fatigue, weight loss and abdominal pain. Malabsorption can also result in anaemia, osteomalacia, neuropathy and oedema. Age at presentation can vary from early childhood to late middle age.

Imaging features of coeliac disease include:
- Small bowel dilatation (due to reduced motility) is the most common imaging finding.
- Reduced number of folds in the jejunum.
- 'Jejunalization' of the ileum – an increased number of ileal folds. This is a response to the reduced mucosal area in the jejunum.
- 'Moulage' sign – dilated small bowel loops with fold effacement, particularly in the jejunum and duodenum.
- Transient intussusception – the cause of abdominal pains.
- Flocculation of the barium contrast due to hypersecretion is not commonly seen with modern barium preparations.

Autoantibodies (e.g. antiendomysial) may be suggestive, but diagnosis is made by demonstration of villous atrophy on jejunal biopsy. This abnormality resolves once gluten is removed from the diet and recurs when it is reinstated. The condition is complicated by an increased risk of lymphoma, adenocarcinoma of the small bowel, oesophageal carcinoma and pharyngeal carcinoma.

Practical tips
- Folds in the jejunum are normally thicker and more numerous than the ileum. Expect to see seven folds per inch in the jejunum and three to four folds per inch in the ileum. A reversal of this pattern should raise suspicion of coeliac disease.
- If the radiological features deteriorate while on a gluten-free diet, raise the possibility of complications such as lymphoma.

Further management
Confirmation of diagnosis is made with endoscopic small bowel biopsy.

ANSWER 70

Observations (70)
Single image from an IVU series shows contrast in the collecting systems and in the bladder. The bladder has an abnormal elongated configuration extending up out of the pelvis. There are bilateral pelvic fractures through the acetabulum. No free contrast is seen leaking from the bladder.

Diagnosis
Pear shaped urinary bladder secondary to pelvic haematoma.

Differential diagnosis
For pear shaped bladder (mnemonic – 'HELP'):
- Haematoma.
- External iliac artery aneurysms.
- Lymphadenopathy.
- Pelvic lipomatosis.

Practical tips
Look for an underlying cause for the abnormal pear shaped bladder appearance – pelvic fractures, curvilinear vascular calcification in the walls of aneurysms, radiotherapy changes in bone/small bowel to suggest underlying malignancy and lymphadenopathy.

Further management
Further treatment will depend on the underlying cause – this is a secondary finding pointing towards an underlying problem.

CASE 71

History
A 58-year-old female with an incidental liver lesion detected on ultrasound.

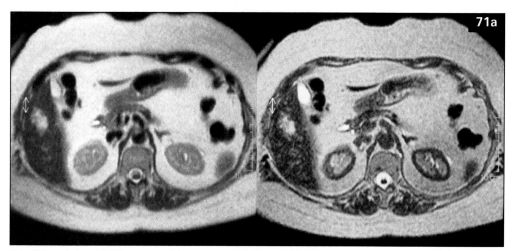

71a T2 weighted MRI scans with a normal and extended TE.

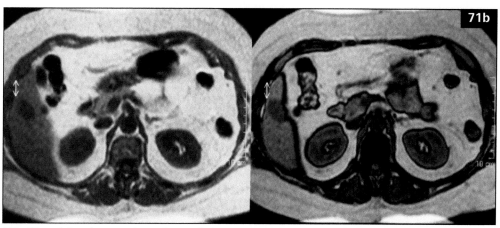

71b T1 weighted scans, in and out of phase.

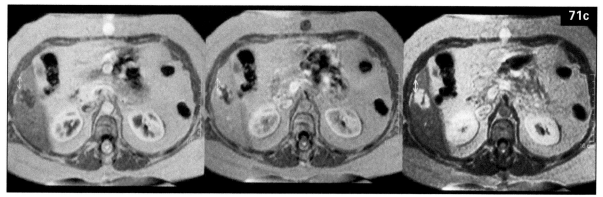

71c T1 weighted scans post IV gadolinium at 30 s, 60 s and 3 min.

ANSWER 71

Observations (71a, 71b, 71c)
T2 weighted images demonstrate a well defined, slightly lobulated mass in the right lobe of liver, which is of increased signal on the normal T2 and ultra-T2 weighted scans (71a). This is the so-called 'light bulb' sign. Axial T1 weighted images (71b) show the lesion to be of reduced signal with no signal change in the liver on out of phase scans to indicate that the lesion represents focal fatty sparing. Dynamic post-contrast images (71c) show peripheral nodular enhancement with centripetal filling in over time. These appearances are diagnostic of cavernous haemangioma.

Diagnosis
Cavernous haemangioma.

Differential diagnosis
For hyperechoic hepatic lesions on US:
- Haemangioma.
- Focal nodular hyperplasia (FNH).
- Adenoma.
- Metastasis.
- Hepatocellular carcinoma.
- Lipoma.

Discussion
Hepatic haemangioma is the most common benign tumour of the liver, affecting up to 20% of the population. They are usually asymptomatic, being incidental findings on imaging studies, however large lesions can present with acute haemorrhage and abdominal pain; 90% are solitary and 90% measure less than 4 cm in diameter. Multiple haemangioma may be associated with Osler–Weber–Rendu syndrome. Some enlargement can be seen during pregnancy.

- Imaging findings on ultrasound: well defined, uniform, hyperechoic lesion is the typical ultrasound appearance (71d). No Doppler signal is seen within the lesion due to the low-velocity flow (71e). Larger lesions can appear hypoechoic and show flow however.
- Imaging findings on CT: lobulated low attenuation lesion, which is frequently peripheral in location. Calcification is not common. Following contrast injection, there is peripheral nodular enhancement with centripetal filling. The lesion usually fills in completely over 3–30 min to become isodense with liver, though larger lesions may show persisting central nonenhancement/scar and small lesions may show immediate uniform enhancement.
- Imaging findings on MRI: haemangiomas show high signal on T2 weighted images that persist on more heavily T2 weighted scans. This is called the 'light bulb' sign and is indicative of cyst or haemangioma. The enhancement pattern with gadolinium is as described for CT.
- Imaging findings on sulphur colloid scan: cold defect.

Usually imaging is sufficient to make the diagnosis but where atypical features are present, biopsy can be undertaken provided there is normal liver between the lesion and liver capsule to prevent haemorrhage.

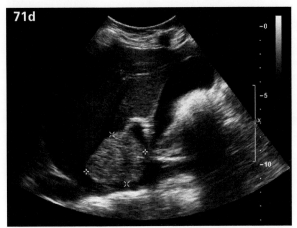

71d Ultrasound appearances of haemangioma are of a well defined, round, hyperechoic lesion.

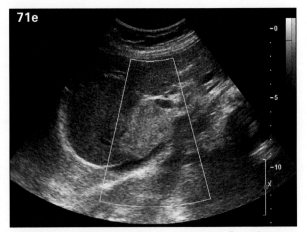

71e No flow is seen within the lesion on Doppler ultrasound.

Answer 71 — **Abdominal Imaging** — Case 72

Practical tips
- MRI is the investigation of choice to characterize suspected haemangioma. A positive 'light bulb' sign indicates that the lesion is either a cyst or a haemangioma. However, depending on the specific circumstances, post-contrast scans may still be required as necrotic or cystic neoplasms can yield a positive 'light bulb' sign.
- Use of IV contrast – obtain pre-contrast scans, then repeat at 30 s (arterial phase), 60 s (portal phase) and 3–5 min (equilibrium phase).
- If the centripetal enhancement is intense and nodular, this is highly specific for the diagnosis of haemangioma.

Further management
These are essentially benign lesions and don't require any further follow-up.

Further reading
Vilanova JC, Barceló J, Smirniotopoulos JG, *et al.* (2004). Hemangioma from head to toe: MR imaging with pathologic correlation. *RadioGraphics* **24**: 367–385.

CASE 72

History
A 43-year-old male presented with central abdominal pain.

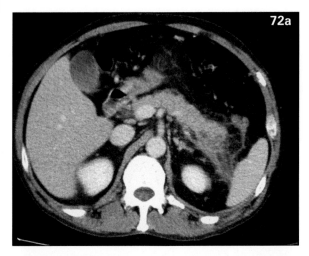
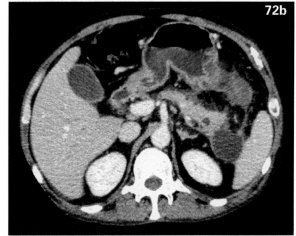
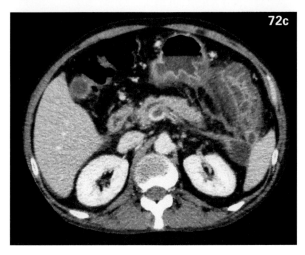
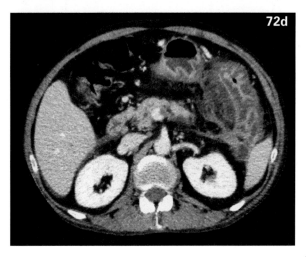

ANSWER 72

Observations (72a, 72b, 72c, 72d)
Several axial CT images of the abdomen with IV contrast enhancement in the portal venous phase are shown. There is significant stranding of the peripancreatic fat indicative of acute inflammation, which is predominantly around the pancreatic tail. Within the pancreatic tail, there is a moderate sized fluid-filled cystic lesion, which would be consistent with a pancreatic pseudocyst in a patient with pancreatitis. The local inflammatory change appears to extend to involve the distal transverse colon at the splenic flexure. In addition, there is central low attenuation within the portal vein extending into the proximal splenic vein in keeping with portal/splenic vein thrombosis. The pancreatic duct is dilated at 4 mm diameter. While the whole gallbladder has not been imaged – no gallstones are seen on these images. The visualized liver edge is smooth and liver has normal attenuation.

Diagnosis
Pancreatitis.

Discussion
Pancreatitis is an acute inflammatory condition. There are two main types of pancreatitis – oedematous and necrotic. Oedematous pancreatitis is the much more common form, characterized by gland oedema, whereas necrotic pancreatitis is rarer and is complicated by pancreatic haemorrhage and necrosis.

Appearances of the pancreas in pancreatitis can therefore be variable, with the pancreas appearing normal, having areas of nonenhancement due to necrosis, having areas of increased attenuation due to haemorrhage, or appearing enlarged and oedematous. Universally, streaking into the surrounding fat due to inflammation is observed.

Causes of pancreatitis include:
- Alcoholism and gallstones are the two most common causes of acute pancreatitis. Assess for signs of alcohol excess by looking for fatty change in the liver (diffuse low attenuation on CT, raised echogenicity on US), cirrhosis (irregular nodular surface to the liver which is atrophic) and portal hypertension (splenomegaly and varices). Assess for gallstones with US initially, then MRCP if there is still uncertainty.
- Infections – hepatitis, mumps.
- Trauma.
- Hypercalcaemia from multiple myeloma, sarcoidosis, amyloidosis.
- Drugs, e.g. steroids, diuretics (frusemide, thiazides), azathioprine.
- Malignancy.

Pancreatitis can be complicated by pseudocyst formation; abscess formation (usually develops 2 weeks after acute inflammation onset); spread of local inflammation to involve bowel loops resulting in strictures, colitis and perforation; portal vein, splenic vein, SMV thrombosis; ascites and chest complications – pleural effusion (usually left sided), empyema, unilateral pulmonary oedema.

In chronic pancreatitis (following several bouts of acute episodes), the pancreas becomes atrophic, there is multifocal calcification, the pancreatic duct becomes dilated and chronic pseudocysts can form (72e).

Practical tips
- Look for the two main causes of pancreatitis – alcohol and gallstones. US is required to look for gallstones and can be used to look for complications, e.g. pseudocyst formation and portal vein thrombosis.
- Look for the main complications of pancreatitis.
- Assessing the pancreas is best done by three phase CT imaging with a pre-contrast and 'pancreatic' phase (~40 s) scan of the pancreas, followed by portal venous phase scans of the abdomen and pelvis. The pre-contrast scan will allow for assessment of calcification in the pancreas to determine whether this is an acute-on-chronic episode. Pancreatic phase scans best assess for areas of necrosis and focal mass lesions. Portal venous imaging allows for assessment of local disease and complications.

Further management
Treatment is usually conservative although necrotizing pancreatitis may well need more aggressive management involving surgery or percutaneous radiologically guided drainage.

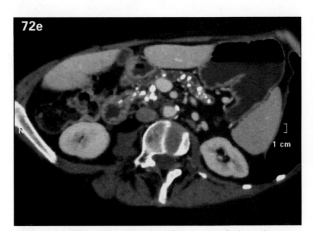

72e Axial CT image showing features of chronic pancreatitis with atrophic pancreas, dilated pancreatic duct and marked calcification.

CASE 73

History
A 34-year-old male presented with scrotal tenderness.

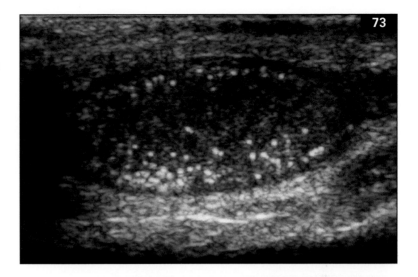

CASE 74

History
A 56-year-old male presented with haematuria and chronic renal failure.

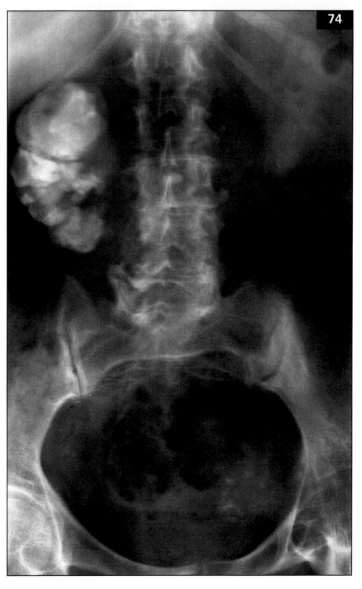

ANSWER 73

Observations (73)
Ultrasound longitudinal image of the right testicle demonstrates multiple small hyperechoic foci, with no posterior acoustic shadowing, distributed evenly throughout the testicle. The testicle is otherwise of normal size and shape. No other focal mass lesion is identified.

Diagnosis
Testicular microlithiasis.

Discussion
Testicular microlithiasis is a condition characterized by failure of clearance of degenerated tubular epithelium from the seminiferous tubules, which subsequently calcify. This is an asymptomatic condition and is an uncommon incidental finding. Image findings on US are of multiple small 1–2 mm hyperechoic foci with no acoustic shadowing, distributed throughout both testes. Atypical appearances of asymmetrical and unilateral foci are also seen. There is an increased risk of testicular germ cell tumour in 40% and therefore follow-up with 6 monthly US is often advised.

Associations include:
- Cryptorchidism.
- Infertility.
- Klinefelter's.
- Down's syndrome.
- Male pseudohermaphrodism.
- Alveolar microlithiasis.

Practical tips
Identifying the distribution of calcific foci is important, since a cluster of calcification within a hypoechoic area suggests tumour or chronic testicular infarction. Infarction can be due to torsion, trauma or severe epididymitis.

Further management
Urological referral with follow-up testicular US at 6 monthly intervals to screen for malignancy.

ANSWER 74

Observations (74)
Single AP abdominal radiograph demonstrates amorphous, putty-like calcification within a shrunken right kidney.

Diagnosis
Renal tuberculosis with autonephrectomy.

Discussion
The urogenital tract is the second most common site to be affected by TB, after the lungs. Renal TB is found in 5–10% of patients with pulmonary TB, but there is only radiographic evidence of pulmonary TB in fewer than 50%. The kidney is usually affected first, via haematogenous spread from a lung/bone/GI focus. There can then be contiguous spread of infection to involve the ureters and bladder. Renal TB is unilateral in 75% of cases and the most common appearance is of a small, shrunken, scarred, nonfunctioning kidney.

Less common appearances are of:
- Cortical scarring.
- Renal pelvis/infundibular strictures resulting in hydrocalycosis and amputated calyx.
- Nephrolithiasis.
- Dystrophic parenchymal calcification.

Ureteral TB is found in 50% of genitourinary TB cases. Radiographic features of involvement include ureteral filling defects, calcification and strictures. Bladder TB presents with a shrunken, scarred, calcified bladder with thickened wall and/or filling defects. Clinical presentation is with frequency, urgency, dysuria, microscopic haematuria and 'sterile' pyuria.

Practical tips
- Urinary tract TB spreads in an antegrade fashion.
- Check chest radiograph for signs of pulmonary TB – but this is only seen in about 50% of cases.

Further management
Medical drug therapy for TB should be initiated.

CASE 75

History
A 57-year-old male patient presented with abdominal pain.

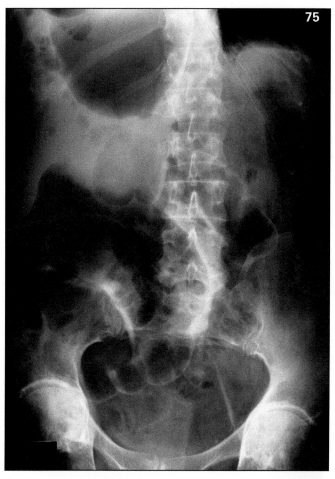

CASE 76

History
A 58-year-old female presented with early satiety.

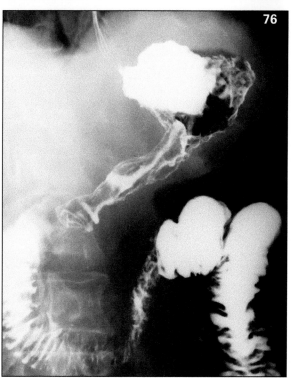

ANSWER 75

Observations (75)
Supine abdominal radiograph shows a positive 'Rigler sign' suggestive of pneumoperitoneum. There is also outlining of the falciform ligament and the left lateral umbilical ligament with a large area of free gas seen overlying the liver. These findings are consistent with pneumoperitoneum.

Diagnosis
Pneumoperitoneum.

Differential diagnosis
Of causes of pneumoperitoneum:
- Trauma.
- Iatrogenic causes, e.g. laparotomy – usually gas should have resolved within 3 days and its presence is suspicious after this; although it can take up to 3 weeks to resolve in some cases. Faster absorption occurs with CO_2 and in obese patients.
- Perforation of abdominal viscus.
- Ruptured pneumatosis intestinalis.
- Rupture of an abscess.
- Extension from chest, i.e. pneumomediastinum, bronchopleural fistula.
- Through female genital tract, e.g. intercourse, waterskiing.

Discussion
There are a variety of signs that aid in the detection of free intraperitoneal gas.

Signs of free gas within the peritoneal cavity on a supine radiograph are:
- 'Football sign' – large round lucency in central abdomen.
- 'Rigler sign' – air on both sides of the bowel wall makes it unusually visible.
- 'Triangle sign' – gas within bowel doesn't normally form edges therefore such unusually shaped collections of air should arouse suspicion of free gas.
- 'Urachus sign' – outline of median umbilical ligament.
- Outlining of falciform ligament as well as the medial and lateral umbilical ligaments.

Practical tips
If there is any doubt about the diagnosis then an erect chest radiograph or a left lateral decubitus film of the abdomen should be acquired.

Further management
Free intraperitoneal gas is suggestive of a perforated viscus and is a surgical emergency – inform the surgical team immediately.

Further reading
Levine MS, Scheiner JD, Rubesin SE, et al. (1991). Diagnosis of pneumoperitoneum on supine abdominal radiographs. *American Journal of Radiology* **156**: 731–735.

ANSWER 76

Observations (76)
Single image from a barium meal examination shows there is poor distension of the entire stomach, which is most evident in the body and antrum, with relative sparing of the cardia. Irregular gastric mucosa is seen within the fundus and body. The duodenum is normal. The appearances are those of linitis plastica and a gastric tumour must be excluded in the first instance.

Diagnosis
Linitis plastica due to gastric carcinoma.

Differential diagnosis
For linitis plastica appearance (mnemonic – 'CALM RAGE'):
- Cancer.
- Amyloidosis.
- Lymphoma – usually non-Hodgkin's type, most common part of GI tract affected.
- Metastases – from lung, breast and melanoma.
- Radiation.
- Alkalis and other corrosives.
- Granulomatous disorders, e.g. Crohn's, TB.
- Eosinophilic enteritis.

Discussion
Gastric carcinoma is the third most common GI malignancy and shows an increased prevalence in Japan. The scirrhous type of the tumour, which produces linitis plastica, accounts for 5–10% of gastric cancer. Diffuse infiltration of tumour causes fibrosis and rigidity with reduction/absence of peristalsis in affected areas. The fundus and body of the stomach are most commonly involved.

Practical tips
Assessment of the stomach on CT is often very difficult due to poor distension; however, contrast investigations are much better due to their dynamic nature.

Further management
Referral to a gastroenterologist for endoscopy +/− biopsy is appropriate.

Further reading
Ba-Ssalamah A, Prokop M, Uffmann M, et al. (2003). Dedicated multidetector CT of the stomach: spectrum of diseases. *RadioGraphics* **23**: 625–644.

CASE 77

History
A 50-year-old female presented with recurrent urinary tract infection.

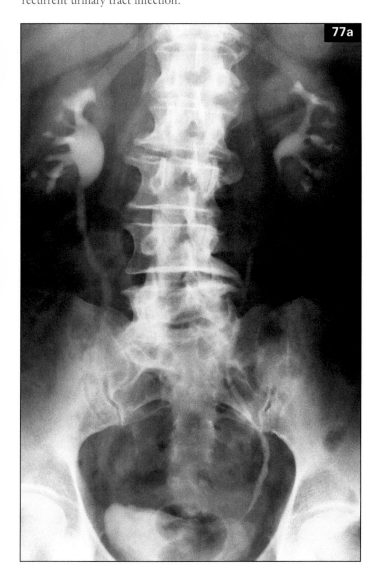
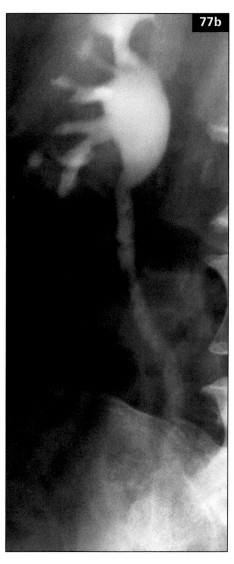

ANSWER 77

Observations (77a, 77b)
This full length film taken at 15 minutes in an IVU series shows multiple small, well defined, smooth rounded filling defects within both ureters.

Diagnosis
Pyeloureteritis cystica.

Differential diagnosis
For radiolucent filling defects in the ureters:
- Radiolucent calculi.
- Transitional cell carcinoma (TCC).
- Pyeloureteritis cystica.
- Blood clots.
- Ureteric polyps.
- Sloughed renal papillae.

Discussion
This is a condition characterized by multiple small subepithelial fluid-filled cysts in the wall of the renal pelvis and ureters extending into the ureteric lumen. There is an association with recurrent urinary tract infections and obstruction, with a predisposition in diabetic patients. The condition is asymptomatic and the lesions are not premalignant. Occasionally it presents with haematuria.

Practical tips
Although any part of the ureter may be involved, there is slight predilection for the upper third.

Further management
Characteristic IVU appearances may well permit a confident diagnosis. However, if there is diagnostic uncertainty then ureteroscopy with biopsy may sometimes be required. Antibiotic treatment may be undertaken, though the response is variable.

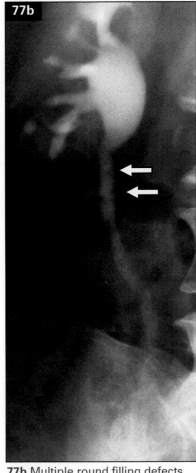

77b Multiple round filling defects.

CASE 78

History
A 52-year-old female with diabetes presented with renal failure.

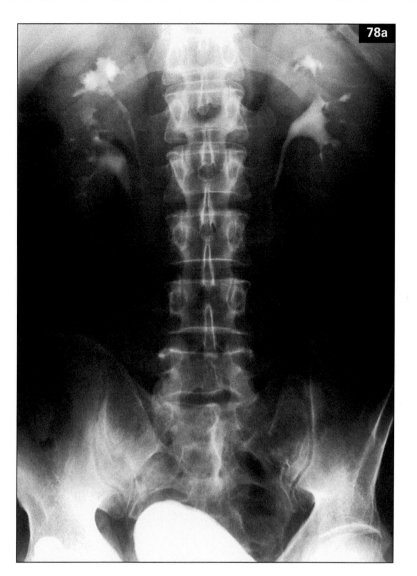

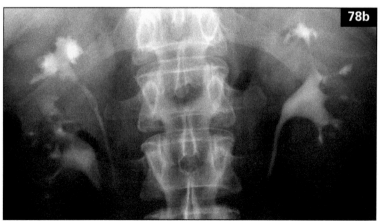

ANSWER 78

Observations (78a, 78b)
Two images from an IVU series are shown. There is evidence of renal papillary swelling and enlargement. The interpolar calyces on the right have a 'ball on tee' appearance with a collection of contrast material in the centre of the papilla. A partial duplex system is also demonstrated on the right. There is a well defined intraluminal non-opaque filling defect in the upper ureter on the right, which represents a sloughed papilla.

Diagnosis
Renal papillary necrosis.

Differential diagnosis
Of causes of renal papillary necrosis (mnemonic – 'SAD ROPE'):
- Sickle cell disease.
- Analgesics.
- Diabetes.
- Renal vein thrombosis.
- Obstructive uropathy.
- Pyelonephritis.
- Ethanol abuse.

Discussion
Renal papillary necrosis is caused by a variety of disease processes that result in ischaemia of the papillary portion of the renal pyramids. There is a progression in radiological appearances as disease progresses. Phases of development:
- Papillary swelling/enlargement.
- Partial papillary sloughing – tract formation communicating with an irregular cavity. On an IVU this is shown by the 'ball on tee' appearance with contrast extending into a centrally cavitated papilla.
- Total papillary sloughing – which gives a 'signet ring' appearance on IVU with the nonopacified sloughed papilla being surrounded by contrast in the calyx/ureter.

Practical tips
- To differentiate between the various causes, identify whether the involvement is unilateral (renal vein thrombosis, obstructive uropathy) or bilateral (systemic causes).
- Diabetes is the most frequent cause (50%).
- A classic 'exam type film' to be aware of is the IVU showing renal papillary necrosis and background bony abnormalities of a condition that has been treated with NSAIDs, e.g. ankylosing spondylitis, or bony changes of sickle cell disease.

Further management
Treatment of the condition requires identification of the underlying cause and control of this disease process.

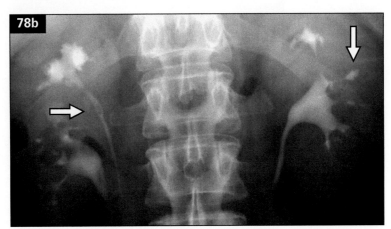

78b Sloughed papilla (left) and 'ball on tee' appearance (right).

CASE 79

History
A 36-year-old immunocompromised patient presented with dysphagia.

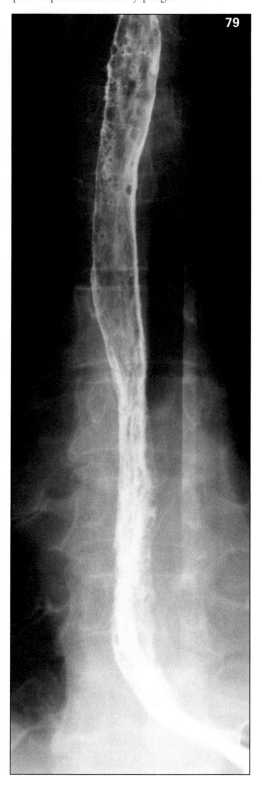

CASE 80

History
A 28-year-old female presented with upper abdominal pain, pyrexia and jaundice.

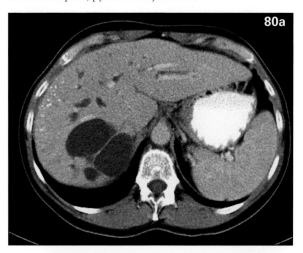

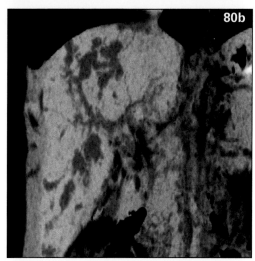

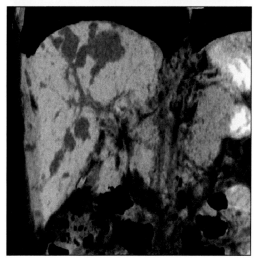

ANSWER 79

Observations (79)
Single image from a barium swallow examination shows a shaggy, ulcerated mucosal pattern in the thoracic oesophagus typical of candidiasis.

Diagnosis
Candida oesophagitis.

Discussion
Candida oesophagitis is the most common cause of infectious oesophagitis with *C. albicans* being the most commonly involved organism. Immunocompromised patients have a predisposition to infection. Presentation is with gradual dysphagia, odynophagia and retrosternal pain. Association with oral infection is seen in up to 80%, characterized by several patchy, white plaques covering the mucosa. In the oesophagus there is predilection for the *upper half of the oesophagus* with the appearance of multiple, shaggy, longitudinal mucosal plaques. There is reduction in primary peristalsis and some narrowing of the lumen due to spasm and oedema. Stricture formation is a rare complication.

Other infective causes of oesophagitis include:
- Herpes oesophagitis – the second most common cause of infectious oesophagitis. Caused by herpes simplex virus (HSV) type 1 and most commonly presenting in males in 2nd–4th decades. Usually involving the mid oesophagus, there are multiple small discrete superficial punctate ulcers. The intervening mucosa is usually of normal appearance.
- Cytomegalovirus (CMV) oesophagitis – presents radiologically with a single or multiple giant flat superficial ulcer(s) near the gastro-oesophageal junction. Less commonly, it can present as discrete small superficial ulcers as are seen in herpes oesophagitis.
- HIV oesophagitis – characterized by giant oesophageal ulcers, difficult to differentiate from CMV oesophagitis.

All affect immunocompromised patients and are rarely seen in immunocompetents.

Practical tips
Do not mistake pseudodiverticulosis of the oesophagus for deep ulceration. This is a benign condition where oesophageal mucous glands become dilated and form flask-shaped outpouchings from the lumen. It is associated with any severe oesophagitis (see Case 38).

Further management
- Always consider immunocompromisation if not already apparent.
- Oropharyngeal candidiasis may be a pointer to the nature of oesophageal ulceration but upper GI endoscopy is still often needed to confirm via biopsies and brushings.
- Antifungal or antiviral drugs for treatment as appropriate.

ANSWER 80

Observations (80a, 80b)
Axial CT image and coronal reformats of the liver with IV contrast in portal venous phase are shown. There are multiple, well defined low attenuation cystic structures seen throughout the liver. These appear to be communicating with the bile ducts and are better demonstrated on the coronal reformatted images (**80b**). No calculi are seen in the ducts. The CT appearances are highly suggestive of Caroli's disease and the clinical details suggest cholangitis has developed.

Diagnosis
Caroli's disease.

Discussion
Caroli's disease is a rare autosomal recessive disorder characterized by multifocal, cystic dilatation of the intrahepatic bile ducts. The differential diagnosis for this condition is polycystic liver disease, however the two can be discriminated by identifying the communication between 'cysts' and bile ducts in Caroli's.

Associations of Caroli's disease:
- Medullary sponge kidney (80%).
- Polycystic kidney disease.
- Congenital hepatic fibrosis.
- Choledochal cyst.

Complications include biliary stasis, stones, cholangitis and hepatic abscess. There is an increased risk of cholangiocarcinoma in patients with Caroli's disease. Biliary cirrhosis and portal hypertension are *not* complications.

Practical tips
Diagnosis is dependent on showing that the cysts communicate with the biliary tree – coronal and sagittal reformats can be essential for this.

Further management
If there is any concern as to whether the cysts are communicating, MRCP (magnetic resonance cholangiopancreatography) is a noninvasive method of clarification.

CASE 81

History
A 42-year-old female presented with pelvic pain and menorrhagia.

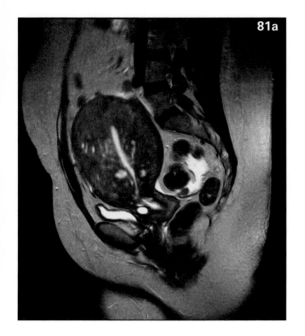
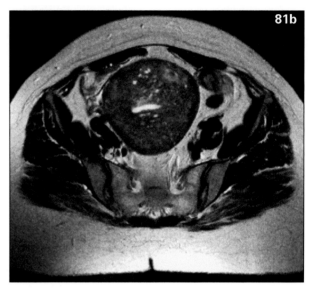

CASE 82

History
A 47-year-old presented with right upper quadrant abdominal pain.

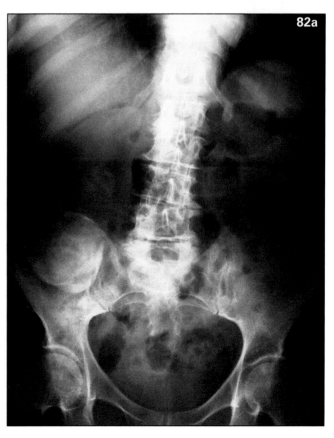

ANSWER 81

Observation (81a, 81b)
Two MRI images are presented – T2 weighted sagittal and axial images through the pelvis. These images show bulky enlargement of the uterus. The junctional zone is widened and poorly defined and there are multiple high signal foci within the myometrium in keeping with ectopic endometrial tissue. These appearances are typical of adenomyosis.

Diagnosis
Adenomyosis.

Discussion
Adenomyosis is a chronic condition affecting women during the reproductive years. There is an increased incidence in multiparous women, suggesting that uterine trauma plays a role in the development of this disease. The disease is characterized by ectopic endometrial tissue spreading into the myometrium resulting in myometrial hyperplasia. The condition is benign and although it is associated with endometriosis, there is no increased risk of developing endometrial/uterine malignancies. The disease can be either focal or diffuse. It can sometimes be difficult on US to differentiate focal forms of the condition from uterine fibroids.

US appearances are of poorly defined hypoechoic areas within the myometrium with multiple small, 2–4 mm, ectopic endometrial cysts seen within the myometrium. There is thickening of the anterior and posterior myometrial walls.

MRI appearances are very similar – myometrial wall thickening; high signal (on T2 weighted images) ectopic endometrial cysts in the myometrium and focal/diffuse thickening of the innermost layer of myometrium known as the junctional zone.

Symptomatically patients present with menorrhagia, pelvic pain and dysmenorrhoea and the condition can lead to infertility.

Practical tips
Widening of the junctional zone with ectopic endometrial cysts are the best MRI features for diagnosis.

Further management
Hysterectomy is the only management option to relieve symptoms.

ANSWER 82

Observations (82a)
Single AP radiograph of the abdomen demonstrates a large mass lesion in the right upper quadrant, which shows curvilinear calcification of the wall. Appearances would best fit with this being a calcified wall of the gallbladder. No discontinuous areas in calcification are seen.

Diagnosis
Porcelain gallbladder.

Differential diagnosis
Similar appearances on US can be due to:
- Emphysematous cholecystitis.
- Gallbladder filled with stones.
- Normal gas-filled bowel.

Discussion
This is an idiopathic condition that was coined to describe the blue discolouration and brittle nature of the gallbladder at surgery. The condition is associated with gallstones in 90% of cases and is more frequently seen in women (sex ratio of 5:1). Patients are usually asymptomatic and diagnosis is made incidentally on plain films or US imaging. Radiographic appearances mirror the histological findings of dystrophic calcification in a chronically inflamed gallbladder. The calcification can be of two types:
- Curvilinear calcification in the muscularis (82b).
- Punctate calcification in the mucosa/glandular spaces.

Imaging features on US are of curvilinear/punctate calcification in the thickened wall of the gallbladder, which can be focal or affecting the whole wall, with minimal acoustic shadowing. On oral cholecystography, the gallbladder is found to be nonfunctioning. The importance of identifying the condition is the risk of developing gallbladder carcinoma, which occurs in 10–20% of cases. Appearances of gallbladder carcinoma in this situation can be of a luminal filling defect, infiltration causing focal wall thickening or a localized fungating mass. Cholecystectomy is therefore recommended even if the patient is asymptomatic.

Practical tips
- Ultrasound and CT scans should be scrutinized for secondary gallbladder malignancy when porcelain gallbladder is noted.
- A discontinuity in the calcification when the whole gallbladder wall appears to be calcified may be a clue to gallbladder carcinoma.

Further management
Cholecystectomy is advised due to the high risk of tumour.

Further reading
Kane R, Jacobs R, Katz J, Costello P (1984). Porcelain gallbladder: ultrasound and CT appearances. *Radiology* 152: 137–141.

Answer 82　　　　　　　　　**Abdominal Imaging**　　　　　　　　　Case 83

82b Axial CT image shows curvilinear circumferential calcification of the gallbladder wall.

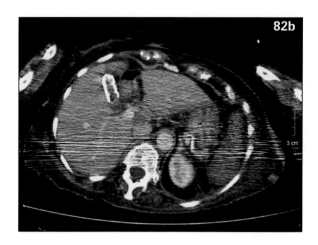

CASE 83

History
A 38-year-old female presented with severe dysmenorrhoea and menorrhagia.

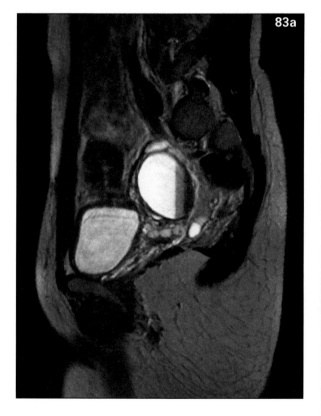

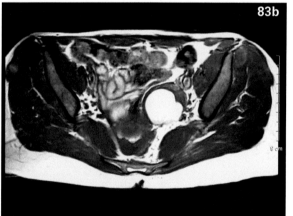

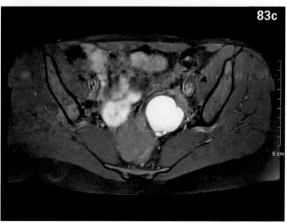

ANSWER 83

Observations (83a, 83b, 83c)
Three MRI images are shown – a sagittal T2 weighted image (**83a**), axial T1 (**83b**) and axial T1 weighted fat suppressed image (**83c**). There is a large 4 cm lesion identified within the left ovary, which is of high signal on both T1 and T2 weighted images and shows no fat suppression. On the sagittal T2 weighted image, there is evidence of layering of the contents of this mass. These appearances would be entirely consistent with blood products and the lesion represents an endometrioma.

Diagnosis
Endometrioma.

Discussion
Endometriosis is a chronic condition characterized by ectopic deposits of endometrium outside the uterine cavity. It affects women in the 4th–6th decades and is characterized by chronic pelvic pain, dysmenorrhoea, menorrhagia and dyspareunia. Common sites for endometrial deposits are the ovaries, fallopian tubes, pouch of Douglas and uterosacral ligaments, however more distal spread can occur to the bladder/bowel wall with even further distal spread to the lungs and pleura. Spread to the GI tract most commonly occurs to the distal sigmoid and the rectosigmoid wall and deposits can result in peritoneal adhesion and subsequent obstruction. Repeated bleeding of the ectopic endometrial deposits results in fibrosis and pain.

Endometrial deposits can be focal or diffuse. In this case, the classical appearance of an endometrioma or 'chocolate cyst' is shown with a 1–5 cm cyst containing layered blood products of high signal on T1 and T2 weighted images. There is no signal loss on fat suppression sequences. The diffuse form is more common, however, with multiple smaller scattered cysts seen in several locations.

Complications depend on the site of the deposits and can result in:
- Infertility (due to involvement of the fallopian tubes causing adhesions/fibrosis).
- Bowel obstruction (due to fibrosis/stricturing of the bowel wall).
- Pneumothorax (due to spread to the pleura).

Practical tips
Endometriomas can be differentiated from dermoid cysts by using a fat suppressed MRI sequence. Both will show high signal on T1 and T2 weighted images but endometriomas will still be high signal on fat suppressed sequences.

Further management
This condition can be difficult to control. Medical management with hormonal suppression of menstruation is often attempted but surgical excision may be required.

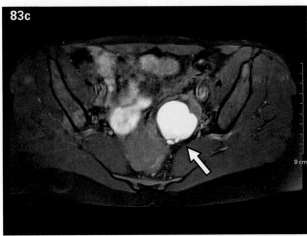

83c Lesion remains high signal on the T1 fat suppressed image suggesting that it represents blood.

CASE 84

History
A 34-year-old female presented with vague abdominal pain.

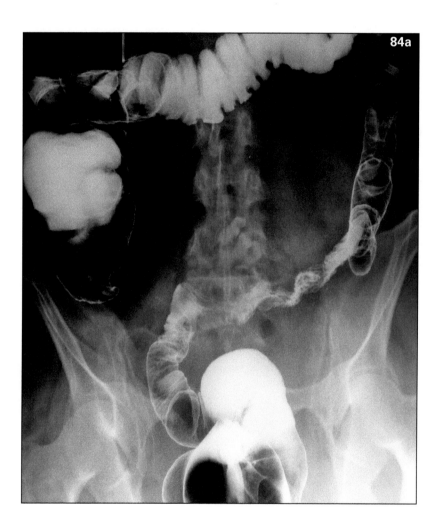

ANSWER 84

Observations (84a)
This single image from a double contrast barium enema shows abnormality of the sigmoid colon with poor distension and apparent external compression of the bowel loops inferiorly. Three well defined calcific densities are seen adjacent to the affected segment and have the appearance of teeth.

Diagnosis
Ovarian dermoid.

Discussion
Ovarian dermoid cysts are benign lesions, which are relatively common, accounting for ~20% of all ovarian neoplasms. These mostly present during the reproductive years, with a mean age of presentation of 30 years. They contain tissue from all three germ cell layers – ectodermal (skin, brain), mesodermal (muscle, fat) and endodermal (mucinous/ciliated epithelium). Tumours are bilateral in ~10%.

Typical appearance is of a unilocular cyst, lined by squamous epithelium and containing sebaceous, fatty material with hair follicles and skin glands arising from the wall. A protuberance into the cavity known as a Rokitansky nodule is usually the site of bone/teeth material.

- Appearances on plain radiograph: teeth occur in 56% of cases and are readily identifiable. Mass effect with bowel loop displacement is often seen (**84b**). The image shows a central lucent density representative of fat in the right side of the pelvis, which is displacing sigmoid colon.
- Appearances on US/CT/MRI: a well defined high echogenicity lesion is identified in the ovary due to high fat content (**84c**). Again teeth are easily identified with posterior acoustic shadowing, within the solid Rokitansky nodule. Fat is readily identifiable on CT and MRI by virtue of its low density and high signal.

Complications are of torsion, rupture and malignant degeneration (seen in 2% of cases).

Practical tips
Some films used in radiological exams rely on the candidate noting an incidental lesion at the edge of the film. Teeth in ovarian dermoids are a classical example of an 'edge of the film' case!

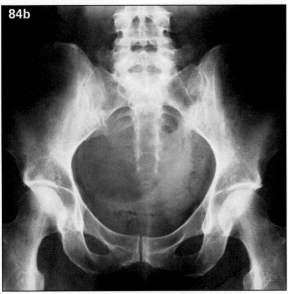

84b Plain radiograph of the pelvis shows lateral displacement of the sigmoid colon due to the lucent central pelvic mass.

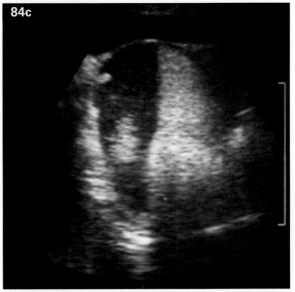

84c Areas of increased echogenicity within the lesion on US represent fat.

Answer 84 — Abdominal Imaging

Further management
- Where there is still clinical concern after ultrasound, MRI is useful in completely characterizing these lesions. Figures **84d–f** are axial T2 weighted (**84d**), T1 weighted (**84e**) and fat saturated (**84f**) axial images of the pelvis showing dermoid cysts in both ovaries. The right most cyst shows signal void posteriorly on all image sequences in keeping with calcification and complete fat suppression confirms the predominant fat content of these lesions.
- Referral to gynaecologist for surgical excision.

Further reading
Outwater EK, Siegelman ES, Hunt JL (2001). Ovarian teratomas: tumor types and imaging characteristics. *RadioGraphics* 21: 475–490.

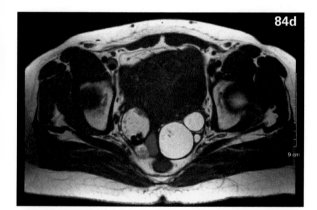
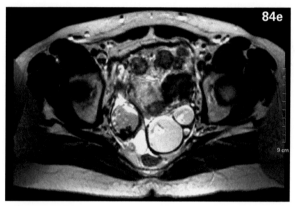
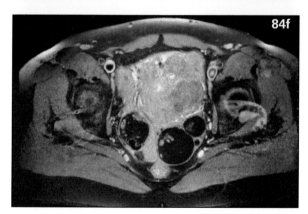

84d–84f Axial T2 weighted (**84d**), T1 weighted (**84e**) and fat saturated (**84f**) axial images of the pelvis showing dermoid cysts in both ovaries. Loss of signal on the fat saturated image confirms the high fat content.

Case 85

History
Incidental liver lesion was noted on abdominal ultrasound scan of a 26-year-old female.

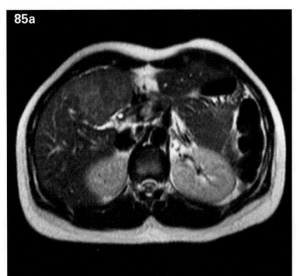

T2 weighted

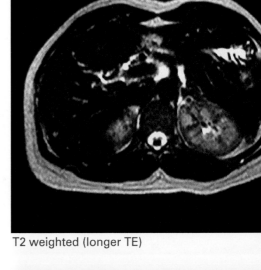

T2 weighted (longer TE)

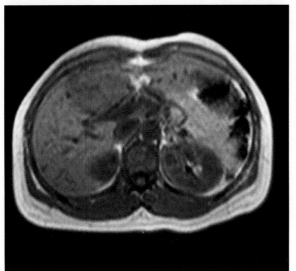

T1 weighted in phase

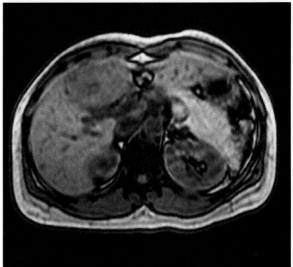

T1 weighted out of phase

Abdominal Imaging — Case 85

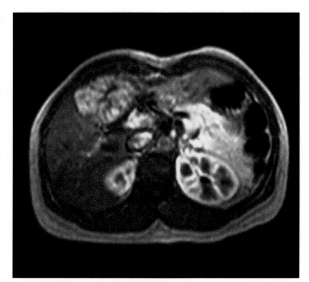
T1 weighted post Gad BOPTA 25 s

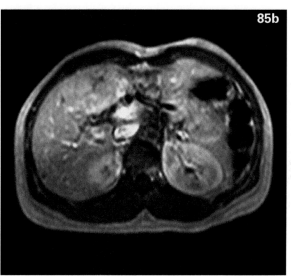
T1 weighted post Gad BOPTA 60 s

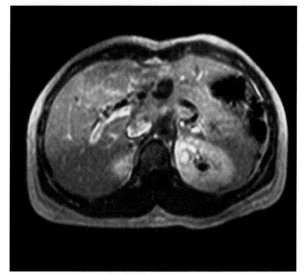
T1 weighted post Gad BOPTA 3 min

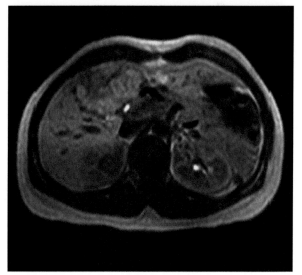
T1 weighted post Gad BOPTA 90 min

ANSWER 85

Observations (85a, 85b)
Selected pre- and post-contrast MRI images of the liver. Pre-contrast images (**85a**) demonstrate a large, well defined lesion in segment 4 of the liver, which is of slightly reduced signal on T1 weighted images. Out of phase T1 weighted images show no significant alteration of liver signal to suggest the area is due to focal fatty sparing. The lesion is slightly hyperintense on T2 weighted scans.

On dynamic post-contrast imaging (**85b**), the lesion shows marked enhancement during early arterial (25 s) phase with a central hypointense scar visible at this stage. There is subsequent wash out of contrast in the portal (60 s) and equilibrium (3 min) phases to become isointense with liver. The central scar shows enhancement in the equilibrium phase.

The contrast agent used is gadolinium BOPTA (Gd-BOPTA) and the image taken at 90 min shows persisting contrast uptake within the lesion indicative of hepatocyte content. These appearances and pattern of enhancement would best fit with the diagnosis of focal nodular hyperplasia.

Diagnosis
Focal nodular hyperplasia (FNH).

Differential diagnosis
For hepatic lesion with central scar:
- FNH.
- Adenoma.
- Hepatocellular carcinoma.
- Haemangioma.
- Fibrolamellar carcinoma.

Discussion
Focal nodular hyperplasia is a benign hepatic lesion that occurs most commonly in young/middle aged women. Usually these patients are asymptomatic, with diagnosis made as an incidental finding, although some patients can present with vague abdominal pain. They are solitary (85–95%) vascular lesions containing normal hepatic elements – Kupffer cells, hepatocytes and bile ducts. Imaging features are very similar to those of hepatic adenomas. Unlike hepatic adenomas, development is not associated with the oral contraceptive pill, though oestrogens can exert trophic effects.

Focal nodular hyperplasia is divided into typical and atypical groups, with approximately 50% in each. Typical lesions show the signal characteristics, enhancement pattern and central scar as described below. Atypical lesions may show signal heterogeneity, with more marked T1 and T2 hyperintensity, and no central scar.
- Imaging features on CT and MRI: classical FNH is isodense on CT, while MRI shows mild T1 hypointensity and mild T2 hyperintensity. There is prominent enhancement in the arterial phase following IV contrast, the central scar being conspicuous at this point due to nonenhancement. Contrast washes out rapidly in the portal and equilibrium phases to become similar to normal liver, though there may be scar enhancement in the equilibrium phase.

Liver specific MRI contrast agents can help further. In this case, a gadolinium agent with additional liver specific properties (Gd-BOPTA) has been used. Most gadolinium chelates in current use are extracellular agents that are excreted via the kidneys. Gd-BOPTA and Gd-EOB-DTPA are two agents currently in use that also show a proportion of hepatic excretion. They behave the same as conventional extracellular agents during the arterial, portal and equilibrium phases of liver MRI, but also illustrate functioning hepatocyte tissue on delayed images. Since FNH contains hepatocytes and abnormal bile ductules, such agents are retained within FNH on delayed images (20 min to 2 h depending on the agent). Other non-gadolinium based liver specific MRI contrast agents can similarly help characterize FNH on the basis of the functioning hepatic tissue elements it contains.
- Imaging features on angiography: these lesions usually have a central supplying artery with centrifugal filling giving a 'spoke wheel' appearance; this can aid differentiation from an adenoma, which has several peripheral supply vessels.
- Imaging features on sulphur colloid scan: usually these lesions show normal activity due to the presence of Kupffer cells.

Practical tips
- Sulphur colloid scans have traditionally been used to help confirm FNH suspected on CT and MRI by virtue of the presence of Kupffer cells. Liver specific contrast agents as described above may now obviate this in many cases.
- Hepatic adenoma is a common differential when FNH is considered and there is evidence that agents such as Gd-BOPTA can help differentiate FNH from hepatic adenoma by demonstrating the presence of functioning liver tissue in the former.

Further management
Differentiation from adenoma and hepatocellular carcinoma can sometimes be difficult even with histological information. Excision is then carried out.

Further reading
Schneider G, Grazioli L, Saini S (2005). *MRI of the Liver*. Springer, New York.

Chapter 3

CENTRAL NERVOUS SYSTEM, HEAD AND NECK IMAGING

CT AND MRI HEAD

As for all imaging, if an abnormality is not obvious at first sight, check all areas systematically:
- Establish if IV contrast has been given.
- Ventricles – check the configuration and size, ensuring the size is appropriate for the other extra-axial CSF spaces such as the sulci.
- Cerebral hemispheres, brainstem and cerebellum – on MRI in particular, there is a lot of information to evaluate for focal masses, signal abnormalities and structural abnormalities! In examination vivas, it may be unrealistic to expect the candidate to quickly detect subtle abnormalities so you may well be given some assistance or just presented with selected images. A rapid evaluation of FLAIR (fluid attenuated inversion recovery) or PD (proton density) sequences may quickly lead you to pathology on MRI.
- Extra-axial spaces – carefully check for normal size, absence of blood or other collections.
- Vessels – check for enhancement on CT and normal flow voids on MRI (including vessels at the skull base).
- The periphery – assess orbits, sinuses, temporal bones/skull base and skull vault.

Everyone has their own blind spots but here are some suggested areas to check when all else seems normal:
- The temporal lobes and posterior fossa on CT – images of the temporal lobes are often degraded by streak artefact and pathology easily missed. The same applies to a lesser extent in the posterior fossa.
- Skull base and petrous bone – pathology can be easily overlooked, especially on MRI where there is a lot to assess.
- Early signs of stroke – the early changes of infarction can be very subtle. Carefully check for subtle focal swelling and reduced grey–white matter differentiation. The latter is best detected by using very 'narrow windows' on CT.
- Venous sinus thrombosis and subdural empyema are two disorders with significant morbidity and mortality that can be easily overlooked. When presented with an apparently normal CT of a patient with a history of convincing acute intracranial pathology, always double check for increased density in the venous sinuses and subtle subdural collections. Administration of IV contrast may help confirm either.
- Haemorrhage – subtle subarachnoid or subdural blood must not be missed. Check carefully for small amounts of subarachnoid blood layering in the occipital horns or around the medulla close to the foramen magnum.
- Pituitary – this is well seen on sagittal MRI scans, so do not forget to check it.

A note on mass lesions:
When confronted with an intracranial mass lesion, assess the following:
- Location – certain tumours have a predilection for certain areas of the brain.
- Age – this has a strong influence on the differential diagnosis. Certain tumours are common in the paediatric age group while metastases always have to be considered in the older adult population.
- Is the mass intra- or extra-axial – that is, does it originate within brain substance or not? The distinction is very important in forming a differential diagnosis and though it seems obvious, can sometimes be difficult to establish on CT in particular. An extra-axial mass causes crowding of the subcortical white matter fronds that extend between gyri. Conversely, an intra-axial mass stretches the grey matter around it and consequently displaces the fronds of white matter apart.
- Mass effect and oedema – check for midline shift and effacement of normal CSF spaces such as sulci and cisterns. If extra-axial CSF spaces are obliterated, there is risk of death due to brain herniation through dural apertures. If you see such features, then indicate the degree of urgency required in seeking neurosurgical evaluation and intervention.
- Assess the enhancement pattern of the lesion. This is often nonspecific but certain patterns such as the intense, homogeneous enhancement of meningioma may allow a confident diagnosis.

CT AND MRI NECK

Cross-sectional imaging of the neck requires excellent anatomical knowledge! Familiarize yourself with the anatomical divisions of the upper aerodigestive tract, the fascial spaces of the neck along which tumour and infection track, and the nodal stations of the neck. With this knowledge, you can make a meaningful interpretation for the ENT surgeon. T2 weighted scans with fat suppression are particularly useful to evaluate at first inspection if these are available, for detecting both primary pathology and nodal disease. Thereafter, simultaneous examination of the T1 weighted scans can help to better delineate the precise anatomical location of disease.

PLAIN RADIOGRAPHS
Skull
There are a very limited number of pathologies that are likely to be shown on a skull radiograph:

Trauma
As well as skull fractures, check for indirect signs of fracture such as fluid levels in sinuses and intracranial air. Remember to look at all the bones on the film – the fracture of odontoid peg at the edge of the lateral skull film is a basic exam type of case.

Calcification
Know the normal intracranial calcifications such as pineal and choroid plexus so that you can differentiate from pathological calcification such as that associated with meningioma.

Pituitary
Size and shape of the pituitary fossa should be assessed.

Vault
Several diffuse processes have characteristic changes on the skull radiograph and make for 'spot diagnoses', e.g. acromegaly, fibrous dysplasia, thalassaemia, hyperparathyroidism and myeloma.

Spine
As always, there are many potential pathologies to see on plain films of the spine but trauma, infection and neoplasia are particularly common.

Trauma
When assessing cervical spine films:
- First ensure that the complete cervical spine has been imaged down to C7–T1 level.
- On the lateral film, look at the anterior spinal, posterior spinal and spinolaminar lines to ensure continuity (i.e. imaginary lines drawn along the anterior and posterior vertebral body cortices and along the anterior limits of the spinous processes). Look at the soft tissues of the anterior cervical space, which should be no greater than a third of the width of a vertebral body for C1–3 and no more than the width of a vertebral body for C4–7. Check the interval between the anterior arch of atlas and the odontoid peg – this should normally be no greater than 3 mm in adults and 5 mm in children.
- On the AP film – look for misalignment of the vertebral spinous processes in a vertical plane, which would suggest a facet joint dislocation. Ensure that the AP 'peg' view adequately excludes a C2 peg fracture.
- When you are suspicious of an unstable fracture, make this clear so that adequate steps are taken to protect the cervical spine until such time as this has been confirmed or excluded with CT.

When assessing thoracic and lumbar films, carefully check alignment and vertebral body height. On the AP film of the thoracic spine, look for widening of the paravertebral stripe suggestive of haematoma.

Malignancy
Bony involvement is one of the most common sites of metastatic tumour spread along with the lungs and liver. Look for focal lucency, sclerosis and destruction. On the AP film, methodically check every pedicle, transverse and spinous process for lytic deposits. As ever, pay attention to the soft tissues – a paravertebral soft tissue mass may guide you to a subtle bony lesion. Do not forget that while myeloma classically produces focal bony lucencies and possible resulting vertebral collapse, a significant number of cases show only diffuse osteopenia, which can mimic osteoporosis.

Infection
Spinal infection is usually centred on the disc and therefore there will be a reduction in disc height with involvement of the superior endplate of the vertebral body below and involvement of the inferior endplate of the vertebral body above. Added soft tissue due to abscess is likely to be seen and in the cervical spine will be seen as a prevertebral soft tissue mass on the lateral cervical spine film; in the thoracic spine this will be seen as a widening of the paravertebral stripe; and in the lumbar region there may be a psoas abscess.

CASE 86

History
A 13-year-old presented with bilateral progressive deafness.

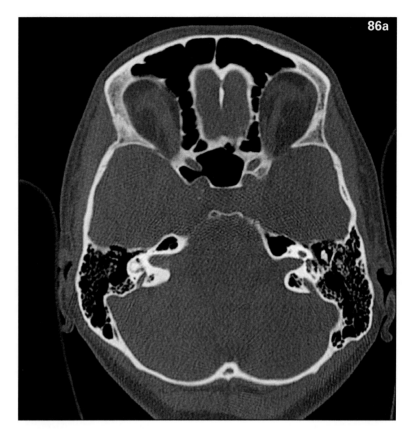

CASE 87

History
A 10-year-old boy presented with recurrent painful enlargement of the parotid gland.

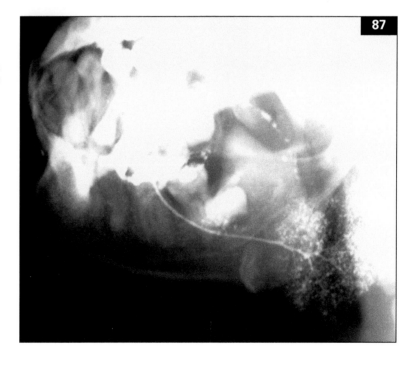

ANSWER 86

Observations (86a)
Single high-resolution axial CT image of the skull at the level of the petrous bone. There is bilateral enlargement of the vestibular aqueduct. Precise measurements have not been documented but the aqueducts are clearly significantly wider than the horizontal semicircular canal seen on the right.

Diagnosis
Enlarged vestibular aqueduct syndrome.

Discussion
Enlarged vestibular aqueduct syndrome presents clinically with sensorineural hearing loss. Hearing is usually present at birth and then deteriorates from age of ~3 years. Deterioration is often in a stepwise manner, associated with episodes of minor head trauma. There is a suggestion of an inherited recessive genetic link and 50% of cases are bilateral. A degree of cochlear dysplasia is present in 75% of cases.

The normal endolymphatic duct originates from the vestibule, via the common crus and extends posterolaterally in the bony vestibular aqueduct to the endolymphatic sac. The endolymphatic sac lies on the posterior aspect of the petrous temporal bone. Enlarged vestibular aqueduct syndrome is diagnosed when the diameter at its midpoint exceeds 1.5 mm. Figure **86b** indicates the dilated aqueduct in this case.

Diagnosis of the condition is important due to the good results achieved with cochlear implantation.

Practical tips
- A quick assessment of the vestibular aqueducts can be made by comparing the diameter at midpoint to the diameter of the adjacent posterior semicircular canal – the aqueduct should not be larger.
- When identified, check the cochlea for evidence of dysplasia.

Further management
- Advise on avoiding head trauma where possible, e.g. no contact sports.
- Hearing can be improved with cochlear implants.

Further reading
Dahlen RT, Harnsberger HR, Gray SD *et al.* (1997). Overlapping thin-section fast spin-echo MR of the large vestibular aqueduct syndrome. *American Journal of Neuroradiology* **18**: 67–75.

Valvassori GE (1983). The large vestibular aqueduct and associated anomalies of the inner ear. *Otolaryngologic Clinics of North America* **16**: 95–101.

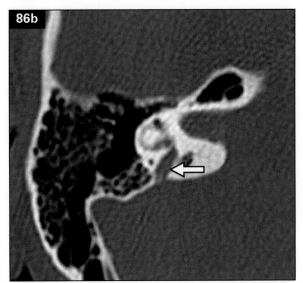

86b Axial CT image demonstrating an enlarged vestibular aqueduct.

ANSWER 87

Observations (87)
Single oblique image from a parotid sialogram with no control film provided for comparison. The parotid duct is of normal calibre with no obstructing stones or stricture. There is, however, florid punctate dilatation of the intraglandular ductules and acini in keeping with punctate sialectasis.

Diagnosis
Juvenile recurrent parotitis (also known as juvenile punctate sialectasis).

Discussion
In adults, recurrent sialadenitis is usually associated with stones or stricture causing duct obstruction. These causes, however, are rare in children and chronic inflammation is most commonly idiopathic in nature. The parotid is affected more than the submandibular gland, perhaps due to a comparatively smaller salivary output. Clinically, episodes present with repeated attacks of swelling of the gland and associated fever. Age of onset is typically 3–6 years, with symptoms usually resolving spontaneously after puberty.

Although sialography is the primary method of diagnosis, US is useful for follow-up as it avoids the radiation burden and invasive nature of sialography. At US, the gland is swollen with a heterogeneous appearance and multiple hypoechoic foci within it. Intraglandular reactive lymph nodes may be noted.

Practical tips
Intraglandular lymph nodes are seen in the parotid but not the submandibular gland, which becomes encapsulated before lymph node development occurs embryologically.

Further management
Although sialectasis most commonly idiopathic, Sjögren's syndrome can also cause this appearance and should be excluded with laboratory investigations.

Further reading
Yam KL, Lau C, Li CK (1997). Primary Sjögren syndrome presenting as recurrent parotitis. *Hong Kong Journal of Paediatrics* (New Series) **2**: 47–50.

CASE 88

History
A 35-year-old male presented with diplopia.

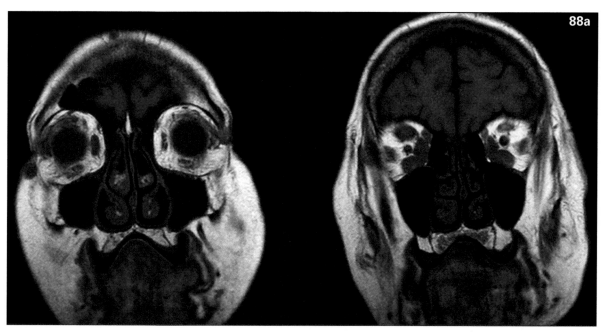

ANSWER 88

Observations (88a)
Coronal T1 weighted MR images of the orbit show marked bilateral swelling of the muscle bellies of the inferior, medial and superior rectus muscles with sparing of the tendinous insertions. This distribution of extraocular muscle swelling is typical of thyroid ophthalmopathy.

Diagnosis
Thyroid ophthalmopathy.

Differential diagnosis
Orbital pseudotumour – usually involves both muscle belly and *tendinous insertion*; is *painful* compared to painless thyroid ophthalmopathy and is more commonly *unilateral*.

Discussion
Thyroid ophthalmopathy is a disease of the orbit characterized by deposition of mucopolysaccharides within the muscle bellies of the intraorbital muscles. It usually presents in adults and is more common in women. The patient is usually hyperthyroid (although 10% of cases are found in euthyroid patients) with ocular presentation within 1 year of hyperthyroid symptom onset. Severity of the eye disease, however, is not related to the severity of the thyroid hormone imbalance.

Radiological features are as follows:
- Majority of cases are bilateral although there is often asymmetrical disease. About 10% are unilateral.
- Inferior and medial rectus are most commonly affected, with the lateral rectus being least likely to be affected.
- Muscle bellies are affected with swollen appearance and relative sparing of the tendinous insertions. Axial CT images (88b) show swollen medial recti with typical sparing of the tendinous insertions.
- Proptosis, lid retraction and reduced eye movements are features.

Usually the disease resolves spontaneously but steroid treatment is prescribed to treat the swelling and to reduce intraorbital pressure, which can otherwise cause optic nerve and ophthalmic vein compression. Surgical decompression is sometimes required when there is acute swelling and threatened visual loss.

Practical tips
The order of muscles involved in thyroid ophthalmopathy is (from most to least frequent) Inferior>Medial>Superior>Lateral>Oblique – Mnemonic = I'M SLO(w).

Further management
Thyroid ophthalmopathy with visual disturbance requires prompt evaluation and treatment given the potential risk to visual function.

Further reading
Hosten N, Sander B, Cordes M, *et al.* (1989). Graves ophthalmopathy: MR imaging of the orbits. *Radiology* **172**: 759–762.

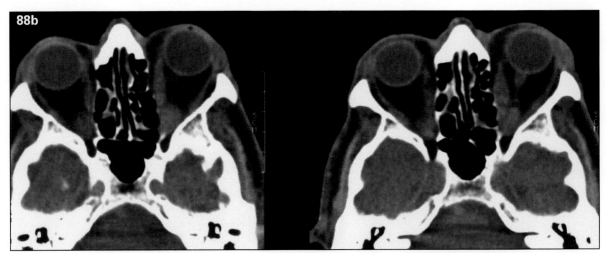

88b Selected axial CT images through the orbits show thickening of the medial rectus muscles with sparing of their tendons.

CASE 89

History
A 21-year-old male presented with positional headaches.

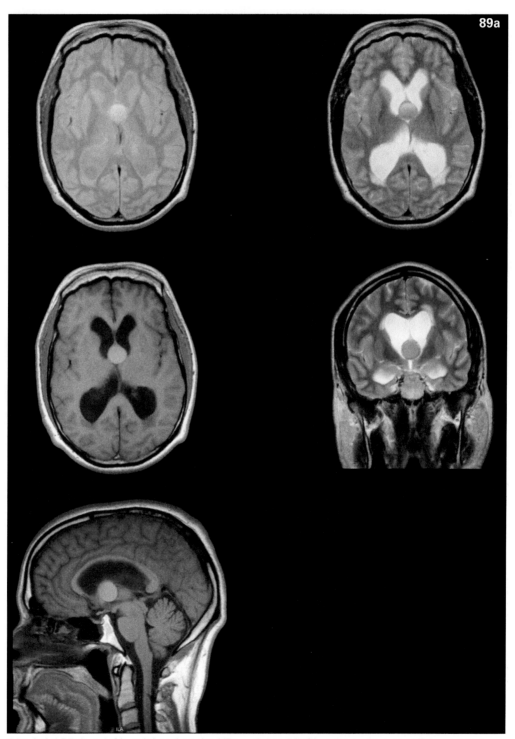

89a Axial PD (top left), axial and sagittal T1 weighted (left), axial and coronal T2 weighted (right) MR images.

ANSWER 89

Observations (89a)
Selected MRI images demonstrate a round lesion in the anterosuperior aspect of the 3rd ventricle. The lesion is mildly hyperintense on T1 weighted images, with variable signal on T2 weighted images and a graduated fluid level appearance. It is likely that the contents are proteinaceous fluid and the findings are consistent with a colloid cyst of the 3rd ventricle.

Diagnosis
Colloid cyst.

Differential diagnosis
For 3rd ventricular lesion:
- Meningioma – these are not usually hyperintense on T1. Meningiomas commonly calcify and show diffuse enhancement with contrast.
- Arachnoid cyst – these are usually isodense on CT and isointense with CSF on MRI.
- Dermoid cyst – usually found in the midline. These contain fat and are therefore usually hypodense on CT and have mixed signal on MRI.
- Ependymoma of the 3rd ventricle – these are very rare. Imaging features include cystic areas, necrosis and calcification and they show diffuse uniform enhancement.
- Basilar tip aneurysm.

Discussion
Colloid cysts account for approximately 0.5–1% of CNS 'tumours'. They usually present in young adults and are more commonly seen in males. The cysts arise from the inferior aspect of the septum pellucidum and extend into the 3rd ventricle. Presentation is usually secondary to obstructed CSF flow at the level of the 3rd ventricle with features of positional headache due to transient obstruction, disturbances of gait, reduced consciousness level and papilloedema. The majority of cysts (80%) contain mucinous material while 20% contain fluid similar to CSF.
- Typical features on CT: well defined thin walled cyst in the 3rd ventricle of slightly increased attenuation with no enhancement (**89b**). Can cause erosion of the sella.
- Typical features on MRI: mucinous material contained within the cyst produces a well defined lesion of increased signal intensity on T1 and T2 weighted images.

Practical tips
- A large basilar tip aneurysm can be mistaken for a colloid cyst on unenhanced CT scan and this requires early identification and treatment.
- Need to assess whether or not there is hydrocephalus – look at the degree of dilatation of the temporal horns of the lateral ventricles and look for depression of the brainstem.

Further management
Although these are benign lesions they can present acutely with CSF flow obstruction resulting in headache, loss of consciousness and death, so a clinical review for evidence of elevated intracranial pressure and neurosurgical review are appropriate.

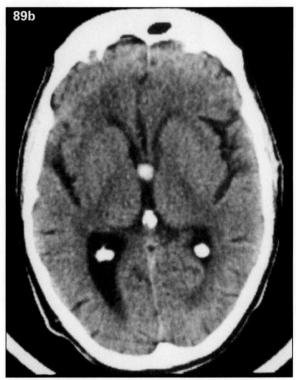

89b Typical CT appearances of a colloid cyst are of a well defined, thin walled cyst in the 3rd ventricle showing increased attenuation without enhancement.

CASE 90

History
A 68-year-old male presented with pyrexia and fits.

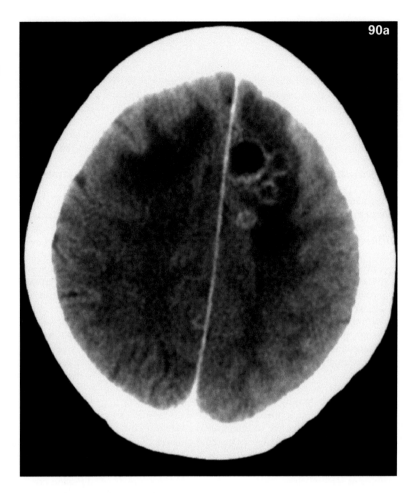

CASE 91

History
A 54-year-old male presented with bilateral visual field blurring.

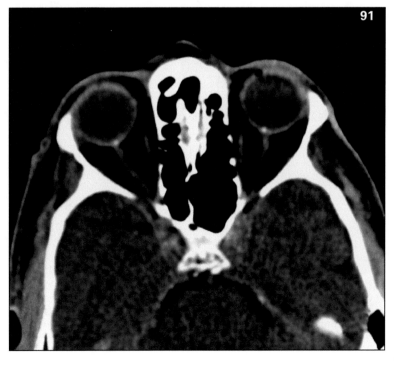

ANSWER 90

Observations (90a)
This contrast enhanced CT image of the brain demonstrates multiple ring enhancing lesions with surrounding vasogenic oedema in the left frontal lobe. Though no lesions are seen in the right hemisphere on this single image, apparent vasogenic oedema in the right frontal lobe suggests that there may be further lesions on this side that are not visualized. The differential diagnosis for ring enhancing lesions is long, but the history of pyrexia points towards cerebral abscesses being most likely.

Diagnosis
Cerebral abscesses.

Differential diagnosis
For ring enhancing CNS lesions:
- Cerebral abscess.
- Metastases.
- Toxoplasmosis.
- Demyelination.
- Lymphoma.
- Multicentric glioma.
- Multiple infarcts.
- Resolving haematomas.

Discussion
Patients who are immunocompromised, on steroids or have diabetes are more susceptible to CNS abscess formation. The most common source of infection is haematogenous spread, though direct spread from infected paranasal sinuses can also occur. Clinical presentation is with headache, seizure and pyrexia. Focal infection preceding abscess formation is cerebritis, and appears as focal low-density change on CT or high T2 signal on MRI (**90b**, **90c**). This proceeds to capsulation/abscess formation at 10–13 days, with the ring enhancement illustrated. When arising via haematogenous spread, the classical location is at the grey–white matter interface, and most commonly in the middle cerebral artery territory. The medial wall is often thinnest (due to better perfusion of the grey matter laterally than the white matter medially) and results in a tendency to rupture on this aspect into the ventricle.

Practical tips
- Differentiation of the above list can be difficult and history is very important to identify immune status, foreign travel and clinical presentation.
- Look for complications of abscesses such as rupture causing meningitis or ventriculitis, radiologically identified by enhancement of these structures or high signal in the sulci on FLAIR MR images.
- Wall enhancement of cerebral abscess is typically uniform – thick, irregular wall enhancement should raise suspicion of cerebral metastases.
- A peripheral ring on the unenhanced scan is more common in metastasis than glioma.
- Assess paranasal sinuses for a primary source of infection and ensure a chest radiograph has been done to look for sources of infection and potential right to left shunts.

Further management
MRI with diffusion weighted imaging can sometimes help differentiate tumour/metastases from abscess. Restricted diffusion of pus in an abscess cavity means that an abscess is high signal on DWI and low signal on ADC (apparent diffusion coefficient) mapping. Opposite findings are seen with necrotic tumours.

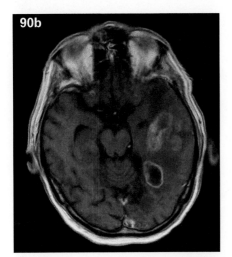
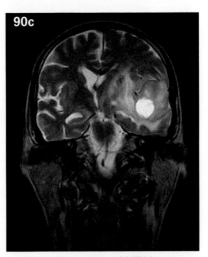

90b, 90c Axial T1 weighted postcontrast and coronal T2 weighted MRI images of left temporal lobe abscesses. The axial T1 postcontrast image shows an enhancing rim with surrounding low signal oedema. The coronal image shows a high signal abscess with significant high signal surrounding oedema causing a moderate degree of mass effect and midline shift.

ANSWER 91

Observations (91)
Axial CT image through the orbits at the level of the optic nerves demonstrates bilateral focal, discrete calcification at the point of union of the retina and optic nerve.

Diagnosis
Optic drusen.

Differential diagnosis
For ocular calcification:
- Neoplasic causes:
    - Retinoblastoma (most common cause, accounting for >50% of cases).
    - Astrocytic hamartoma.
    - Choroidal osteoma.
- Infection:
    - Toxoplasmosis.
    - Rubella.
    - Cytomegalovirus (CMV).
    - Herpes simplex.
- Other:
    - Optic drusen.
    - Phthisis bulbi.
    - Retinal detachment.
    - Retinopathy of prematurity.
    - Hypercalcaemic states – hyperparathyroidism, sarcoidosis, chronic renal failure.

Discussion
Optic drusen are focal accumulations of hyaline material in the region of the optic nerve head, which commonly calcify. Aetiology is thought to be either a developmental abnormality or a degenerative process and it is histopathologically separate from retinal drusen deposits that can be a normal finding or associated with age related macular degeneration. Clinically, patients are usually asymptomatic but can present with reduced visual acuity, migraine-like headaches and pseudopapilloedema. Diagnosis is made by the absence of adverse imaging features such as abnormal enhancement, optic nerve thickening, mass effect or posterior globe solid lesions. Ocular ultrasound can be particularly useful in evaluating, and confirming this is not actually papilloedema. Optic disk haemorrhage is a very rare complication. The majority of cases (75%) are bilateral.

Practical tips
- Bilateral calcification does not necessarily suggest a benign disease process. The nonheritable form of retinoblastoma (66%) presents at ~24 months with usually unilateral disease; but the heritable form (33%) presents at ~12 months with often (66%) bilateral disease.

Further management
Ophthalmological assessment is required to confirm the diagnosis and check visual fields and acuity.

CASE 92

History
A young adult male presented with headaches and paralysis of upward gaze.

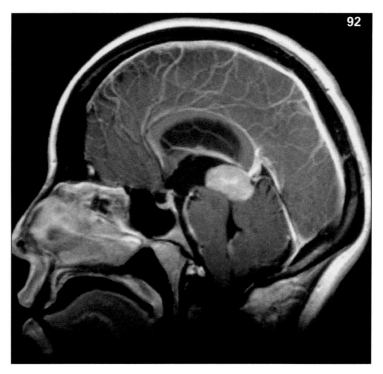

ANSWER 92

Observations (92)
This midline sagittal T1 post-contrast MR image demonstrates a large, slightly lobulated but well defined mass in the pineal region. The mass enhances homogeneously, compresses the superior colliculus and causes dilatation of the 3rd ventricle. The most likely diagnosis is a pineal germinoma causing Parinaud's syndrome and obstructive hydrocephalus.

Diagnosis
Pineal germinoma.

Differential diagnosis
Of pineal region masses:
- Germ cell tumours (>50%):
  - Germinoma.
  - Teratoma – extremely heterogeneous mass. Occurs in young children.
  - Choriocarcinoma.
  - Embryonal cell tumour.

- Pineal parenchymal tumours (25%):
  - Pineocytoma – well demarcated, calcified, slow growing tumour in middle aged adults.
  - Pineoblastoma – similar to medulloblastoma. Affects young children. Enhances avidly and is not usually well circumscribed.

- Others:
  - Meningioma.
  - Epidermoid or dermoid.
  - Arachnoid cyst – CSF density/signal.
  - Pineal cyst – common; fluid density or signal though contents can be proteinaceous on MRI.
  - Lipoma.

Discussion
The pineal gland is a midline structure situated behind the 3rd ventricle and responsible for biorhythm. It is calcified in most people over the age of 15 years and in almost all elderly. Germ cell tumours are the most common tumours of the pineal region, accounting for over 50% of all pineal masses. The most common subtype is germinoma, which is histologically similar to testicular seminoma. Pineal germinomas are well defined midline masses that are much more common in males than females. They are normally seen in children and young adults. The lesion enhances avidly. Due to the anatomical location of the pineal gland these lesions compress the aqueduct of Sylvius producing hydrocephalus. The superior colliculus of the brainstem may also be compressed producing Parinaud's syndrome: paralysis of upward gaze. Less common germ cell tumours of the pineal gland include teratomas, which are mostly seen in young children. Choriocarcinomas and embryonal cell tumours are even less common and are highly malignant.

Practical tips
- The pineal region is in the midline and masses in this region may compress the aqueduct of Sylvius, so always look for associated hydrocephalus.
- When the normal calcification in the pineal gland exceeds 1 cm in diameter a pathological pineal process should be suspected.
- Calcification in germinoma when present is central, in pineoblastoma peripheral.
- In young children think of teratoma (which are very heterogeneous masses), pineoblastoma and a vein of Galen aneurysm.
- In young adults, the most common solid lesion is a germinoma.

Further management
Surgery is difficult due to the central location in the brain. The main role for surgery is in obtaining a biopsy and possibly debulking of tumour to relieve obstructive symptoms. However, germinomas are extremely radiosensitive and therefore radiotherapy is the mainstay of treatment.

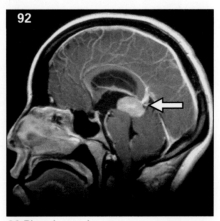

92 Pineal germinoma.

CASE 93

History
A 35-year-old male patient presented with headache.

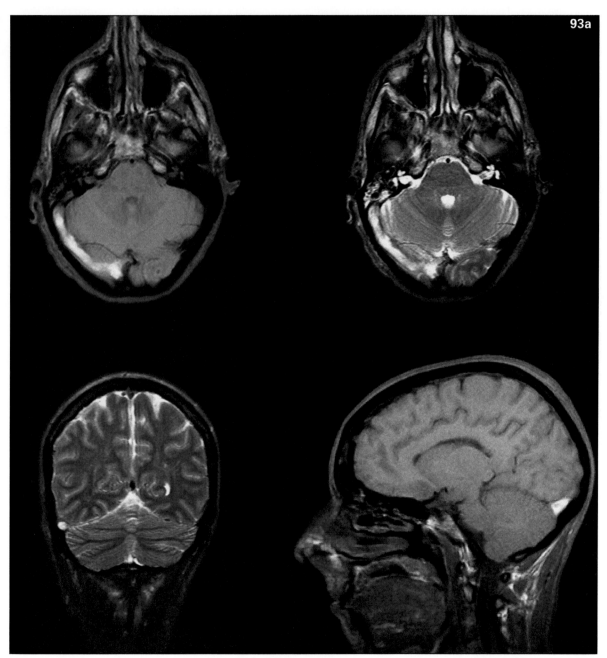

93a PD and T2 weighted axial (top), T2 weighted coronal and T1 weighted sagittal (bottom) images.

Answer 93 — CNS, Head and Neck Imaging

ANSWER 93

Observations (93a)
Selected MR images of the brain demonstrate hyperintensity in the right transverse sinus on the T1 and T2 weighted images with an absence of the normal venous sinus flow voids. There is high-signal abnormality seen within the right mastoid air cells on T2 weighted images, which is intermediate signal on T1 imaging – this is likely to indicate infection/inflammatory change. Appearances are consistent with a diagnosis of venous sinus thrombosis secondary to mastoiditis. No intracerebral/cerebellar haemorrhage or infarct is demonstrated on these images.

Diagnosis
Venous sinus thrombosis.

Discussion
There are a variety of underlying causes of venous sinus thrombosis, which include trauma, infection, idiopathic and hypercoagulable states, i.e. oral contraceptive pill, antiphospholipid syndrome, paraneoplastic tumour syndromes, antithrombin III deficiency. Presenting symptoms can often be very nonspecific, meaning that diagnosis is often only made radiologically. Symptoms include headache, nausea, vomiting and drowsiness. The superior sagittal sinus is most commonly affected, followed by transverse and sigmoid sinuses.

Radiological appearances are:
- Uncontrasted CT may show a hyperdense venous sinus due to thrombus (Figure **93b** shows a thrombosed superior sagittal sinus). Contrast enhanced CT shows a filling defect within the triangular lumen outlined by a small rim of contrast – the 'empty delta' sign.
- MRI demonstrates an absence of flow void within the venous sinus, with local effects of oedema, subcortical infarction, sulcal effacement and haemorrhage.
  - In the acute phase, thrombus can appear as isointense on T1 weighted imaging and hypointense on T2 weighted imaging. This hypointensity on T2 can sometimes be mistaken for flow void and therefore phase-contrast MRA, which shows flow, is better at identification.
  - In a chronic thrombosis, the venous sinus appears hyperintense on T1 and T2 weighted images due to extracellular methaemoglobin.
- Venous infarcts are identifiable by their nonconformity with arterial territories and haemorrhagic tendency. Figure **93b** demonstrates a venous infarct that does not conform to the anatomical area supplied by the vessels of posterior circulation.

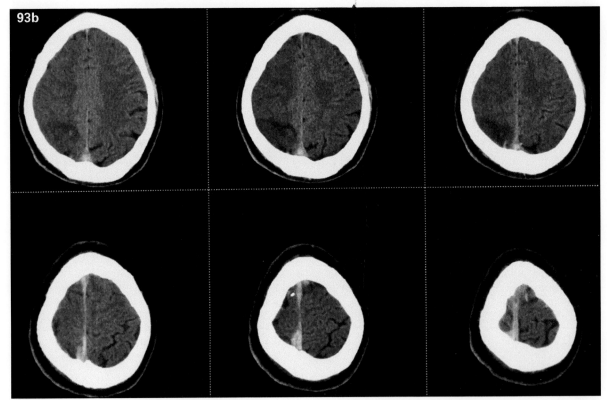

93b Selected axial CT images demonstrate a focal area of low attenuation involving grey and white matter with appearances consistent with an infarct. The distribution, however, does not conform to arterial territories since this represents a venous infarct.

Practical tips
- Venous sinus thrombosis can present in a very nonspecific manner and has significant morbidity and mortality untreated. When assessing scans of acutely 'neurologically unwell' patients, always keep it in mind and check the scan carefully. Similarly, beware of dismissing infarcts that show features as described above without questioning the possibility of an underlying venous sinus thrombosis.
- The appearances of thrombus on MRI are complex and vary with the age of thrombus. Moreover, patent venous sinuses can show absence of flow void when imaged in certain planes. Making the diagnosis of venous sinus thrombosis from MRI can therefore be complicated. Modern multidetector CT scanners have sufficient speed and spatial resolution to image the venous sinuses and provide an alternative that can be easier to interpret, thrombus appearing as a filling defect in the lumen of the otherwise enhanced venous sinus. Figure **93c** is a coronal reformat of a CT venogram showing thrombus in the left transverse sinus as an 'empty delta' sign.

Further management
Usual treatment involves anticoagulation.

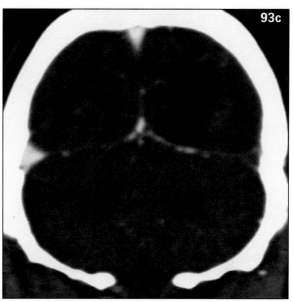

93c Coronal reformat CT image shows thrombus in the left transverse sinus.

CASE 94

History
A 57-year-old male presented with tinnitus and hearing loss.

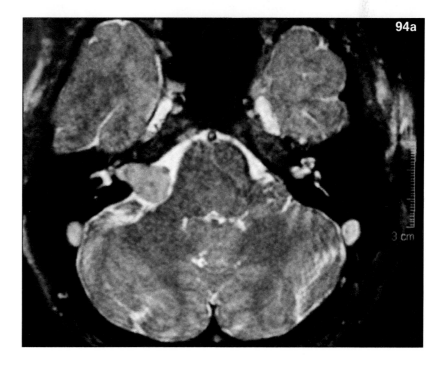

ANSWER 94

Observations (94a)
Single T2 weighted MR image of the brain at the level of the internal auditory meatus. There is a large, well defined soft tissue mass lesion in the right cerebellopontine (CP) angle with extension into the internal auditory canal. Widening of the canal is seen. No dural tail is evident. Acoustic neuroma is most likely.

Diagnosis
Acoustic neuroma.

Differential diagnosis
Of CP angle lesions:
- Acoustic neuroma accounts for 75% of CP angle masses.
- Meningioma is the most likely differential at 10% (94b). Lesions are extra-axial and tend to be extracanalicular and commonly calcify. Dural tails are seen in up to 60% of tumours on MRI.
- Epidermoid – 5% of CP angle lesions.
- Arachnoid cyst.
- Posterior circulation aneurysm.
- Metastases.

Discussion
Acoustic neuromas are the most common tumours of the CP angle and internal auditory canal. They typically arise from the vestibular division of the 8th nerve and should perhaps be more accurately termed vestibular schwannomas. These lesions present in the 4th–7th decades and are more frequently seen in females. Presentation occurs at a younger age in patients with type 2 neurofibromatosis, with presentation in the 2nd decade. Bilateral acoustic neuromas are virtually pathognomonic of neurofibromatosis type 2, while solitary tumours are seen in up to 25% of cases. Presentation is with symptoms of sensorineural hearing loss, tinnitus, vertigo and dizziness.

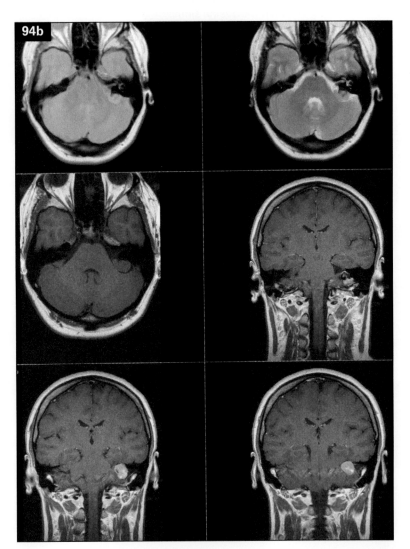

94b Axial PD, T2 and T1 weighted images with three post-contrast coronal images demonstrate a well defined, extracanalicular, uniformly enhancing lesion in the left CP angle representing a meningioma.

Answer 94

Imaging features:
- 80% arise *in* the internal auditory canal (IAC).
- 80% cause enlargement/erosion of the IAC.
- Lesions extend into the CP angle.
- Larger tumours (>3 cm) have central areas of necrosis and haemorrhage.
- Calcification is not a feature.
- On CT lesions are usually isodense with uniform enhancement.
- On MRI, lesions are low signal on T1, high signal on T2 and show uniform enhancement with gadolinium.

Practical tips
- Distinguishing the main CP angle masses from each other:
  - Both acoustic neuroma and meningioma show uniform enhancement so this is unhelpful.
  - Acoustic neuroma – expands the IAC, causing flaring of the porus acousticus. May be bright on T2 unlike meningioma. Makes an acute angle with petrous bone.
  - Meningioma – dural tail of enhancement, obtuse angle with petrous bone. Relatively little tissue in the IAC compared to acoustic neuroma.
  - Epidermoid vs arachnoid cyst – both appear to follow the density and signal of CSF on CT and T1 and T2 weighted MRI. However, the epidermoid shows increased signal on PD, FLAIR and diffusion weighted MRI.

- Detection of acoustic neuroma is largely done with MRI when possible – thin section T2 weighted sequences are used in the main, with contrast reserved for difficult cases. When contraindicated, use contrast enhanced CT.
- A subgroup of acoustic neuroma show relatively rapid growth that necessitates treatment while others show extremely slow growth and can be managed more conservatively. Following initial diagnosis, a repeat scan after approximately 6 months may help identify the subgroup that is going to grow rapidly and those that can be managed more conservatively.
- Neurofibromatosis type 2: bilateral acoustic neuroma is a recognized diagnostic criterion for this condition, also known as the MISME syndrome (multiple inherited schwannoma, meningioma and ependymoma). In the 'real world' most acoustic neuromas are unrelated to neurofibromatosis type 2. However, in exam vivas (and certainly when bilateral), have a high index of suspicion for the meningioma elsewhere on the scan.

Further management
Therapeutic options involve surgical excision, stereotactic radiation and conservative management. Which one depends on the particular circumstances of each patient, but also whether the tumour is fast growing or not. A repeat scan a few months after the first can help identify the group of faster growing lesions that require a more aggressive approach.

CASE 95

History
A 30-year-old male: orthopantomogram (OPG) done for dental assessment.

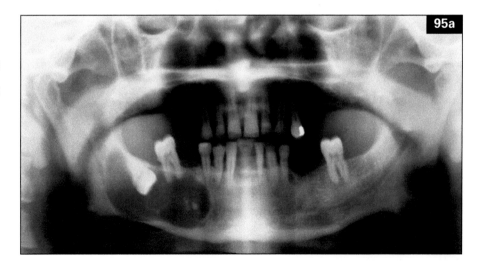

ANSWER 95

Observations (95a)
The OPG shows multiple missing teeth in the upper jaw and to a lesser extent the lower jaw too. In the right body of the mandible, there is a well circumscribed, thin walled, unilocular lucency measuring several centimetres in diameter. There is no associated bony destruction. The cyst is associated with the crown of an unerupted molar and appearances are consistent with a dentigerous cyst.

Diagnosis
Dentigerous cyst.

Differential diagnosis
Of cystic mandibular lesion:
- Periapical/radicular cyst.
- Dentigerous cyst.
- Odontogenic keratocyst.
- Ameloblastoma.
- Aneurysmal bone cyst.
- Simple bone cyst.
- Metastasis/myeloma.
- Brown tumour.
- Fibrous dysplasia.
- Many other 'small print' lesions – nasopalatine cyst, Pindborg's tumour, Stafne's bone cyst, median mandibular cyst, etc.

Discussion
Dentigerous cysts arise from the crown of an unerupted tooth. The typically affected age group is 10–30 years, with a male predominance. The cysts are slow growing and usually an incidental finding, but occasionally cause pain, swelling or become secondarily infected. The majority occur in the posterior mandible. They are variable in size, and have a thin walled, unilocular appearance. *The association with an unerupted crown is the key to diagnosis.*

The differential diagnosis of cystic lesions of the mandible is very long but most of the causes are so rare that they can be dismissed most of the time. The emphasis will consequently be on common lesions and important rare ones. It is best to assess lesions according to visible association with dentition, unilocular vs multilocular nature and age of the patient. Note that although not visibly dentition related, lesions such as ameloblastoma and odontogenic keratocyst do arise from dental-related tissue.

Dentition-associated cysts:
- Periapical/radicular cyst – secondary to pulp necrosis of a carious tooth. *Unilocular cyst associated with the root of a tooth.* Can be destructive when large, but not expansile. Most common lesion seen. Likely to be painful.
- Dentigerous cyst – *unilocular cyst associated with the crown of an unerupted tooth.*

No visible association with teeth:
- Ameloblastoma/adamantinoma – rare, locally aggressive (but non-metastasizing) lytic tumour that is slow growing and often painless. This is *an expansile, multiloculated cyst with 'bubbly' appearance* (though 20% unilocular). Can be associated with unerupted molar tooth. Thinned cortex and no matrix mineralization. Contrast enhanced CT/MRI may show enhancement of soft tissue elements and possibly an enhancing mural nodule. Five times more common in mandible than maxilla. Typical age group *30–50 years.* Figure **95b** is an OPG in an adult patient with ameloblastoma showing a lytic expansile lesion of the right side of the mandible with areas of internal septation producing a 'soap bubble' appearance. The lesion is locally aggressive and has destroyed several right lower teeth roots.
- Odontogenic keratocyst (OKC) – *multiloculated or unilocular cyst often near site of 3rd lower molar; expansile* extending along the mandible; sclerotic rim; may displace teeth. Same age and sex group as dentigerous cyst; 50% are symptomatic with swelling, growth rate is rapid and recurrence rate after curettage is high. Multiple OKCs are a feature of Gorlin–Goltz (basal cell naevus) syndrome, an autosomal dominant condition characterized by multiple cutaneous basal cell carcinomas.
- Aneurysmal bone cyst (ABC) – *multilocular cyst with 'soap bubble' appearance in posterior mandible.* Appearances are therefore very similar to ameloblastoma but ABC occurs primarily in those under 20 years of age.
- Fibrous dysplasia – 'ground glass' *matrix with calcification.*
- Metastases and myeloma – don't forget these in the older patient.

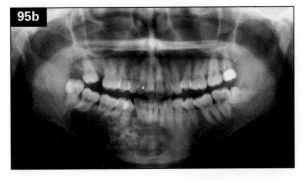

95b OPG shows large lytic ameloblastoma in the right mandible with areas of internal septation producing a 'soap bubble' appearance.

Answer 95

Practical tips
The cystic mandibular lesion – ask yourself:
- Any relation to tooth?
- Multilocular or unilocular?
- Age of patient?

Multilocular cyst:
- <30 years = ABC or OKC.
- Multiple = OKC with Gorlin syndrome.
- >30 years = ameloblastoma.
- 'Ground glass' contents – OKC or fibrous dysplasia (but matrix calcification in the latter).

Unilocular cyst with dental association:
- Associated with tooth apex and pain = periapical cyst.
- Associated with unerupted tooth = dentigerous cyst (<30 years and associated with crown) or ameloblastoma (>30 years).

Unilocular cyst with no dental association:
- <30 years = OKC, simple bone cyst.
- >40 years = ameloblastoma, metastases or myeloma.

If brown tumour is suspected look for other signs of hyperparathyroidism such as resorption of the lamina dura of the teeth producing 'floating teeth' and generalized demineralization of the mandible and maxilla.

Further management
Though often asymptomatic, dentigerous cyst can cause pain and swelling and may predispose to pathological fracture. Surgical excision (including the unerupted tooth) may therefore be undertaken.

Further reading
Scholl R, Kellett H, Neumann D, Lurie A (1999). Cysts and cystic lesions of the mandible: clinical and radiologic-histopathologic review. *RadioGraphics* **19**: 1107–1124.

CASE 96

History
A 30-year-old patient presented with headaches and suspected sinusitis.

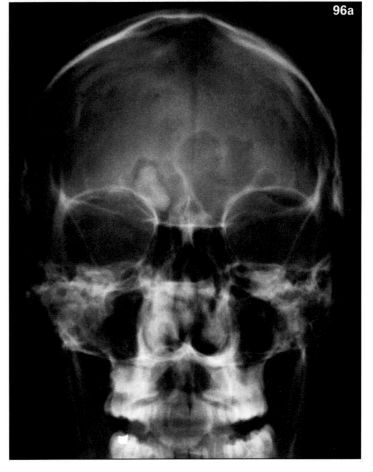

ANSWER 96

Observations (96a)
This occipitomental radiograph shows a large calcified lesion in the right frontal sinus. The lesion has very well defined margins and a slightly lower density centre. No fluid is seen within the sinus and there is no evidence of local bony destruction. The appearances are those of a frontal sinus 'ivory osteoma'.

Diagnosis
Ivory osteoma.

Discussion
Osteomas are benign tumours of membranous bone. These are round, well defined lesions of bony density that are usually found incidentally. They are commonly found in the paranasal sinuses, particularly the frontal and ethmoid sinuses. Other common sites include the calvarium and mandible. A CT coronal reconstruction (**96b**) in the same patient confirms that the lesion lies within the right frontal sinus.

Practical tips
- When multiple osteomas are seen always consider Gardner's syndrome and investigate the family history and for the presence of colonic polyposis.
- Paranasal sinus osteomas may cause local pressure erosion. A coronal CT reconstruction (**96c**) demonstrates a left ethmoid sinus osteoma eroding the lamina papyracea and extending into the left orbit. Background sinus inflammatory changes are present.

Further management
Incidental finding requiring no further management.

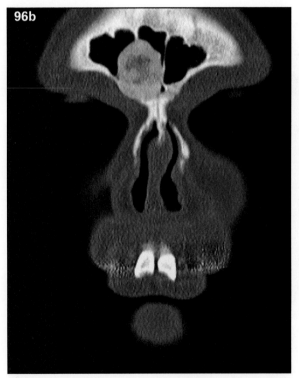

96b Coronal CT reconstruction demonstrating a right frontal sinus osteoma.

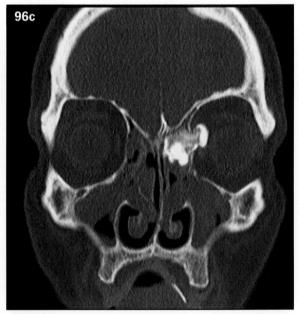

96c Coronal CT reconstruction showing an osteoma of the left ethmoid sinus extending into the left orbit.

CASE 97

History
A 39-year-old female presented with transient visual loss; and an episode of ataxia 6 months ago.

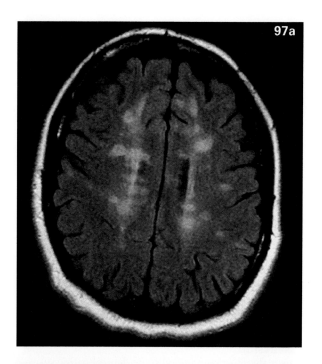

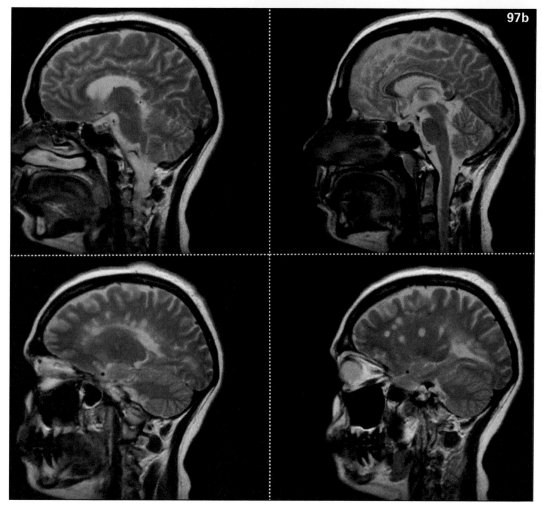

Answer 97

Observations (97a, 97b)
Selected MR images of the brain – FLAIR axial and T2 weighted sagittal – are presented. These scans show multiple focal ovoid signal abnormalities in the periventricular white matter, which are orientated perpendicular to the long axis of the ventricles. Further lesions involve the corpus callosum. No associated oedema. No evidence of hydrocephalus. Given the clinical details, it is likely that the patient has multiple sclerosis and is currently experiencing optic neuritis.

Diagnosis
Multiple sclerosis (MS).

Differential diagnosis
Of white matter lesions on MRI:
- Acute disseminated encephalomyelitis (ADEM).
- Vasculitis.
- Ischaemic disease (97c).
- Migraine.
- Neurosarcoid.

Discussion
This is the most common chronic demyelinating disease and is characterized by multiple lesions spread in time and space. Typically, it has a remitting/relapsing course. The onset of symptoms is usually in the 3rd–4th decades and there is a slightly increased predominance in females. Increased prevalence is noted in areas of temperate climate. Clinical presentation is with focal neurological signs, commonly including optic neuritis.

Imaging features are:
- Lesions are classically periventricular in location, oval in shape, with their long axis perpendicular to the lateral ventricle walls – 'Dawson's fingers'.
- Common locations for plaques include periventricular white matter, corpus callosum, internal capsule, centrum semiovale, optic nerve/tracts, cerebellum. Lesions on the inferior aspect of the corpus callosum are characteristic.
- Acute lesions can have mild surrounding oedema and can enhance with contrast.
- Chronic lesions have no mass effect/oedema and don't enhance.
- Lesions are hyperintense on T2, hypo/isointense on T1.

Multiple sclerosis is also the most common demyelinating process affecting the spine – the cervical spine being most frequently affected. It is characterized by plaques orientated along the axis of the spinal cord.

Further clinical evaluation involves:
- Lumbar puncture with CSF analysis for oligoclonal bands.
- Electrophysiological studies.

Practical tips
- Focal white matter signal abnormalities in cerebral white matter (sometimes referred to as unidentified bright objects – UBOs) are common incidental findings on MRI with several aetiologies. Making a specific diagnosis of demyelination is often not possible from imaging alone though multiple lesions involving the corpus callosum are characteristic for MS. Coexisting lesions in the brainstem, cerebellum and spinal cord also increase specificity.
- Be wary of making a conclusive diagnosis of MS from MRI unless features are highly specific and there is a supporting history – the consequences for the patient are significant. Often, one can only offer a differential diagnosis for 'UBOs' that includes MS.

Further management
MRI of the spinal cord is frequently also undertaken to complete assessment. Though MRI findings may be highly suggestive, careful neurological assessment is required to correlate the imaging findings with clinical and laboratory findings before making the diagnosis.

Further reading
Runge VM, Price AC, Kirshner HS, *et al.* (1986). The evaluation of multiple sclerosis by magnetic resonance imaging. *RadioGraphics* **6**: 203–212.

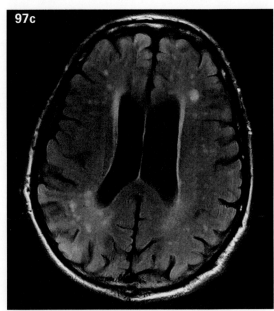

97c Single axial MRI FLAIR image shows periventricular high signal with scattered high signal white matter foci. Appearances are of age-related small vessel disease.

CASE 98

History
A 51-year-old male presented with chronic headaches.

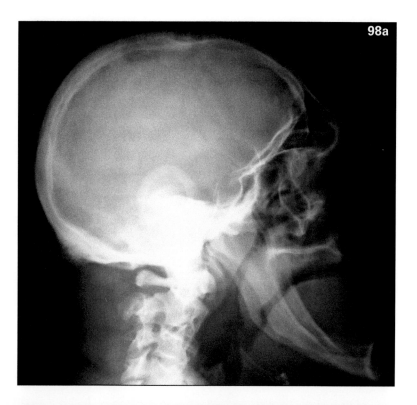

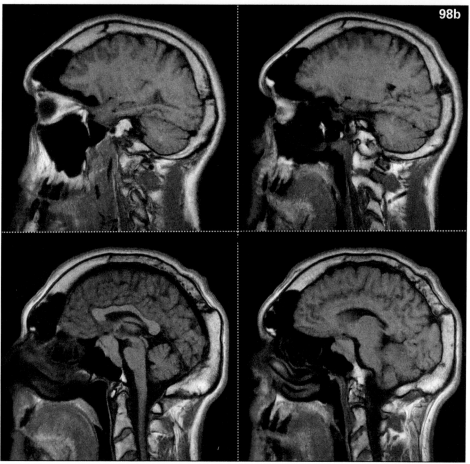

ANSWER 98

Observations (98a, 98b)
This lateral image of the skull (**98a**) shows elongation of the jaw (prognathism), frontal bossing, enlargement of the frontal sinuses and thickening of the calvaria. There is marked enlargement of the pituitary fossa with evidence of expansion but no erosion.

Selected sagittal T1 weighted images (**98b**) of the brain confirm the plain film findings of enlargement of the frontal sinuses, frontal bossing and thickening of the calvaria. There is a mass lesion within the pituitary fossa with appearances consistent with pituitary macroadenoma. Enlargement of the tongue is also noted.

Diagnosis
Acromegaly.

Discussion
Excess growth hormone secretion by the anterior lobe of the pituitary gland results in a variety of musculoskeletal abnormalities.

Plain radiographic image findings are:
- Enlargement of the sella (**98c**).
- Mandibular enlargement.
- Increase in size of the frontal sinuses with prominence of the supraorbital ridge.
- Enlarged hands with spade-like appearances of the terminal phalanges (**98d**).
- Thickening of the calvaria.
- Dural ectasia and posterior vertebral body scalloping.
- Increased heel pad thickness(>25 mm) (**98e**).
- Premature osteoarthritis (OA).

Practical tips
Normal dimensions of the pituitary fossa on lateral skull films are a length of <15 mm and height of <12 mm.

Further management
Management of this condition is both medical (somatostatin/bromocriptine) and surgical (transsphenoidal hypophysectomy).

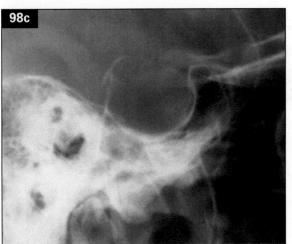

98c Magnified image from plain skull radiograph shows enlargement of the sella.

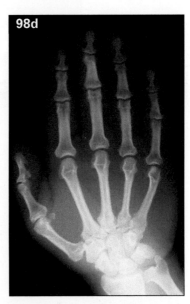

98d Radiograph of the hand shows marked soft tissue enlargement giving it a spade-like appearance. In addition there is widening of the terminal tufts.

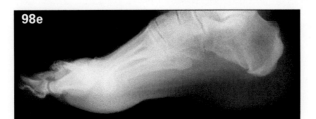

98e Soft tissue lateral radiograph demonstrates thickening of the heel pad, which measures >25 mm in thickness.

CASE 99

History
A 22-year-old female presented with visual field defects.

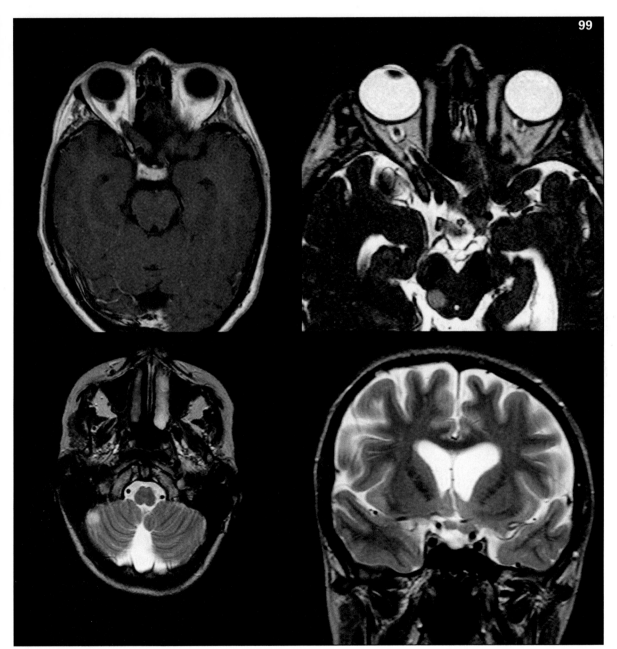

99 T1 weighted axial (top left), thin section T2 weighted axial orbits (top right), axial and coronal T2 weighted (bottom) MR images.

ANSWER 99

Observations (99)
The axial images of the orbit show fusiform enlargement of the posterior right optic nerve, which also involves both sides of the optic chiasm. The coronal scan confirms thickening of the posterior aspect of both optic nerves. Axial T2 weighted images also show a round focus of high signal in the right cerebellar hemisphere and a second lesion in the posterior aspect of right midbrain that produces convexity to the margins of the cerebral peduncle. The appearances are likely to indicate optic nerve glioma involving the chiasm and both optic nerves along with hamartomas in the cerebellum and midbrain due to neurofibromatosis type 1. No cutaneous neurofibromas are seen on these images.

Diagnosis
Optic chiasm/nerve glioma due to neurofibromatosis type 1 (NF1).

Differential diagnosis
For optic nerve thickening:
- Optic nerve glioma – 80% under 20 years, variable enhancement, calcification rare, buckling of nerve, often asymptomatic.
- Meningioma of optic nerve – middle aged women, 'tramtrack' enhancement, calcification in 20–50%, straight nerve, visual impairment early.
- Sarcoidosis.
- Multiple sclerosis.
- Lymphoma, leukaemia and metastatic disease.
- Intracranial hypertension – enlarges the perineural CSF space.

Discussion
Optic nerve glioma typically presents in childhood, only 20% manifesting beyond the age of 20. Relatively slow growing and benign in children, lesions presenting in adults often show more rapid malignant growth with intracranial spread. Though often asymptomatic, presentation can be with visual loss and strabismus. Bilateral tumours herald NF1. The tumour causes fusiform or tubular enlargement of the optic nerve sheath complex and shows variable enhancement with IV contrast. The majority of lesions occurring in the orbital portion of the nerve do not extend intracranially. Some optic nerve gliomas have extensive associated thickening of the surrounding meninges, termed arachnoidal hyperplasia, which is often seen in patients with NF – on T2W MRI, this is seen as a central low-signal tumour surrounded by a higher-signal rim that can look like a dilated perineural CSF space.

Approximately 25% of patients with optic glioma have NF1 and it is one of the diagnostic criteria listed for the condition, of which two or more are required: six or more 'café-au-lait' patches; two or more Lisch nodules; two or more neurofibromas or one plexiform neurofibroma; axillary freckling; optic glioma; bone dysplasia or pseudarthrosis; first degree relative with NF1. In this case, the coexisting lesions in the cerebellum and midbrain lead one to the overall diagnosis of NF1. These high T2 signal foci are seen in the brainstem, basal ganglia, cerebral peduncles, cerebellum and the supratentorial white matter. They are usually thought of as representing hamartomas and often decrease in size with age. NF1 also predisposes to astrocytoma in the cerebrum, brainstem and cerebellum and telling the difference may be difficult. If a lesion enlarges over time or shows enhancement, then the possibility of astrocytoma must be considered. Prominent choroid plexus calcification and hydrocephalus due to aqueduct stenosis are other intracranial features.

NF1 is sporadic in 50% and autosomal dominant in 50% (chromosome 17).

Practical tips
- T1 weighted post-contrast scans of the orbit should be performed with fat suppression in view of the adjacent orbital fat.
- Meningioma is the main differential diagnosis for optic nerve thickening and the features listed above may help distinguish the two.
- Whenever NF1 enters the differential for any radiological study, always check for evidence of cutaneous nodules that 'clinch the diagnosis'.

Further management
Treatment depends on the size of tumour along with the age and general condition of the patient. Options include surgery, radiotherapy and chemotherapy.

CASE 100

History 1
A 73-year-old male presented with acute onset of dysphagia, right sided Horner's syndrome and ataxia, with left sided sensory disturbance.

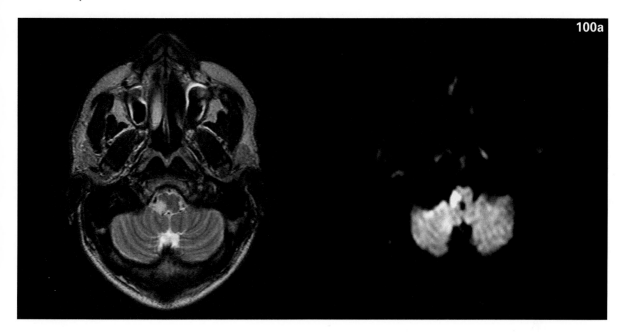

History 2
A 69-year-old female with diabetes and hypertension presented with sudden onset right oculomotor palsy and left sided ataxia and tremor.

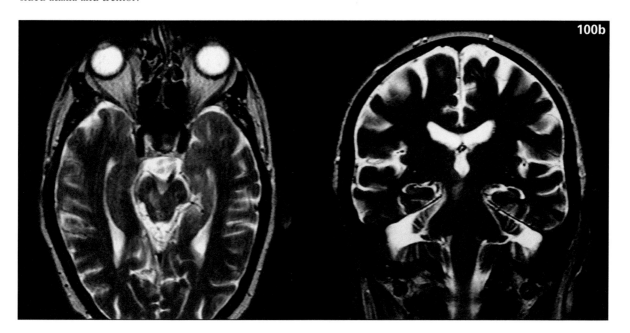

ANSWER 100

Observations 1 (100a)
Axial T2 weighted image demonstrates high signal in the lateral aspect of right medulla. This is bright on the DWI indicating restricted water molecule diffusion probably from cell swelling due to acute infarction. Together with the clinical details, findings are consistent with lateral medullary syndrome due to infarction in the territory of the right posterior inferior cerebellar artery (PICA).

Observations 2 (100b)
These axial and coronal T2 weighted images show a focus of increased signal in the right side of the midbrain. There is no associated mass effect and the lesion lies in the region of the red nucleus. The clinical symptoms are compatible with an infarct affecting the red nucleus and causing Claude's syndrome.

Diagnosis 1
Right PICA infarction (Wallenberg's syndrome).

Diagnosis 2
Right midbrain infarction affecting the red nucleus (Claude's syndrome).

Discussion
There are various specific patterns of brainstem infarction, often having unusual eponyms. Others include Weber's, Nothnagel's, Millard–Gubler and Foville's syndromes.

Wallenberg's syndrome is due to PICA occlusion and presents with ipsilateral ataxia, dysphagia, facial pain and temperature sensory impairment and Horner's syndrome, with contralateral impairment of pain and temperature sensation in the body and limbs. The PICA is the first major intracranial branch of the vertebrobasilar system and supplies the dorsolateral medulla, cerebellar vermis and posterolateral cerebellar hemisphere. It arises from the distal vertebral artery just below the basilar artery origin. As well as thrombosis, infarction can result from dissection of the vertebral artery.

Claude's syndrome is due to a lesion of the red nucleus, of which infarction is one example. The consequences are ipsilateral oculomotor palsy and contralateral tremor and ataxia.

Practical tips
- These are examples of comparatively rare and very specific infarcts but they do make for an interesting test of neuroanatomy understanding!
- DWI depicts reduction in Brownian motion of water molecules. Cytotoxic oedema in acute infarction will produce this and present high signal on the DWI scan. It is very sensitive, depicting infarcts just 30 min or so from onset.
- The DWI image also has inherent T2 weighting (T2 'shine through'), that is, the signal is a combination of T2 weighted and reduced diffusion. As such, it may not distinguish an older infarct (T2 hyperintense) from a recent one (reduced diffusion) as both will appear bright. An alternative depiction that can differentiate acute and nonacute infarcts is the apparent diffusion coefficient (ADC) map. This has no T2 component and shows reduced diffusion (i.e. acute infarct) as low signal. An older infarct that is also bright on DWI by virtue of T2 'shine through' will be bright on ADC.
- Ischaemia is not the only cause of reduced diffusion. Others include seizure, trauma, hypoglycaemia, abscess.

Further management
DWI is more sensitive in the early detection of infarction when compared to CT. However, when thrombolysis is being considered, CT is more than adequate to exclude a haemorrhage alone.

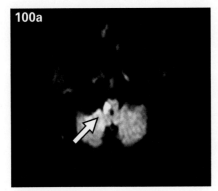

100a High signal in lateral aspect of right medulla.

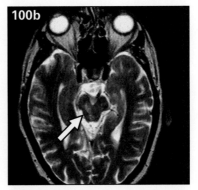

100b Right midbrain high signal.

CASE 101

History
A 32-year-old male presented with poorly controlled epilepsy.

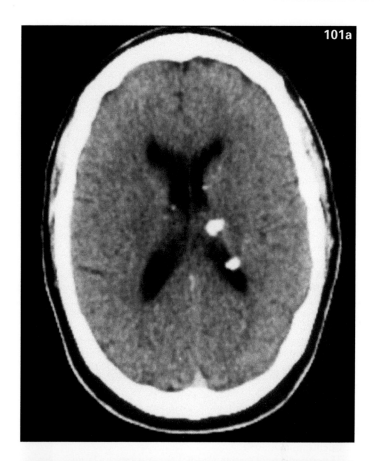

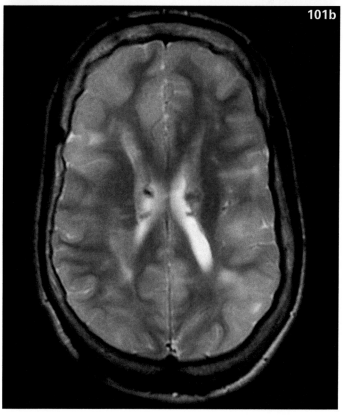

ANSWER 101

Observations (101a, 101b)
The axial CT image of the brain (**101a**) shows several small calcified lesions in the subependymal region of the body of the lateral ventricles. The T2 weighted MR image of the brain (**101b**) confirms several small subependymal nodules with associated low signal representing calcification. These appearances are consistent with subependymal hamartomas. There are abnormal widened gyri in the left parietal lobe and right frontal lobe seen on the MR image, which are likely to indicate cortical hamartomas.

Diagnosis
Tuberous sclerosis.

Discussion
Tuberous sclerosis is an inherited autosomal dominant disorder of the neuroectoderm that is characterized by multisystem abnormalities. The classical triad of features are mental retardation, seizures and adenoma sebaceum.
  CNS features:
- Subependymal hamartomas – most commonly seen along the ventricular surface of the caudate nucleus. Multiple small subependymal lesions which calcify in 80%. Figure **101c** shows another case where nodules have not calcified, but produce a 'wavy' border to the ventricle walls.
- Cortical tubers – appearances are of large widened atypical gyri with reduced attenuation centres on CT. They are usually multiple and can show rim calcification in 50%.
- Heterotopic grey matter islands – these appear as large hypodense focal islands of tissue within the cerebral white matter.
- Giant cell astrocytomas – occur around the foramen of Monro, and can cause hydrocephalus. Malignant potential is low.

Multisystem involvement:
- Ocular – ocular phakomas, optic nerve gliomas.
- Renal – angiomyolipoma, cysts, increased risk of renal cell carcinoma.
- Respiratory – lymphangiomyomatosis-like features with cystic lung disease, spontaneous pneumothoraces and chylothorax.
- Cardiovascular – rhabdomyoma, aortic aneurysms.
- Skin – adenoma sebaceum (red/brown small flat skin lesions distributed symmetrically over nose and cheeks), shagreen patches, ash leaf lesions, subungual fibromas.

Practical tips
- The phakomatoses (neurocutaneous disorders), of which tuberous sclerosis is an example, make great exam cases because of the multitude of radiological signs to 'piece together' – know them well!

- Distinguishing tubers/hamartomas from giant cell astrocytomas: tubers and subependymal hamartomas can show some enhancement on MRI but CT is not usually sensitive enough to show this. Because giant cell astrocytomas show more enhancement, this may be appreciable on CT and should arouse suspicion.

Further management
Tuberous sclerosis has a high mortality with 70% dying before the age of 24 years. A multidisciplinary team approach is required with follow-up imaging involving MRI brain, renal ultrasonography (monitoring angiomyolipomas and looking for renal cell carcinomas) and echocardiography (50% of patients have rhabdomyomas).

Further reading
Altman NR, Purser RK, Post MJ (1988). Tuberous sclerosis: characteristics at CT and MR imaging. *Radiology* **167**: 527–532.

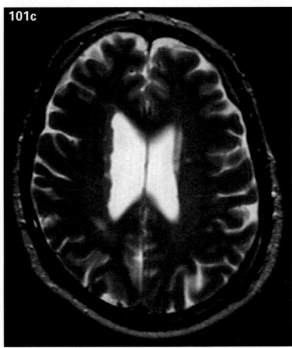

101c Subependymal nodules have not calcified in this case.

CASE 102

History
Adult patient presented with recent onset of seizures.

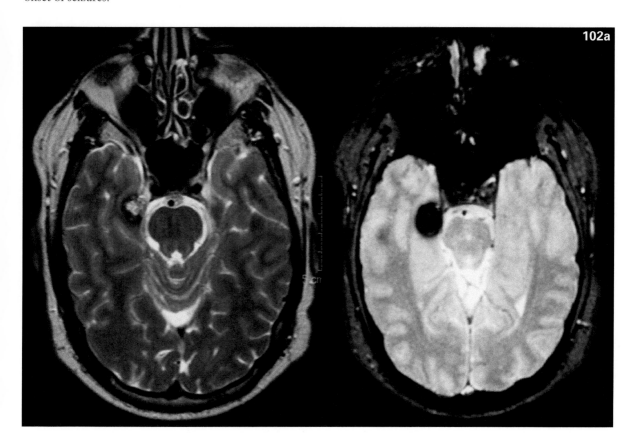

Answer 102

Observations (102a)
Axial T2 (left) and gradient echo T2 (right) images demonstrate a lesion in the medial right temporal lobe with a very low signal rim representing haemosiderin. This is characteristically more prominent on the gradient echo T2 sequence with 'blooming' artefact. The centre of the lesion shows T2 hyperintensity and the overall shape is round. The features are consistent with a cavernoma.

Diagnosis
Cavernoma (cavernous angioma or cavernous malformation).

Discussion
Vascular malformations are a common cause of parenchymal brain haemorrhage and should be excluded when young patients present with spontaneous haemorrhage. They develop from congenitally abnormal vascular connections, which may increase in size with time.

Radiological features of vascular malformations are:
- Arteriovenous malformations (AVMs) are the most common type and are essentially an abnormal collection of arteries connected directly to veins with no intervening capillaries (**102b**). The vast majority are supratentorial. On CT they are of mixed density and may have calcifications. Enhancement is also seen. However, the classical appearance is found on MRI where flow voids with complex flow patterns are seen. Figure **102c** demonstrates an example on an axial T2 weighted image with an AVM in the right frontal lobe producing the characteristic tangle of flow voids.
- Cavernous malformations (cavernomas) are thin walled sinusoidal vessels representing congenital hamartomas. Unlike other vascular malformations, there is no brain parenchyma between the vascular spaces. The appearances on CT are rather nonspecific but MRI shows very characteristic features, as illustrated. The central high signal represents methaemoglobin and the outer low signal rim haemosiderin. They present with focal seizures or small parenchymal haemorrhages.
- Venous angiomas are usually asymptomatic and are anomalous veins that drain the normal brain. Classically, an enhancing stellate venous malformation is seen extending to the ventricular or cortical surface.

Practical tips
- AVMs typically have a tangle of low-signal flow voids on MRI best seen on T2 and PD weighted imaging.
- 10% of AVMs develop an associated aneurysm so always look for this.
- Gradient echo T2 is an excellent technique for identifying haemosiderin on MRI, which is often seen in vascular malformations.

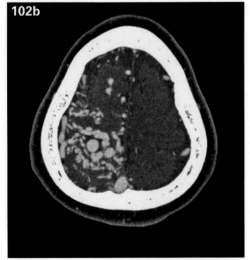

102b Large right cerebral AVM demonstrated on a CT cerebral angiogram.

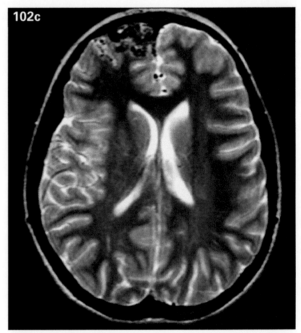

102c Axial T2 MRI demonstrates right frontal AVM with characteristic flow voids.

Answer 102

- Haemosiderin will also be seen in an old haemorrhage not necessarily involving an underlying vascular malformation. Figure **102d** demonstrates an old haemorrhage in the left internal capsule/thalamus and it would be easy to confuse this with cavernoma from the axial image. However, an old haemorrhage collapses to form a slit-like cavity unlike the rounded shape of cavernoma, and the coronal scan illustrates this difference. Note also the local volume loss due to gliosis resulting in some enlargement of the adjacent left lateral ventricle.

Further management
Often these are asymptomatic and can be monitored with imaging to assess change in growth. There is, however, an up to 2% risk of bleeding and surgery/stereotactic radiosurgery are treatment options.

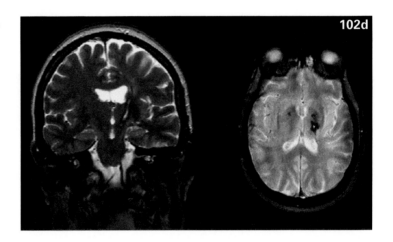

102d Coronal T2 and axial gradient echo T2 MRI demonstrating old haemorrhage in left internal capsule.

CASE 103

History
A 65-year-old male presented with swelling and impaired vision of the left eye.

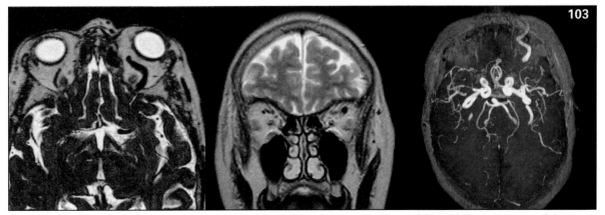

103 Axial and coronal T2 weighted scans of orbits (left/middle) and a 'time of flight' MR angiogram of the intracranial circulation (right).

ANSWER 103

Observations (103)
T2 weighted images demonstrate dilatation of the left superior ophthalmic vein with presence of flow void and no focal compressive mass lesion. The 'time of flight' MRA demonstrates normal arterial intracranial anatomy with signal in the dilated left ophthalmic vein indicating fast flow. The findings are in keeping with a left caroticocavernous fistula.

Diagnosis
Caroticocavernous fistula.

Differential diagnosis
For superior ophthalmic vein distension:
- Cavernous sinus thrombosis.
- Superior ophthalmic vein thrombosis.
- Pseudotumour.
- Graves' disease.
- Obstructive orbital mass.

Discussion
Fistulous communication between the internal carotid artery and the cavernous sinus can arise secondary to head trauma or rupture of an internal carotid artery aneurysm. The condition often occurs spontaneously, however, due to atherosclerosis. In addition, fistulae can occur with dural branches of the external carotid artery. Orbital bruit is found in ~50% of patients due to turbulent arterial blood flow. The increased arterial pressure in the venous system and orbital vein congestion result in the symptoms of:
- Pulsatile proptosis.
- Chemosis.
- Reduced visual acuity due to impaired retinal perfusion – severe/rapid visual loss requires angiographic investigation and fistula closure as an emergency to preserve function.
- Cranial nerve palsies – most commonly 6th and 3rd nerves. This is thought to be due to either impaired venous drainage of the nerve or direct compression of nerves by distended veins.
- Contralateral symptoms are seen in ~10% due to the presence of connections between the two cavernous sinuses.

Imaging features on MRI are:
- Dilated superior ophthalmic vein with flow void.
- Enlargement of the cavernous sinus.
- Swelling of the extraocular muscles, which can result in limited eye movements.

Angiography shows early opacification of the superior ophthalmic vein when contrast is injected into internal carotid artery. Early opacification of the veins communicating with cavernous sinus may also be noted.

Practical tips
- Early radiological changes are of enlarged oedematous extraocular muscles and dilatation of the superior ophthalmic vein.
- More chronic changes are of enlargement of the superior orbital fissure and sellar erosion.
- Clinically, pulsatile exophthalmos suggests this condition.

Further management
When imaging features of a caroticocavernous fistula are associated with decreased visual acuity, emergency treatment is required to relieve intraocular pressure.

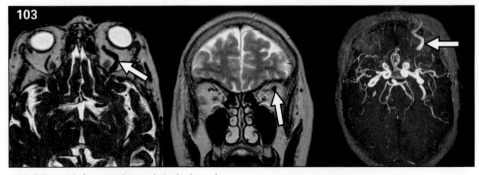

103 Dilated left superior ophthalmic vein.

CASE 104

History
A 32-year-old male presented with headaches and new onset epilepsy.

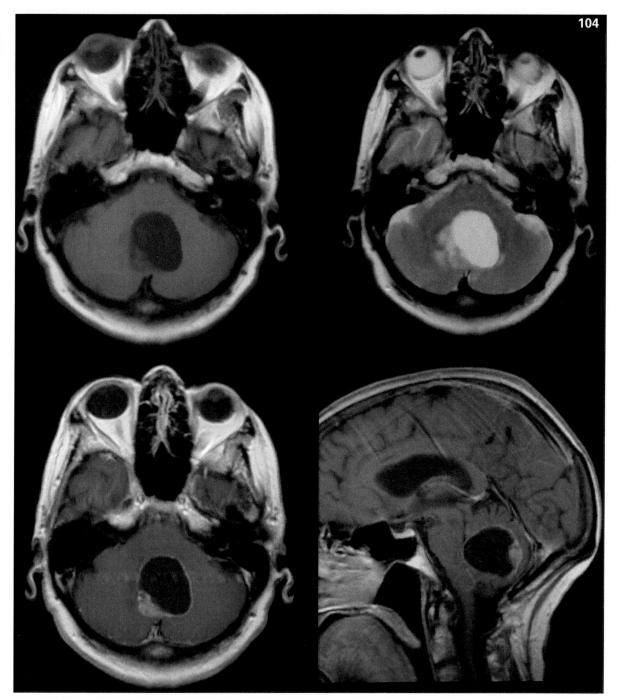

104 MRI T1 and T2 weighted axials (top) and T1 weighted post IV gadolinium axial and sagittal (bottom).

ANSWER 104

Observations (104)
Selected MR images of the brain show a large lesion in the cerebellum, which is predominantly cystic in nature (hyperintense on T2 and hypointense on T1 weighted images). Following IV contrast there is enhancement of the wall of the cystic component and an associated solid nodule posteriorly. Sagittal image shows some fullness of the lateral ventricles and obstructive hydrocephalus is likely with compression at the level of the 4th ventricle.

Diagnosis
Haemangioblastoma.

Differential diagnosis
- Juvenile pilocytic astrocytoma – can be very difficult to differentiate from a haemangioblastoma. This is the most common infratentorial tumour in children. There is an association with neurofibromatosis type 1. Lesions are of an identical appearance, with a predominant cystic component and enhancing solid peripheral nodule.
- Metastasis.
- Atypical medulloblastoma.

Discussion
Haemangioblastoma is a benign vascular tumour affecting the CNS. It is the most common primary infratentorial tumour in adults. The majority (80%) present in adults in the 3rd–6th decades, although there is an association with von Hippel–Lindau (VHL), which sees these tumours presenting in childhood and in this case may be multiple.

Typical appearance is of a well defined cystic lesion containing fluid of CSF density with a solid peripheral nodule, showing uniform avid enhancement. There is commonly haemorrhage or necrosis in the solid nodule but it rarely calcifies. In up to 30% of cases the lesions can be entirely solid with no cystic component.

Practical tips
When forming a differential for the posterior fossa cystic mass with enhancing peripheral nodule, the following generalizations apply:
- Children – pilocytic astrocytoma > haemangioblastoma.
- Younger adults – haemangioblastoma most common.
- Older adults – consider cystic metastasis.

Further management
When haemangioblastoma is suspected, don't forget to raise the possibility of VHL (4–20% of haemangioblastoma occur in the context of VHL and multiple lesions are diagnostic of VHL). VHL is an autosomal dominant (AD) inherited condition characterized by a predisposition to develop a spectrum of tumours including haemangioblastomas, cardiac rhabdomyomas, renal cell carcinomas, pheochromocytomas, pancreatic cystadenocarcinomas, islet cell tumours and haemangioblastomas, liver haemangiomas and retinal angiomas.

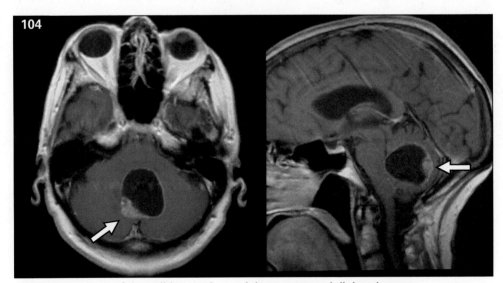

104 Enhancement of the solid posterior nodule on post-gadolinium images.

CASE 105

History
A 28-year-old male of no fixed abode, presented with a short history of confusion and limb weakness.

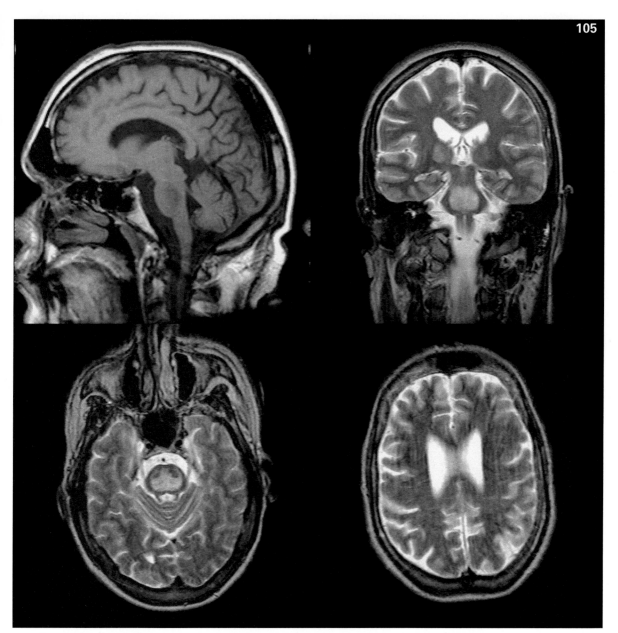

105 T1 sagittal (top left) and T2 weighted images (top right and bottom).

ANSWER 105

Observations (105)
The selected images demonstrate diffuse cerebral atrophy exceeding that expected for the patient's young age. There is a large focal area of signal abnormality in the central pons that is hyperintense on T2 weighted and hypointense on T1 weighted scans. There is no associated mass effect. The signal changes would fit with central pontine myelinolysis and the clinical details and cerebral atrophy suggest that chronic alcohol abuse may be the underlying cause.

Diagnosis
Central pontine myelinolysis.

Differential diagnosis
- Pontine glioma.
- Infarction.

Discussion
Central pontine myelinolysis results from the destruction of myelin sheaths, classically in patients with rapidly corrected hyponatraemia. Cases are reported in patients with:
- Chronic alcohol abuse.
- Chronic liver disease.
- Severe malnutrition.
- Wilson's disease, chronic renal failure, diabetes, acute myelogenous leukaemia.

In the case demonstrated there is diffuse global cerebral atrophic change suggestive of chronic alcohol abuse.

Clinically this results in pseudobulbar palsy, tetraplegia, convulsions, acute confusion and progression to coma. It is most commonly confined to the pons but changes can also be seen in the basal ganglia, caudate, thalamus and subcortical white matter. Radiological presentation is with fairly well defined low attenuation lesions on CT in the central pons. On MRI, lesions are of low intensity on T1 and high signal intensity on T2 imaging.

Practical tips
Standard MR/CT imaging can be normal for up to 14 days after symptom onset, lagging considerably behind the clinical presentation. Restricted diffusion on DWI, however, is found within 24 hours.

Further management
- Early MRI appearances can be similar for a basilar infarct and MRA can be useful to look for arterial thrombus.
- Search for underlying cause if not readily apparent.

Further reading
Ruzek KA, Campeau NG, Miller GM (2003). Early diagnosis of central pontine myelinolysis with diffusion-weighted imaging. *American Journal of Neuroradiology* **25**: 210–213.

Stadnik TW, Demaerel P, Luypaert RR, *et al.* (2003). Imaging tutorial: differential diagnosis of bright lesions on diffusion-weighted MR images. *RadioGraphics* **23(1)**: e7.

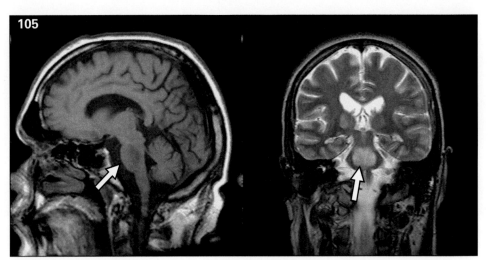

105 Focal area of reduced signal on T1 weighted (left) and increased signal on T2 weighted (right) images.

CASE 106

History
A 49-year-old female patient presented with headaches.

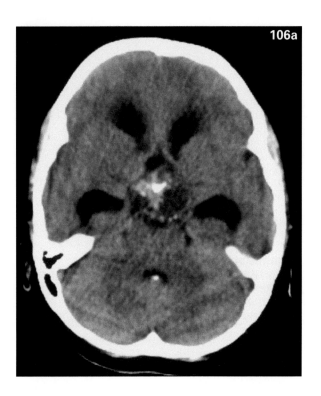

CASE 107

History
A 2-year-old female presented with developmental delay.

(see page 188 for case answer)

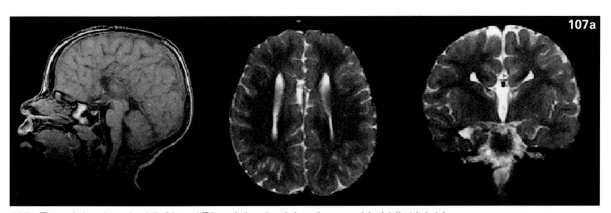

107a T1 weighted sagittal (left) and T2 weighted axial and coronal (middle/right) images.

ANSWER 106

Observations (106a)
This non contrast enhanced CT image demonstrates a large midline mass extending into the 3rd ventricle, which has both solid and cystic components with central calcification. There is dilatation of the temporal and anterior horns of the ventricles but normal appearance to the 4th ventricle – findings are in keeping with obstructive hydrocephalus at the level of the 3rd ventricle secondary to a mass lesion. The mixed density and calcification are very suggestive of a craniopharyngioma and MRI is suggested to further evaluate.

Diagnosis
Craniopharyngioma.

Differential diagnosis
Of suprasellar/intrasellar mass lesion:
- Pituitary macroadenoma.
- Craniopharyngioma.
- Rathke cleft cyst.

Other masses in the sellar region include meningioma, metastases, chordoma and internal carotid artery aneurysm.

Pituitary macroadenoma is the most common lesion involving the sellar and suprasellar regions. Microadenomas (20%) are defined as being less than 10 mm in size and usually present with symptoms due to hormonal secretion. Macroadenomas (80%) measure over 10 mm in size and are usually endocrinologically inactive. They present with symptoms secondary to mass effect such as hydrocephalus, bitemporal hemianopia from optic chiasm compression, involvement of cranial nerves travelling in the adjacent cavernous sinus (3, 4, 5a and 6) and hypopituitarism resulting from compression of normal pituitary tissue.

Compared to craniopharyngioma, pituitary macroadenomas are predominantly solid and show more intense uniform enhancement. Calcification is rare, unlike craniopharyngioma. Suprasellar extension produces the 'snowman' configuration due to waisting at the level of the diaphragm sellae. Figure 106b shows pre- and post-contrast T1 weighted images of a pituitary macroadenoma with such features.

Rathke cleft cyst is the other main differential diagnosis, with 70% involving sellar and suprasellar regions. It is a benign cyst arising from remnants of Rathke's pouch and can be differentiated by the following features: more regular and ovoid shape, smaller size (<2 ml), cystic with no, or minimal enhancement of the thin wall.

Discussion
Craniopharyngioma account for ~4% of intracranial neoplasms, with a slight predominance in males, and two peaks of increased incidence:
- Firstly in children in 1st–2nd decades, where they account for 50% of suprasellar tumours.
- Secondly in adults in 5th–6th decades.

These are benign tumours arising from remnants of Rathke's pouch. They grow from a suprasellar origin into the base of the 3rd ventricle. Intrasellar extension occurs in 21%. Involvement of the bony sella can be seen on plain radiographs and on CT bone window images. These demonstrate appearances of J-shaped sella, enlarged sella and then ultimately erosion and destruction.

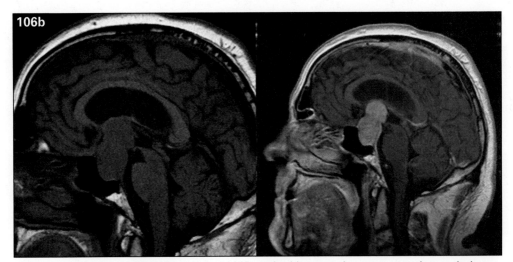

106b Pre- and post-contrast T1 weighted MR sagittal images demonstrate a large pituitary adenoma with uniform enhancement with contrast and with no cystic elements or signal voids to suggest calcification.

Answer 106 — CNS, Head and Neck Imaging

- Typical CT appearances are shown in this case with solid and cystic elements and calcification (which is seen in ~90% of cases). Following contrast there is enhancement of the solid components and the cyst wall.
- Typical MRI findings reflect CT features with a cystic component following fluid signal (although high signal may be seen on T1 weighted images depending on protein/blood content). The solid component is isointense on T1 and shows enhancement with gadolinium contrast.

Figure 106c shows T1 sagittal pre- and post-IV contrast (right) and T2 axial and sagittal images (left). These illustrate a large suprasellar lesion with intrasellar extension. There are solid and cystic elements with enhancement of the solid components and cyst wall. Complications of obstructive hydrocephalus, pituitary stalk and optic chiasm compression can be appreciated.

Practical tips
Look for the complications of mass lesions in this area:
- Hydrocephalus and optic chiasm compression.
- Lateral extension to involve the cavernous sinus (seen in up to 10% of pituitary macroadenomas), which can lead to thrombosis and cranial nerve palsy. Lateral extension beyond the lateral wall of the internal carotid is rare with Rathke cleft cyst and may help differentiate it from the other two conditions listed.

Further management
Treatment is surgical +/– postoperative radiotherapy.

Further reading
Choi SH, Kwon BJ, Na DG, *et al.* (2007). Pituitary adenoma, craniopharyngioma, and Rathke cleft cyst involving both intrasellar and suprasellar regions: differentiation using MRI. *Clinical Radiology* 62: 453–462.

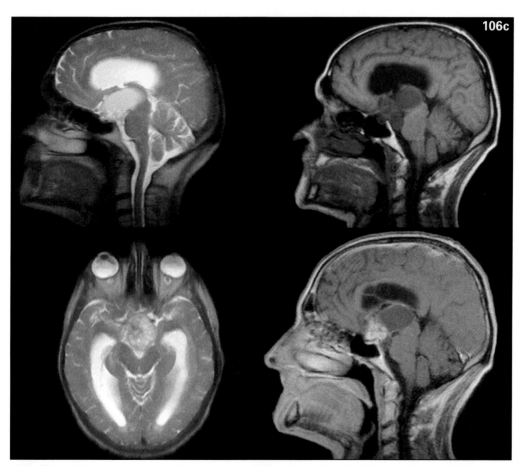

106c T1 sagittal pre- and post-IV contrast and T2 axial and sagittal images demonstrate a large suprasellar lesion with solid and cystic elements with enhancement of the solid components and cyst wall. The lesion is causing obstructive hydrocephalus, pituitary stalk and optic chiasm compression.

ANSWER 107

Observations (107a)
T1 sagittal and T2 axial and coronal images of the brain demonstrate complete agenesis of the corpus callosum with no callosal tissue identified. There is increased separation of the lateral ventricles on the axial images creating a 'bat's wing' appearance. Coronal image demonstrates elevation of the 3rd ventricle.

Diagnosis
Agenesis of the corpus callosum.

Discussion
The corpus callosum usually develops by 20 weeks' gestation. The genu and the body of the corpus callosum develop first and the posterior body and splenium develop later. The rostrum is the last part of the corpus callosum to develop. Identifying the parts of the corpus callosum present can help to differentiate between dysgenesis (absent genu/splenium) and destruction, most commonly due to ischaemia (genu present but may be atrophic). Corpus callosal agenesis is usually associated with reduced intellectual function and can be associated with a variety of CNS abnormalities including hydrocephalus, midline lipoma, Dandy–Walker cysts, interhemispheric arachnoid cysts, neuronal migration disorders and Arnold–Chiari malformation.

Classical imaging appearances on CT/MRI are with:
- 'Bat's wing' appearance of the lateral ventricles due to parallel lateral ventricles with marked separation (107b).
- 'High riding' 3rd ventricle – can be seen at the level of the lateral ventricles.
- Enlarged foramen of Monro.

Prenatal detection can be made by US investigation. Diagnosis cannot usually be made before 22 weeks' gestation. Equivalent image findings are of:
- Absence of the septum pellucidum.
- Dilated/elevated 3rd ventricle.
- Enlargement of the occipital horns of the lateral ventricles.

Practical tips
Differentiating between dysgenesis and ischaemic damage is done by determining which parts of the corpus callosum are abnormal. With ischaemic injury the rostrum will be present but atrophic.

Further management
Sometimes this finding is made incidentally on brain imaging in later life and no further investigation is required.

Further reading
Babcock DS (1984). The normal, absent, and abnormal corpus callosum: sonographic findings. *Radiology* 151: 449–453.

Davidson HD, Abraham R, Steiner RE (1985). Agenesis of the corpus callosum: magnetic resonance imaging. *Radiology* 155: 371–373.

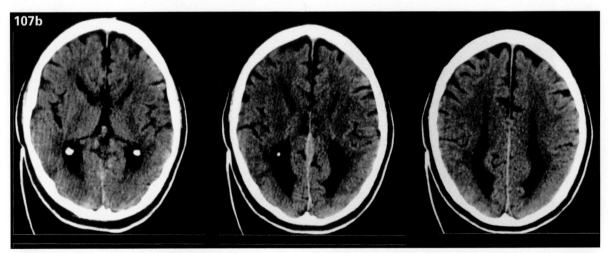

107b Axial CT images of the brain demonstrating 'bat's wing' appearance of the lateral ventricles in a patient with agenesis of the corpus callosum.

CASE 108

History
A 38-year-old female presented with left sided tinnitus and hearing loss.

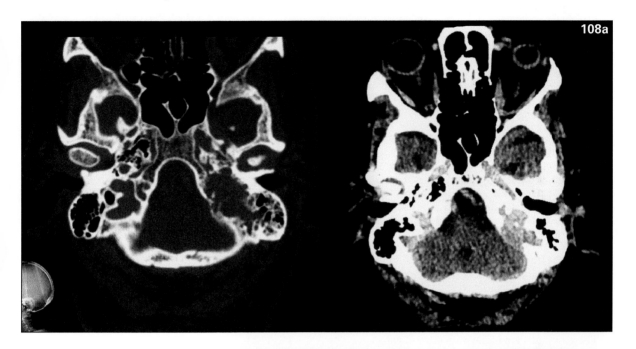

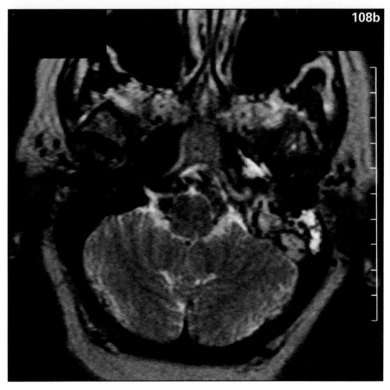

ANSWER 108

Observations (108a, 108b)
Axial CT images (**108a** – axial CT scan at skull base with IV contrast, seen on bone and soft tissue windows) of the brain demonstrate a poorly defined enhancing lesion in the jugular foramen, which is extending superiorly to involve the middle ear and is causing permeative erosion of the petrous temporal bone at the jugular foramen. The T2 weighted MR image (**108b**) confirms this mass lesion, which appears hyperintense with serpiginous flow voids indicating vascular flow.

Diagnosis
Glomus jugulotympanicum tumour.

Description
Glomus jugulare tumours are paragangliomas and are the most common jugular foramen lesion. Typically, these lesions are solitary with a peak incidence in the 5th–6th decades and increased incidence in females. There are familial associations in which multiple paragangliomas present in conditions such as multiple endocrine neoplasia (MEN).

Glomus jugulare tumours usually extend intracranially and can involve the middle ear, as demonstrated here. Clinical presentation may be related to involvement of the 9th, 10th and 11th cranial nerves. When there is extension to involve the middle ear (glomus jugulotympanicum) then pulsatile tinnitus is the classical presentation.

These tumours are highly vascular and enhance avidly with contrast on CT and MRI. On CT, permeative bone erosion is classical, differing from the coarser lytic destruction seen with skull base metastases. Vascular flow voids and foci of haemorrhage are better demonstrated on MRI – flow produces black signal voids and haemorrhage produces hyperintense foci on T1 weighted images. This combination of black holes and white dots leads to the so-called 'salt and pepper' appearance commonly described.

Angiography is sometimes required for smaller tumours that don't demonstrate the classical imaging appearances, and reveals a hypervascular lesion with a dense reticular tumour stain.

There is a small risk of malignant transformation seen in ~2% of cases.

Practical tips
When suspected on MRI, CT can still help make a more conclusive diagnosis in many cases by demonstrating the classical permeative pattern of erosion at the jugular foramen.

Further management
Depending on the size of the tumour and the intracranial extension, a combined ENT/neurosurgical procedure is performed.

Further reading
Caldemeyer KS, Mathews VP, Azzarelli B, Smith RR (1997). The jugular foramen: a review of anatomy, masses, and imaging characteristics. *RadioGraphics* **17**: 1123–1139.

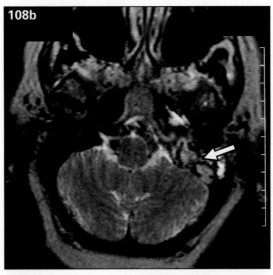

108b Hyperintense mass lesion with flow voids.

CASE 109

History
A 24-year-old female presented with chronic headaches and visual loss.

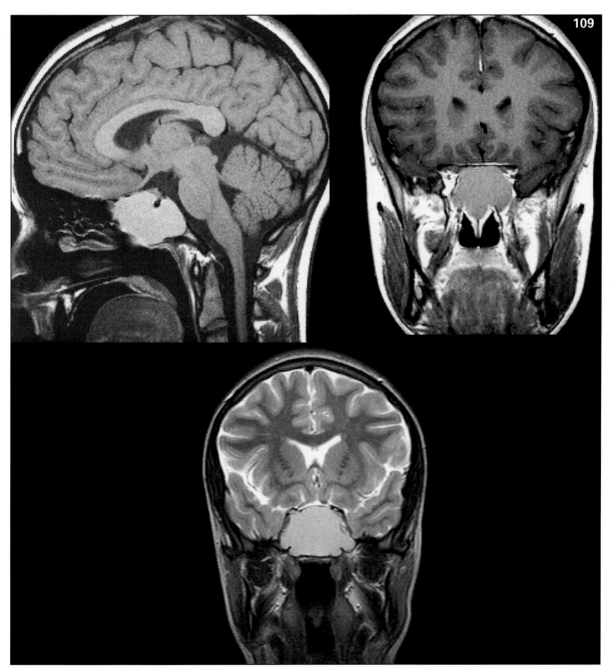

109 T1 weighted sagittal and coronal (top) and T2 weighted coronal (bottom) MR images.

ANSWER 109

Observations (109)
These selected MR images show an expanded sphenoid sinus filled with abnormal signal rather than air. The contents show mild uniform hyperintensity on T1 weighted and T2 weighted images. The walls of the sinus appear smooth and intact with no obvious evidence of destruction. The findings are consistent with a mucocele of the sphenoid sinus, the signal indicative of proteinaceous fluid contents. Sagittal T1 and coronal T2 images demonstrate displacement of the optic nerves by the expanded sinus, presumably causing compression of the anterior optic pathway given the history of visual disturbance.

Diagnosis
Sphenoid sinus mucocele.

Discussion
A mucocele arises due to chronic obstruction of a sinus, which then becomes filled with mucus. This collection acts like a slow growing mass causing expansion of sinus bony walls without frank bony destruction. Vessels and other structures are displaced rather than being encased, as with a tumour. Usually these lesions are asymptomatic until they become large when they can cause optic nerve compression, proptosis and headache. Secondary infection of the mucocele can supervene, but this is a rare complication. Ninety per cent of lesions are found in the frontal and ethmoid sinuses with sphenoid sinus mucoceles being only rarely seen.

Appearances on MRI are variable depending on the fluid/protein content of the mucocele but important imaging findings are of a nondestructive, slow growing lesion.

Practical tips
- CT is good for showing bony expansion with the absence of bone erosion.
- MRI is good for identifying the extent/size of the lesion and looking for complications of optic nerve compression (usually from posterior ethmoid lesions) and proptosis (usually from frontal and anterior ethmoid sinuses).
- T1 hyperintensity within a lesion on any MRI study often helps to rapidly limit the differential diagnosis as there are a limited number of things that are bright on T1 imaging, i.e. fat, blood, proteinaceous fluid, paramagnetic contrast agents.

Further management
Referral to ENT for consideration of endoscopic sinus surgery.

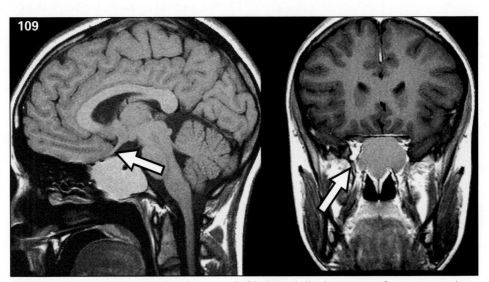

109 Superior displacement of optic nerve (left); lateral displacement of cavernous sinus by large sinus mucocele (right).

CASE 110

History
A 68-year-old female presented with worsening headaches.

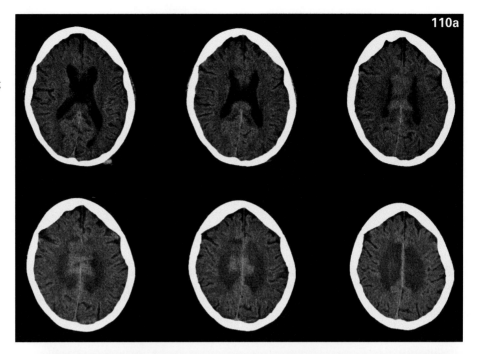

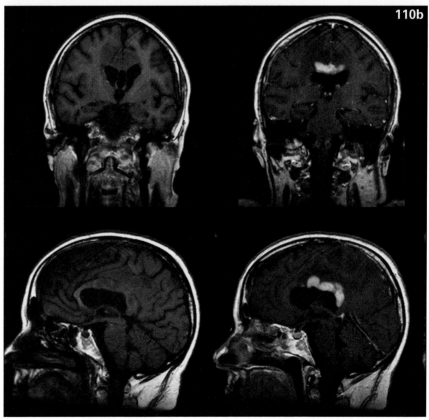

ANSWER 110

Observations (110a, 110b)
The selected plain CT images (**110a**) show a poorly defined, hyperdense midline lesion extending across the body of the corpus callosum. There is no significant surrounding oedema.

Pre- and post-contrast T1 weighted MR images (**110b**) from the same patient show a multilobulated lesion with uniform enhancement crossing the midline in the body of the corpus callosum. No further lesions are seen within the brain parenchyma. Incidental note is made of cavum septum pellucidum. The findings are of a 'butterfly' tumour in the corpus callosum.

Diagnosis
Butterfly glioblastoma multiforme (GBM).

Differential diagnosis
For lesions crossing the midline in the corpus callosum:
- GBM.
- Lymphoma.
- Demyelinating disease – multiple sclerosis.

Discussion
This is the most common and the most malignant primary brain tumour. It accounts for >50% of brain tumours with a wide age distribution peaking at the 7th–8th decades. The most common location is within the white matter of centrum semiovale with increased incidence in the frontal lobes. Other patterns of distribution include callosal extension giving this appearance of a butterfly glioma, posterior fossa lesions and multifocal distribution (seen in 2–4%).

Tumours spread by direct extension involving white matter tracts, such as the corpus callosum and cerebral peduncles or via the CSF (<2% of cases). Haematogenous spread can also very rarely occur.

Typical imaging appearances of a butterfly glioma are of a poorly defined lesion that enhances uniformly. Cyst formation, necrosis and haemorrhage are seen in about 5% of cases and calcification is rare and usually associated with chemo/radiotherapy. The corpus callosum is made up of dense, tightly packed white matter tracts and therefore mass effect and vasogenic oedema are minimal. Hemispheric glioblastomas conversely have quite marked mass effect and surrounding oedema.

Practical tips
GBM and lymphoma are the two likeliest diagnoses for butterfly lesions involving the corpus callosum. Although difficult to differentiate radiologically, cavitation and necrosis are relatively uncommon in lymphoma (except in AIDS patients).

Further management
- T2 hypointensity is sometimes present with CNS lymphoma and therefore this image sequence can sometimes help to differentiate lymphoma from glioblastoma.
- Neurosurgical evaluation.

Further reading
Bourekas EC, Varakis K, Bruns D, *et al.* (2002). Lesions of the corpus callosum: MR imaging and differential considerations in adults and children. *American Journal of Radiology* **179**: 251–257.

Rees JH, Smirniotopoulos JG, Jones RV, Wong K (1996). Glioblastoma multiforme: radiologic-pathologic correlation. *RadioGraphics* **16**: 6.

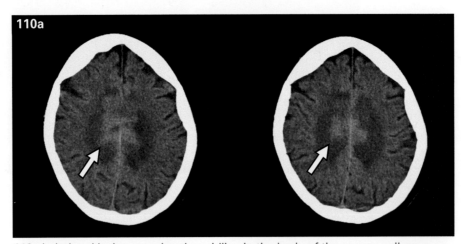

110a Lobulated lesion crossing the midline in the body of the corpus callosum.

CASE 111

History
A 33-year-old male presented with lower back pain.

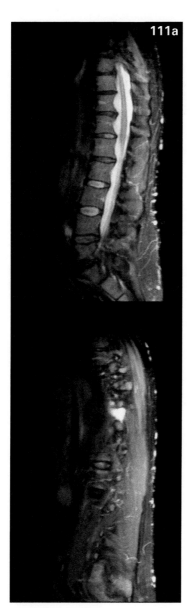
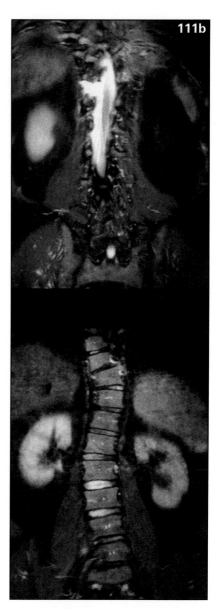
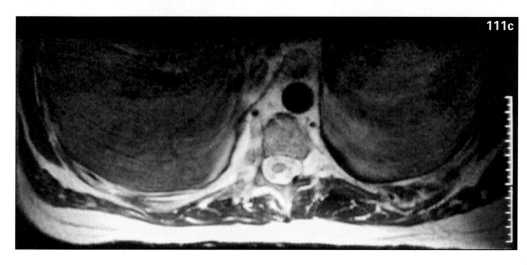

ANSWER 111

Observations (111a, 111b, 111c)
These STIR sagittal (**111a**), STIR coronal (**111b**) and T2 weighted axial (**111c**) images of the spine demonstrate posterior vertebral scalloping, particularly at the T11, T12 and L2 levels. There is also a thoracic scoliosis. At approximately T10 level, coronal images show a right sided high-signal lesion projecting laterally from the spinal canal, presumably through the intervertebral foramen. This follows CSF signal and is probably a lateral thoracic meningocele. The axial T2 weighted image shows a second lateral thoracic meningocele on the left side, in a similar region of the spine. The combination of findings is strongly suggestive of neurofibromatosis type 1 and multiple high-signal cutaneous nodules on the sagittal images confirm this diagnosis.

Diagnosis
Neurofibromatosis type 1 (NF1).

Discussion
Neurofibromatosis type 1 is a neurocutaneous disorder, of which 50% is inherited in an autosomal dominant manner and 50% is sporadic. Classical features in the spine include:
- Lateral thoracic meningocele (dysplasia of the meninges resulting in diverticula of the thecal sac, which extends through the neural foramina).
- Posterior vertebral scalloping – also due to dural ectasia.
- Neurofibromas – enhancing dumbbell-shaped lesions.
- Scoliosis and kyphosis.
- Enlarged vertebral foraminae – due to neurofibroma or lateral meningocele.
- Hypoplasia of the pedicles, transverse and spinous processes.

Practical tips
- Always look for the presence of subcutaneous nodules on the image when NF1 is suspected.
- It may be difficult to differentiate between a lateral thoracic meningocele and a 'dumbbell' neurofibroma. However, on MRI the former will be of CSF density on all sequences, i.e. high signal on T2, whereas the latter will have a hyperintense periphery on T2 with a hypointense core.
- In a case such as this, one might also comment that there are no obvious adrenal masses or renal asymmetry (implying association with phaeochromocytoma and renal artery stenosis, respectively).

Further management
Neurofibromas can undergo malignant transformation in 2–3%; therefore a rapid rate of growth or new onset pain should be thoroughly investigated.

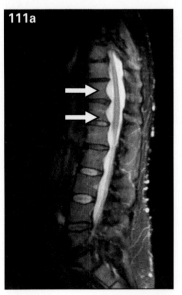

111a Posterior vertebral scalloping.

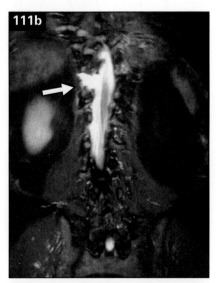

111b Lateral thoracic meningocele.

CASE 112

History
A 22-year-old female had had persistent headache for several days. There was no history of trauma.

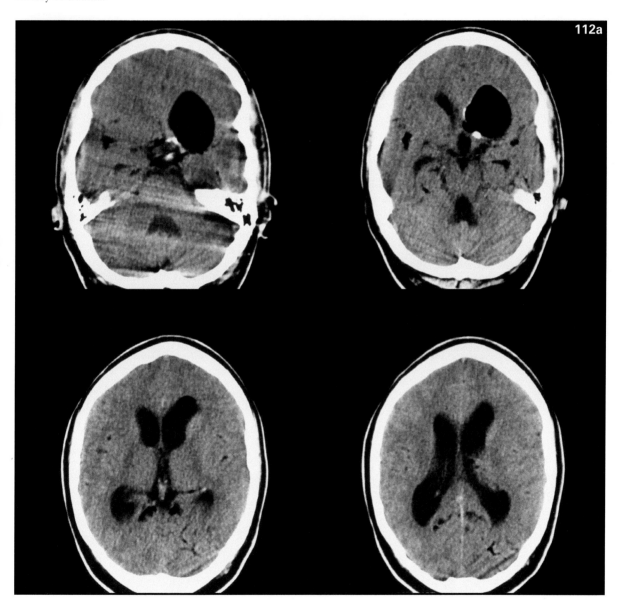

ANSWER 112

Observations (112a)
Selected unenhanced axial CT images of the brain show a well defined low attenuation lesion in the left frontal lobe causing minimal mass effect. The contents are of lower attenuation than CSF but given the absence of trauma it is unlikely that this is due to intracranial air. It is likely that instead, it represents fat, which could be easily confirmed by adjusting the CT windows or taking a direct density measurement. A calcified nodule is seen at the posterior aspect of the lesion with further mural calcifications elsewhere. Further small locules of fat are seen in the anterior horn of the left lateral ventricle and several sulci.

Diagnosis
Ruptured dermoid cyst.

Discussion
Dermoid cysts are fairly uncommon CNS lesions, usually presenting before the 4th decade. They arise due to inclusion of epithelial elements at the time of closure of the neural tube and therefore contain ectodermal and mesodermal components, i.e. hair, sebaceous glands and skin. Dermoids are usually located near the midline and can be found within brain parenchyma, ventricles, CSF spaces or within bone. Development and growth are very slow and presentation is therefore late.
- Typical appearances on CT: low-density lesions containing fat with no contrast enhancement. Mural or focal central calcification can be seen.
- Typical appearances on MRI: well defined lesion which is high signal intensity on T1 weighted imaging with signal void at points of calcification. No enhancement with contrast.

Cyst rupture leading to chemical meningitis is an occasional complication, as in this case. Release of fat globules can produce fat-fluid levels with CSF. Figure 112b demonstrates typical appearance of a dermoid with a fat-containing lesion of high signal on T1 weighted imaging. Some strands of mesodermal tissue are noted within it. A fat-fluid level is seen in the lateral ventricle due to rupture into the subarachnoid space.

Practical tips
- Posterior fossa dermoids are usually found in the midline and show no contrast enhancement on CT/MRI.
- On T1 weighted MRI high signal is produced by:
  - Fat.
  - Blood products (methaemoglobin).
  - Proteinaceous fluid.
  - Contrast.

Further management
MRI is better than CT for identifying rupture of a dermoid cyst and the consequent chemical meningitis.

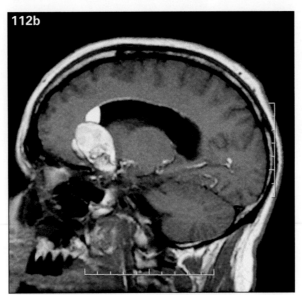

112b Sagittal T1 weighted image of the brain shows rupture of the midline dermoid cysts with a fat-CSF level seen in the lateral ventricle.

CASE 113

History
A 45-year-old patient presented with confusion developing over 1 week.

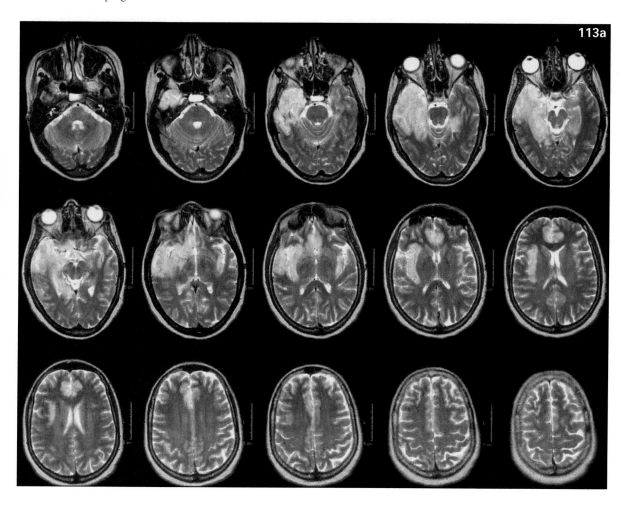

ANSWER 113

Observations (113a)
These T2 weighted axial brain images show a diffuse increase in signal affecting the right temporal lobe. This involves grey and white matter, extending to the cortical surface. Sulci in the affected area are effaced. Similar signal changes extend along the cingulate gyrus and also affect the contralateral temporal lobe to a lesser extent. The duration of the history and distribution of involvement are in keeping with encephalitis, most likely due to herpes simplex virus.

Diagnosis
Herpes simplex (HSV) encephalitis.

Differential diagnosis
Right middle cerebral territory infarct.

Discussion
Encephalitis is the term generally used to describe a diffuse cerebral inflammatory process of viral aetiology. Clinical presentation is with confusion, headache and seizures progressing to coma. Fever is almost always present. The most common organism is HSV, infection being either primary or due to virus reactivation. The resulting cytotoxic oedema manifests as high signal on T2 weighted, FLAIR and DWI MRI. The temporal lobe is typically affected, often with the inferior frontal lobe and cingulate gyrus. Unlike other viral infections, the basal ganglia are usually spared.

Practical tips
- HSV encephalitis has high mortality and morbidity rates but is treatable with acyclovir so a high index of suspicion is needed, especially on CT, which may well be the first imaging done – signs of oedema and swelling are likely to be comparatively subtle compared to MRI (if present at all).
- Bilateral temporal lobe involvement is virtually pathognomonic of HSV infection. Features that are atypical and should arouse suspicion of other organisms include basal ganglia involvement and isolated involvement of other lobes without temporal lobe involvement.
- Cytotoxic oedema (seen in stroke and encephalitis) extends to the periphery of the brain whereas vasogenic oedema (seen with tumours, abscess, etc.) affects white matter only.
- Without clinical history, one might mistake the MRI changes of HSV encephalitis for a middle cerebral artery (MCA) infarct. However, note that the posteromedial temporal lobe affected by HSV is spared in an MCA infarct as this territory is supplied by the posterior cerebral artery (PCA). Figure 113b shows a typical MCA infarct with low attenuation change in the right temporal lobe but sparing the area described posteromedially (this scan also happens to show a hyperdense MCA due to thrombus). For comparison, Figure 113c shows a PCA infarct with the posteromedial temporal lobe affected.
- Neonatal herpes-related encephalitis is due to HSV type 2, probably acquired via the genital tract perinatally. The imaging features are different from those due to HSV type 1 described above.

Further management
Urgent treatment with antiviral drugs – mortality in untreated HSV encephalitis can be as high as 65%.

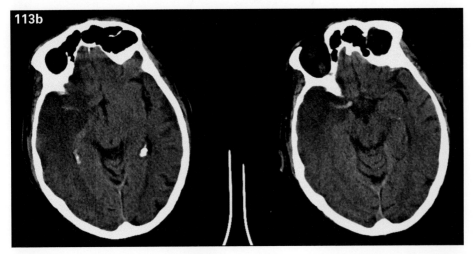

113b Axial plain CT brain shows a right middle cerebral artery territory infarct with hyperdense artery sign.

113c Axial plain CT brain shows a PCA infarct with low attenuation in the posteromedial temporal lobe.

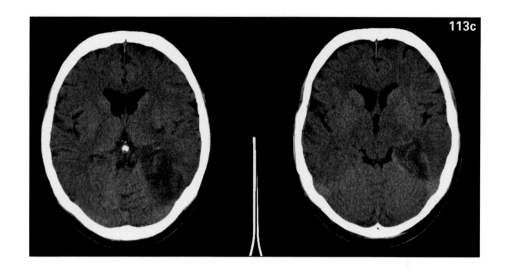

CASE 114

History
A 36-year-old male was brought to A&E in cardiorespiratory arrest. No other history is available.

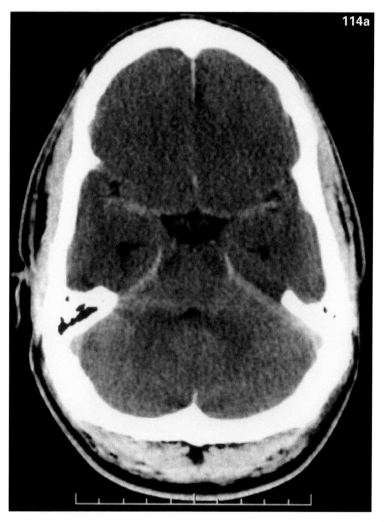

ANSWER 114

Observations (114a)
This single CT image shows diffuse low-attenuation change in the frontal and temporal lobes and brainstem with loss of the grey–white matter differentiation. The cerebellum is better preserved. Generalized sulcal effacement indicates cerebral swelling.

This widespread reduction in brain density makes the normal cerebral vessels and dural reflections appear spuriously conspicuous. Close inspection confirms that this is a perceptual 'abnormality' – the basal cisterns are of normal CSF density so there is not acute subarachnoid haemorrhage. The findings are suggestive of global cerebral ischaemia and oedema.

Diagnosis
Global cerebral anoxia.

This particular case turned out to be secondary to asthma-induced cardiorespiratory arrest.

Discussion
Global ischaemia can occur following prolonged hypoxia, which may be secondary to fitting, aspiration, smothering, strangulation, etc. The CT findings are distinctive, with loss of grey–white matter differentiation and changes due to cerebral oedema including sulcal effacement. Generalized low density of the cerebral cortex develops. The cerebellum is more resistant to hypoxia and therefore appears of high density in comparison with the low-density cerebral cortex; the so-called 'reversal sign' (see also Case 163).

The conspicuity of the vessels and dura may lead one to the erroneous diagnosis of acute subarachnoid haemorrhage (SAH) on first inspection. An example of a real SAH is shown (**114b**) – note high density in the suprasellar cistern representing acute haemorrhage and the normal density cerebral cortex with preserved grey–white matter differentiation. There is also dilatation of the temporal horns of the lateral ventricles indicating early obstructive hydrocephalus. Trauma is the most common cause of SAH. CT is 90% sensitive in the detection of SAH in the first 24 hours following presentation. However, this decreases to 50% at 1 week and continues to fall thereafter. Small SAH may not be seen on CT and will only be detected on lumbar puncture (LP) as xanthochromia. The cause of 75% of spontaneous SAH is berry aneurysms and these are mostly found sprouting from the circle of Willis. An example of a large SAH in a patient with a ruptured aneurysm is shown (**114c**). Note the extensive amount of blood filling the sulci and Sylvian fissures. Blood has also entered the ventricular system and can be seen in the 3rd and 4th ventricles. The large aneurysm appears to arise from the origin of the left middle cerebral artery.

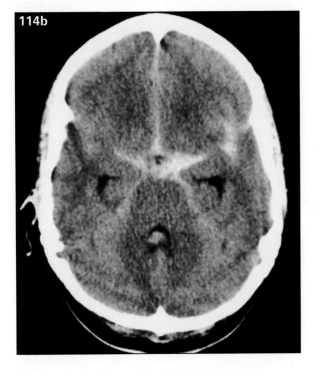

114b Axial plain CT of brain showing SAH with blood in suprasellar and basal cisterns.

Answer 114   CNS, Head and Neck Imaging

Practical tips
- Don't mistake cerebral anoxic change for SAH in the unconscious patient – check that the hyperdensity really is in the subarachnoid space and not a perceptual illusion from cerebral anoxia.
- Always remember that a normal CT scan does not exclude SAH, especially as the time interval from onset of symptoms increases. If the CT is normal, LP looking for xanthochromia is required (this may be evident in CSF after 2–4 hr but can only be conclusively excluded if the LP is done at least 12 hr after onset).
- Remember that SAH can be secondary to trauma as well as leaking aneurysm, etc.
- When SAH is present, the site of aneurysm is likely to be where there is most blood!
- CT remains the primary imaging modality for suspected SAH. Conventional T1 and T2 MRI scans are unhelpful. FLAIR MRI may show high signal in the CSF spaces but such changes are also seen in meningitis, i.e. it is not specific for SAH. However, MRI may be useful in detecting evidence of chronic small subarachnoid bleeds as low signal along the leptomeninges on gradient recalled T2 weighted scans.

Further management
Regarding suspected SAH, a negative CT alone is insufficient to exclude the diagnosis. LP (looking for xanthochromia) is required in cases where CT is normal. This should be delayed for at least 12 hr from the onset of headache as false negatives may occur before this time.

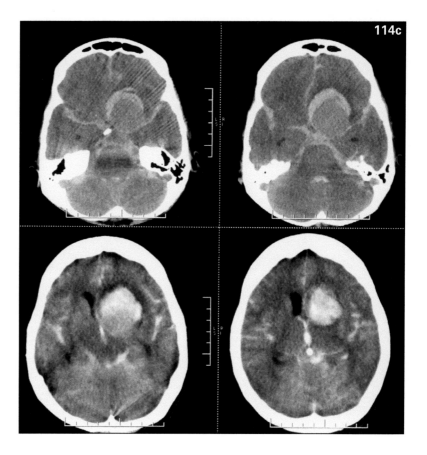

114c Axial plain CT brain demonstrating large SAH with large aneurysm arising from the left middle cerebral artery.

Chapter 4

MUSCULOSKELETAL IMAGING

Much of the advice given here relates to the plain radiograph, though the fundamental principles can often be applied to CT and MRI too. When analysing a musculoskeletal film, check the bones, the joints and the soft tissues. There may be obvious abnormalities at first inspection but, as always, a systematic check of all three areas will ensure nothing is missed.

In the real world, the radiologist is usually made aware of a history of trauma but this may not be provided in a viva. There are certain diagnoses that must not be missed on the chest radiograph (e.g. tension pneumothorax) and abdominal film (e.g. viscus perforation) due to the gravity of the consequences for the patient (and the viva candidate, who will fail as a result!). Similarly in MSK imaging, fractures must not be missed. One should therefore always be 'on guard' for subtle fractures when nothing else is apparent, especially those such as the unstable cervical spine injury where the consequences of nonrecognition are serious.

Musculoskeletal imaging is one area in particular where there are many 'Aunt Minnie' diagnoses – disorders with classical appearances that rely on recall from previous experience rather than a systematic analysis. In the real world, some such conditions are important to recognize so as to avoid unnecessary further investigation. In a viva, they represent easy points for those who have spent time preparing well!

BONES
When a bony abnormality is identified, the first thing to establish is whether you are dealing with a focal lesion or a diffuse abnormality. Fundamentally, a diffuse process affecting several bones implies a systemic problem be that metabolic, inflammatory, congenital, etc. A focal bone lesion implies a local disease process with a very different differential diagnosis.

The focal bone lesion is a common problem in radiology, especially the radiology viva. There are several features to assess and pieces of information to assimilate to produce a differential diagnosis; the main three are as follows.

Aggressive vs benign
This is a very important decision with regards to clinical management of focal bone lesions. Note the use of the term 'aggressive' rather than 'malignant' – while malignant bone lesions are often aggressive, nonmalignant pathology such as infection can also behave in an aggressive manner. Thus, not all aggressive lesions are malignant!

Aggressive bone lesions often represent tumour or infection and show features such as:
- Poor definition of edges suggesting rapid growth and an aggressive nature. The radiological term for poorly defined borders is a 'wide zone of transition'.
- 'Moth eaten'/permeative bone destruction.
- Cortical destruction.
- Associated periosteal reaction – particular patterns of periosteal reaction point to an aggressive underlying lesion. The following examples are those classically described but like most things in medicine, are not absolute associations!
    - Multilamellated reaction, e.g. active osteomyelitis, Ewing's sarcoma and osteosarcoma.
    - Spiculated perpendicular 'hair on end' reaction, e.g. Ewing's sarcoma.
    - Divergent 'sunburst' appearance, e.g. osteosarcoma, metastases, Ewing's sarcoma, TB.
- Associated soft tissue swelling/extension.

Benign lesions typically show features such as:
- Well defined borders/narrow zone of transition, perhaps with marginal sclerosis.
- Intact cortex (unless there has been a pathological fracture).
- No associated soft tissue mass.
- Periosteal reaction absent or of benign pattern.

Assessment of periosteal reaction is one feature that may help assess whether a focal lesion is benign or aggressive, but it is worth noting that periosteal reaction does not automatically mean there is an underlying bone lesion. There are a few systemic conditions that cause periosteal reaction on normal underlying bone. The key here is to note features such as normal underlying bone, multiple bones affected or symmetrical distribution.

Location
As well as the obvious question of which bone is affected, the part of the bone affected (epiphysis, metaphysis or diaphysis) also helps one to narrow down the differential diagnosis. For example, an aggressive lesion with a permeative appearance in the diaphysis of a young patient might be a Ewing's sarcoma but the same type of appearance in the metaphysis would raise the possibility of osteosarcoma instead. An expansile lesion seen within the pelvis would have a different differential to an expansile lesion seen in the axial skeleton.

Age

Age is vitally important in forming a differential diagnosis for focal bone lesions, as the probability of many lesions varies dramatically between young and older people. For the purposes of radiological assessment of focal bone lesions, one might consider less than 30 years of age as being young and over 40 as older! For example, many benign bony lesions such as simple bone cyst and aneurysmal bone cyst are really only seen in the younger age group. Similarly, there are certain primary bone malignancies also seen primarily in this age group, e.g. Ewing's sarcoma. Conversely, metastases are relatively common in the older age group and consequently often enter the differential diagnosis.

JOINTS

Arthropathy is a very common radiological problem in the real world and in examinations. Pattern recognition of the more common varieties is aided by exposure to as many films as possible but thereafter, first principles can be used when in doubt.

The 'do-not-miss' lesion involving the joints is septic arthritis – be suspicious of this when presented with a case in which there is a single joint showing features of joint space narrowing, erosion of bone on both sides of the joint and soft tissue swelling.

Subchondral sclerosis, geodes and osteophytosis are features of degenerative disease, while osteopenia, soft tissue swelling and erosions are common features of inflammatory arthropathy. Joint space loss is seen in both, so is not usually helpful in discriminating the two.

Other features to assess are the distribution – axial vs appendicular skeleton, small vs large joints, distal vs proximal, synovial vs nonsynovial joints, symmetrical vs nonsymmetrical. Age and gender may also be very helpful to know. The distribution and nature of erosions are often typical for various disorders and the radiologist must be familiar with these aspects of the various erosive arthropathies. Sometimes there is no definite best fit diagnosis and one can only state the features supporting the various possibilities and the importance of correlation with clinical and laboratory features.

Other points to consider:

- Syndesmophytes in the spine indicates a seronegative arthropathy, commonly associated with the HLA-B27 antigen. These include ankylosing spondylitis, psoriatic arthropathy, Reiter's syndrome and inflammatory bowel-related arthropathy.
- Rheumatoid arthritis has classical features of bilaterally symmetrical, proximal arthropathy with marginal erosions and deformity but it is often difficult to make a definite diagnosis from radiographs alone.
- Don't forget the crystal arthropathies – well defined erosions with sclerotic borders are typical of gout.
- The 5 Ds of neuropathic joint – destruction, disorganization, dislocation, debris, density (sclerosis).

SOFT TISSUES

Though more readily assessed on MRI, it is easy to forget the soft tissues on plain films. However, swelling around a bone may guide you to underlying fracture or osteomyelitis, while swelling around a joint may point to arthropathy or intra-articular fracture for example.

CASE 115

History
A 13-year-old male presented with pain in his left arm following a fall.

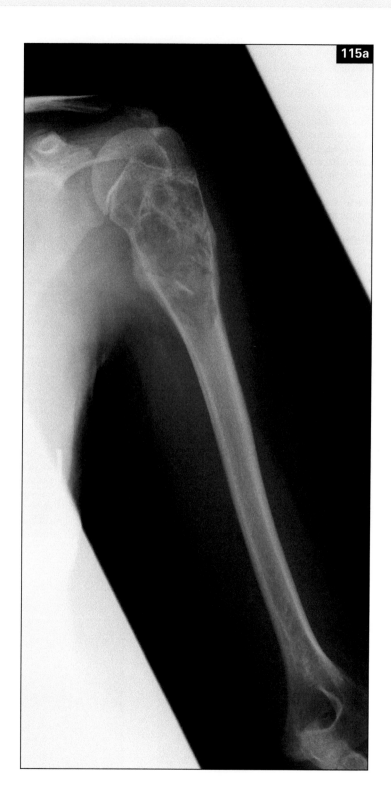

ANSWER 115

Observations (115a)
This radiograph demonstrates a well defined lucent lesion of the proximal metaphysis of the left humerus. The lesion is centrally located with slight thinning of the cortex, mild expansion and several internal septae. It has a narrow zone of transition. There is a pathological fracture through the lesion with associated periosteal reaction and a 'fallen fragment' sign. The features are consistent with a benign lesion, specifically a simple bone cyst.

Diagnosis
Simple bone cyst (SBC).

Differential diagnosis
The 'fallen fragment' sign is supposedly very specific for SBC, but otherwise, possibilities include:
- Aneurysmal bone cyst (ABC) – 10–30 year olds. Occurs in the metaphysis +/– epiphysis. Like a simple bone cyst it is a well defined lucency with an intact cortex. This is typically an expansile lucent lesion. An example is shown in the pelvis of a child (**115b**).
- Giant cell tumour (GCT) – seen in 20–35 year olds. Subarticular, eccentric location within epiphysis (metaphysis if growth plate open). Cortical destruction can occur and rarely metastases to the lungs.
- Brown tumour.
- Fibrous dysplasia.
- Enchondroma.

Discussion
Simple (unicameral) bone cysts are benign lesions usually (75%) located in the proximal humerus and femur. They occur in patients aged 5–15 years and are more commonly found in males (ratio 3:1). Typical imaging features are demonstrated with the lesion seen in the metaphysis, however they gradually migrate to the diaphysis as the bones grow (**115c**). They are asymptomatic unless pathological fracture occurs and a small fragment of bone is identifiable within the cyst – the 'fallen fragment' sign. Periosteal reaction is not seen unless there is a fracture. A fluid-fluid level may be seen on CT/MRI. Most spontaneously regress.

Practical tips
A detailed discussion of all the possible focal lucent bone lesions is beyond the scope of this case discussion and the reader is advised to consult the relevant chapter in one of the many excellent textbooks available. However, a few words of advice can be given on how to approach the problem and some basic guidelines regarding this case:
- Know the age of the patient (this may be obvious from the radiograph, for example if there are unfused epiphyses). Over the age of 40, metastases and myeloma become common and can show benign features so often end up high on the list of possibilities. Conversely, a young age immediately skews the differential towards benign pathology.
- Does the lesion have aggressive or nonaggressive features? Bear in mind that aggressive does not necessarily mean malignant as certain pathologies such as infection can look aggressive. Aggressive features include cortical destruction/breakthrough, the presence of lamellated, spiculated or 'hair on end' periosteal reaction and a wide zone of transition (i.e. poorly defined margins). Permeative lesions (multiple small holes with no perceptible border and a wide zone of transition) also tend to indicate malignancy. Shown as an example is the pelvic radiograph (**115d**) in an elderly female with metastases from breast carcinoma; these lytic deposits are affecting the majority of the right hemipelvis, the left ilium and both femoral necks. In fact, there is a pathological fracture of the left femoral neck. Note how the lesions have a wide zone of transition and evidence of cortical destruction with aggressive periosteal reaction, i.e. all the features of an aggressive pathology. This contrasts markedly with the nonaggressive features of the ABC (**115b**).

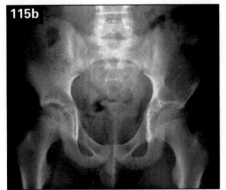

115b AP pelvis in a child with an aneurysmal bone cyst of the left iliac bone characteristically appearing as a lucent expansile lesion with a narrow zone of transition.

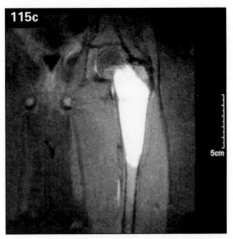

115c Sagittal T2 weighted MRI image shows a well defined high signal cystic lesion in the proximal left femur.

- Which bone is affected and is it epiphyseal, metaphyseal or diaphyseal? Certain pathologies tend to have characteristic locations.
- Differentiating SBC from ABC – both affect a similar age group and location and show benign features with possible expansion, cortical thinning and fluid levels on MRI. However, the SBC has a more central location within the affected bone, is less expansile and may show a pathognomonic 'fallen fragment'.
- GCT in the fused skeleton is subarticular and eccentric with no marginal sclerosis – when all these features are present in the correct age group, the diagnosis is clear.
- Infection can look aggressive or benign so is always worth bearing in mind depending on clinical history. Similarly, fibrous dysplasia has such varied appearances that it frequently enters the differential diagnosis for the focal benign bone lesion!

Further management
None is necessary. Most spontaneously regress with age. Pathological fractures commonly occur and may need fixation.

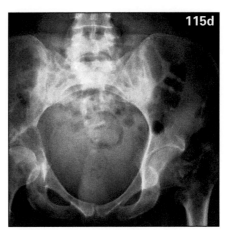

115d AP pelvis in a female with widespread lytic metastases and a pathological fracture of the left femoral neck. Note the cortical destruction and the wide zone of transition of the majority of the lesions.

CASE 116

History
A 40-year-old male patient with left hip pain.

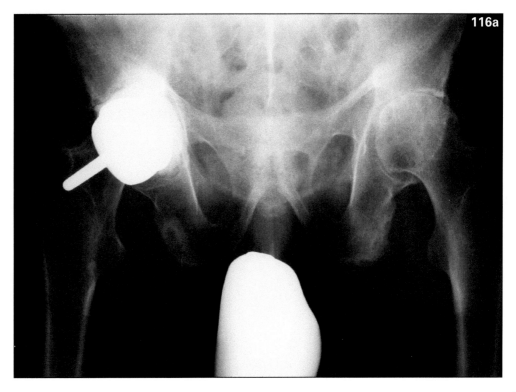

ANSWER 116

Observations (116a)
There is right femoral head resurfacing in this patient. Arthropathy of the left hip is seen with loss of joint space and subchondral cysts. Sacroiliac joints are not well demonstrated but there is the suspicion of fusion along with ossification in the midline along the interspinous ligaments. There is also arthropathy at the pubic symphysis and 'whiskering' at the ischial tuberosities in keeping with enthesopathy. The features are characteristic of ankylosing spondylitis.

Diagnosis
Ankylosing spondylitis.

Differential diagnosis
Of sacroiliitis on plain film:
- Ankylosing spondylitis.
- Inflammatory bowel disease.
- Hyperparathyroidism – tends to cause sacroiliac joint widening due to bone resorption.
- Rheumatoid.
- Gout.
- Psoriatic arthropathy.
- Reiter's syndrome.
- Osteoarthritis (OA).
- Infection – TB.

Discussion
Ankylosing spondylitis is an autoimmune seronegative arthropathy primarily affecting young males and predominantly involving the spine. Syndesmophyte formation and ossification of spinal ligaments leads to ankylosis and stiffness. Bilateral symmetrical sacroiliitis is seen and enthesopathy causes calcification at sites of ligamentous insertion, described on plain films as 'whiskering'. An early sign of the disease is inflammation at the site of attachment of the anterior longitudinal ligament to the vertebral bodies and discs giving rise to erosions at the anterior disco-vertebral margin. This finding is termed a Romanus lesion, examples of which are shown affecting the 3rd and 4th lumbar vertebrae in a young adult patient (116b).

The peripheral skeleton is affected in 20% of patients and commonly involves the hips. The disease is associated with ulcerative colitis, aortic insufficiency and apical lung fibrosis.

There are several causes of sacroiliitis, which can sometimes be differentiated by looking for ancillary signs and the degree of symmetry if bilateral. Generally, most causes are bilateral except for infection and OA. However, Reiter's and psoriasis in particular are more likely to be asymmetrically bilateral.

One final condition worth mentioning is osteitis condensans ilii, a chronic stress reaction occurring in young multiparous females, presumably due to pelvic instability. This produces focal sclerosis along the inferior margin of the joint on the iliac side only. The joint space itself is spared.

Practical tips
On the pelvic radiograph showing sacroiliitis:
- Unilateral disease – infection or OA.
- Bilateral but asymmetrical disease – consider Reiter's and psoriasis. Figure 116c shows a case of Reiter's with sacroiliitis worse on the left.

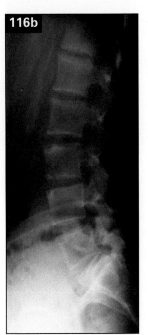

116b Lateral lumbar spine radiograph demonstrates lucent lesions of the anterosuperior aspects of the L3 and L4 vertebrae. These represent Romanus lesions in a young adult with early onset ankylosing spondylitis.

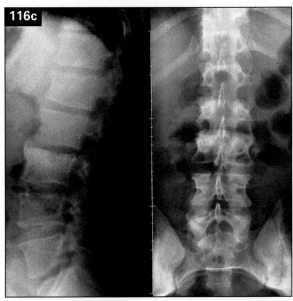

116c AP and lateral lumbar spine radiographs showing sacroiliitis worse on the left side with erosions and sclerosis.

- Bilateral symmetrical disease:
  - Spondylitis, syndesmophytes and periosteal 'whiskering' point to ankylosing spondylitis.
  - Look for bowel wall thickening or a stoma as a marker of inflammatory bowel disease (Figure 116d shows bilateral sacroiliitis and thickened distal sigmoid colon in a patient with ulcerative colitis).
  - A femoral haemodialysis line or peritoneal dialysis catheter may be present in patients with hyperparathyroidism secondary to renal failure.

- Iliac involvement only at the inferior joint margin in a female patient is osteitis condensans.

Further management
Treatment of ankylosing spondylitis is supportive, one in five patients progressing to significant disability. Ulcerative colitis and aortitis are associations. One per cent of patients develop upper zone lung fibrosis, which can be complicated by superinfection with aspergillus. Death may occur from cervical spine fracture or aortitis.

Further reading
Levine D, Forbat S, Saifuddin A (2004). MRI of the axial skeletal manifestations of ankylosing spondylitis. *Clinical Radiology* **59**: 400–413.

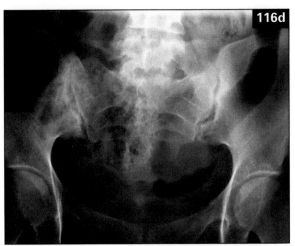

116d AP pelvis of a patient with ulcerative colitis. There is bilateral sacroiliitis with an oedematous thick walled sigmoid colon.

CASE 117

History
A 13-year-old male presented with pain in his left hip.

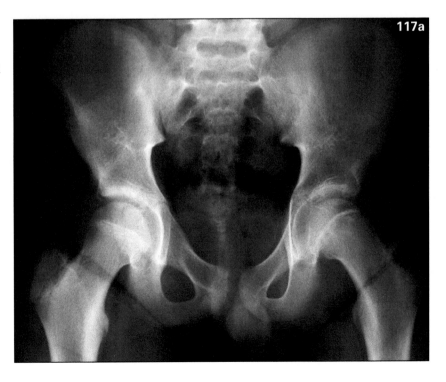

ANSWER 117

Observations (117a)
This AP radiograph in an unfused skeleton shows widening of the growth plate of the left hip with a slight decrease in height of the left femoral epiphysis compared to that on the right. Also, Klein's line does not intersect the femoral epiphysis on the left. The appearances are consistent with a slipped left upper femoral epiphysis. A frog lateral should be done to check if there is a subtle slip on the right.

Diagnosis
Slipped upper femoral epiphysis (SUFE).

Discussion
Atraumatic fracture through the hypertrophic zone of the physeal plate results in a slipped capital femoral epiphysis. It is the most common abnormality of the hip in adolescence with an incidence of 2 in 100,000. It is thought to occur due to widening of the epiphyseal plate during growth spurt with change in the orientation of the physis leading to an increase in shear forces. Affected patients tend to be overweight teenaged males. The mean age affected is 13 years for boys and 11 years for girls, corresponding to the growth spurts. The condition is associated with delayed skeletal maturation after adolescence and is bilateral in 20%. Hip pain is the most common presenting symptom with knee pain affecting a quarter of all cases.

Radiographs show:
- Apparent reduction in height of the femoral epiphysis.
- Irregularity of the growth plate.
- Klein's line does not intersect the femoral epiphysis.

The apparent reduction in epiphyseal height on the AP radiograph is due to the direction in which it slips, most commonly posteromedial. The line of Klein is drawn along the superior edge of the femoral neck and should intersect part of the epiphysis in a normal hip. Figure **117b** shows Klein's lines drawn on this child's film – note how the left line fails to intersect the epiphysis. These features may all be very subtle on the AP radiograph and therefore a frog lateral should always be performed when the diagnosis is suspected. The frog lateral will often accentuate the findings and may also confirm a subtle slip in the contralateral hip. The frog lateral in this case (**117c**) confirms the slip, which is more obvious than on the anteroposterior film.

Practical tips
When assessing radiographs of children's hips, the likely pathologies can be easily predicted from the child's age: 4–8 years – Perthe's; 8–17 years – SUFE.

Further management
If untreated, slipped capital femoral epiphysis can result in avascular necrosis (AVN) of the femoral head with consequent osteoarthritis, a debilitating condition when acquired at such a young age. The risk of AVN increases the larger the degree of slip and the longer the delay to surgery. It is therefore of paramount importance that it is not missed on imaging. Treatment involves pinning the epiphysis to the femoral neck, sometimes with osteotomy to correct any rotational deformity. Prophylactic pinning of the contralateral hip is often performed due to the risk of bilateral disease.

Further reading
Boles C, El-Khoury G (1997). Slipped capital femoral epiphysis. *RadioGraphics* **17(4)**: 809–823.

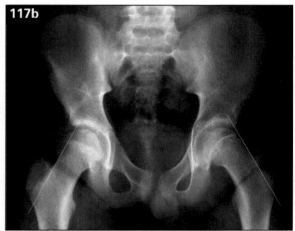

117b Pelvis radiograph shows Klein's lines drawn on it. The left line fails to intersect the epiphysis suggesting slip.

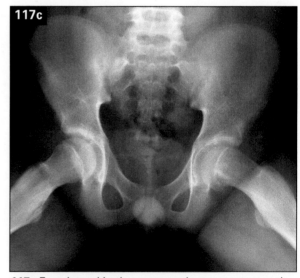

117c Frog lateral in the same patient accentuates the slipped left femoral epiphysis.

CASE 118

History
A male patient presented with pain in amputation stump.

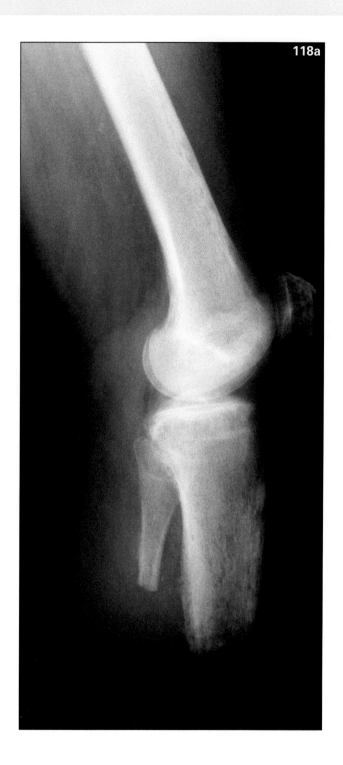

ANSWER 118

Observations (118a)
A below knee amputation has previously been performed. There is a permeative lucency with a wide zone of transition affecting the tibial stump. Periosteal reaction is visible along the posterior cortex and there is also a hint of this along the fibula. Furthermore, faint lucencies are suspected along the anterior cortex of the distal femur. These are the appearances of an aggressive lesion.

The reason for amputation and the time interval since have not been stated – this would help clarify the likely diagnosis. From the radiological findings alone, the main possibilities are that the amputation was for a distal malignancy such as bone lymphoma that has now recurred, or that the current findings are due to osteomyelitis in the stump following amputation for an unrelated reason. However, suspected involvement of the distal femur without joint destruction favours the former option.

Diagnosis
Lymphoma recurrence following amputation.

Differential diagnosis
Of permeative bone lesions:
- Metastases.
- Myeloma.
- Lymphoma.
- Leukaemia.
- Osteomyelitis.

Discussion
Another example of a lymphoma is seen affecting the right tibia of a patient in Figure 118b; a permeative lesion is present with evidence of cortical destruction.

Permeative bone destruction on radiography indicates the presence of aggressive pathology with rapid growth potential. The permeative lesion has a diffuse lytic 'moth eaten' appearance (118c). The zone of transition is wide, in other words the lesion is poorly demarcated and imperceptibly merges with uninvolved bone, unlike benign lesions where the zone of transition to normal bone is narrow. Periosteal reaction may or may not be present. The finding of a permeative lesion on imaging usually indicates malignant pathology; however, infection can produce the same appearance.

Practical tips
This is an example of a viva type film where there is no definite or 'spot' diagnosis to be made – it is simply a case of presenting a reasoned approach to a sensible differential diagnosis, then stating how this could be narrowed down using clinical information or further investigations.

Further management
Recurrence of lymphoma may entail further surgery and/or radiotherapy. MRI may be helpful to assess the local extent more accurately.

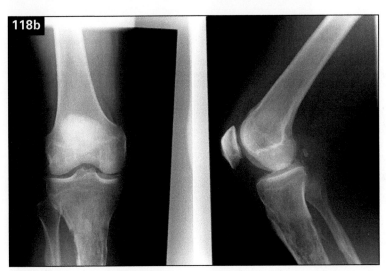

118b AP and lateral images of the tibia show a permeative lesion is present with evidence of cortical destruction.

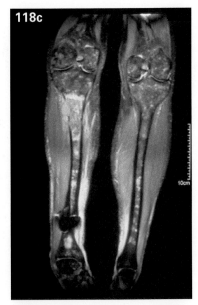

118c Fat Saturated coronal MRI image from the same patient as **118b** shows an aggressive lytic bone lesion with a wide zone of transition and permeative bone destruction breaching the cortex of the tibia.

CASE 119

History
A 4-year-old boy presented with a suspected chest infection.

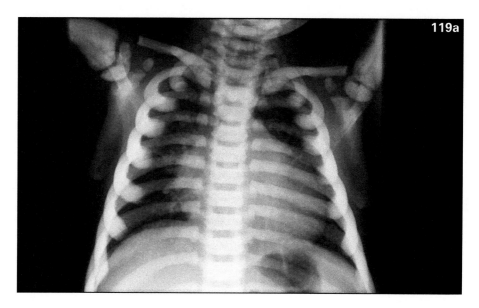

CASE 120

History
A 62-year-old female presented with neck pain.

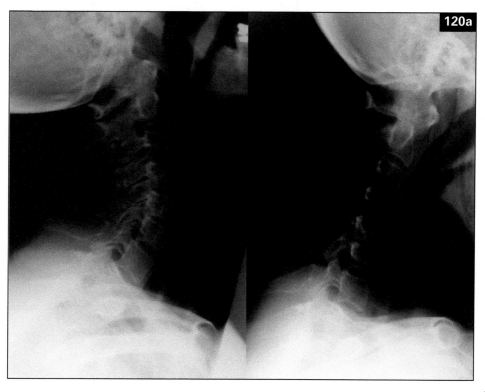

ANSWER 119

Observations (119a)
There is diffuse osteosclerosis of the visible skeleton. Subtle widening of the dia-metaphysis of the proximal humeri are noted, suggestive of Erlenmeyer flask deformity. There is no lung abnormality. The findings are consistent with osteopetrosis.

Diagnosis
Osteopetrosis.

Differential diagnosis
Of osteosclerosis in children:
- Osteopetrosis.
- Pyknodysostosis.
- Renal osteodystrophy.
- Hypervitaminosis D.
- Hypervitaminosis A.
- Fluorosis.

Of Erlenmeyer flask deformity (mnemonic – 'Lead GNOME'):
- Lead.
- Gaucher's.
- Niemann–Pick disease.
- Osteopetrosis.
- Metaphyseal dysplasia (Pyle's) and craniometaphyseal dysplasia (same as Pyle's disease but there is a history of cranial nerve palsies).
- 'E'matological!! – thalassaemia.

Discussion
Osteopetrosis (known as marble bone disease) is a rare hereditary disorder of defective osteoclast function with failure of proper reabsorption and remodelling leading to sclerotic and structurally brittle bones. In adults, the disease has an autosomal dominant inheritance and is asymptomatic in half of patients. Symptomatic patients have recurrent fractures and occasionally cranial nerve palsy due to narrowing of the neural foramina at the skull base (the calvaria is often spared). Erlenmeyer flask deformity of the long bones may be seen due to lack of tubulization. Erlenmeyer flask deformity is a descriptive term used to describe the distal expansion of long bones, particularly the femora, that is seen in a number of skeletal diseases (named after the wide-necked laboratory flask bearing the name of this German chemist). A radiograph of the right femur of the same 4-year-old boy (**119b**) shows the characteristic Erlenmeyer flask deformity with diffuse osteosclerosis. Other associated features on plain radiography include 'bone within bone' appearance and 'sandwich vertebrae' (sclerotic endplates). The infantile autosomal recessive form is the severe type associated with stillbirth whereas the adult type is associated with normal life expectancy.

Practical tips
For osteosclerosis in children:
- Erlenmeyer flask deformity, 'sandwich vertebrae' and 'bone within bone' appearance point to osteopetrosis.
- Pyknodysostosis is associated with multiple wormian bones. As with osteopetrosis, pathological fractures may be seen (**119c**). A hand radiograph in another

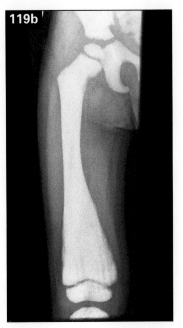

119b Radiograph of femur in same child shows diffuse osteosclerosis with widening of the distal femoral diametaphysis, i.e. Erlenmeyer flask deformity.

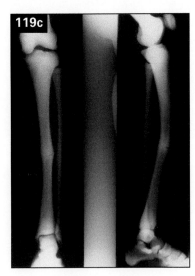

119c Diffuse osteosclerosis with a pathological fracture of the tibia in a patient with pyknodysostosis.

patient with pyknodysostosis (**119d**) demonstrates diffuse sclerosis with classical 'pointed chalk' terminal phalanges.
- Look for a haemodialysis line in renal osteodystrophy.
- Fluorosis (**119e**) is associated with ligamentous insertion calcification.

For Erlenmeyer flask deformity:
- Diffuse sclerosis indicates osteopetrosis.
- Pyle's disease will demonstrate sclerosis of the diaphysis and lucency of the widened metaphysis.
- Gaucher's disease will be associated with generalized osteopenia and pencil-thin cortices. There may also be signs of avascular necrosis of the femoral or humeral heads and massive hepatosplenomegaly may be seen on abdominal radiographs.
- Thalassaemia is associated with coarsened trabeculation producing a 'cobweb' appearance.
- Lead poisoning causes dense metaphyseal bands.

Further management
The only treatment available for osteopetrosis is bone marrow transplantation. Patients are more prone to fractures than the normal population.

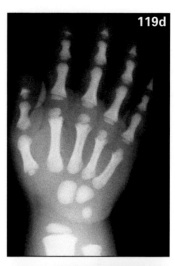

119d Pyknodysostosis hand showing osteosclerosis with pointing of the distal phalanges producing a 'pointed chalk' appearance.

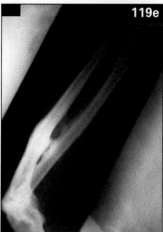

119e Forearm of a patient with fluorosis showing diffuse osteosclerosis and prominent ligamentous insertion calcification.

ANSWER 120

Observations (120a)
Lateral flexion and extension views of the cervical spine are shown. On flexion there is significant atlantoaxial joint subluxation. The odontoid peg is not clearly demarcated and is likely to be partially eroded. The remainder of the cervical spine is quite well preserved. The most likely diagnosis in a patient of this age is rheumatoid arthritis.

Diagnosis
Atlantoaxial subluxation in a patient with rheumatoid arthritis (RA).

Differential diagnosis
Of atlantoaxial subluxation:
- RA.
- Psoriatic arthropathy.
- Juvenile idiopathic arthritis.
- Ankylosing spondylitis.
- Systemic lupus erythematosus (SLE).
- Down's syndrome.
- Morquio's syndrome.
- Retropharyngeal abscess in a child.

Discussion
Atlantoaxial subluxation occurs when the distance between the posterior aspect of the arch of the atlas and the anterior aspect of the odontoid peg exceeds 3 mm in adults and 5 mm in children. Erosion and destruction of the odontoid peg may also be seen, particularly when the process is caused by an inflammatory arthropathy. Several causes are described in the differential diagnosis list but RA is the most common cause in adults. Synovitis with pannus formation causes erosion of the odontoid peg and atlantoaxial ligaments and consequent subluxation. This

(*cont.*)

can be more readily seen on MRI: a T1 weighted sagittal image (**120b**) shows synovial destruction of the odontoid peg and subluxation at midcervical spine level causing compromise to the spinal cord. Eventually 'cranial settling' can occur whereby the odontoid process can project into the skull base due to significant disease of the atlanto-occipital and atlantoaxial joints.

The hallmark of RA is bilateral symmetric arthropathy of more than three joints. Typically, the second and third metacarpophalangeal and the third proximal interphalangeal joints are involved early in the course of the disease. Bilateral and symmetric involvement of foot joints is another typical manifestation of RA (**120c**). The radiological features seen in RA affecting the extremities include:
- Periarticular soft tissue swelling.
- Periarticular osteoporosis.
- Marginal erosions.
- Ankylosis.
- Subluxation and dislocation.
- Subchondral cysts.
- Bilateral symmetrical distribution.
- Widening of joint space early on, with narrowing later in disease.
- Arthritis mutilans late in disease.

Practical tips
- Look for other signs of RA in the neck.
- Bamboo spine suggests ankylosing spondylitis.
- Posterior vertebral scalloping and anterior vertebral beaks in Morquio's.
- Soft tissue swelling in a child – consider abscess.

Further management
Clinical assessment and measurement of serum markers such as rheumatoid factor are required. To confirm the findings on plain radiography one might consider MRI of the cervical spine to assess the soft tissue component of the disease. Atlantoaxial subluxation may be managed surgically or conservatively with a stiff collar depending on the particular circumstances. The anaesthetist is often particularly interested in excluding this complication in rheumatoid patients as it presents an obvious hazard during preoperative airway intubation.

Further reading
Sommer O, Kladosek A, Weiler V, *et al.* (2005). Rheumatoid arthritis: a practical guide to state-of-the-art imaging, image interpretation, and clinical implications. *RadioGraphics* **25**: 381–398.

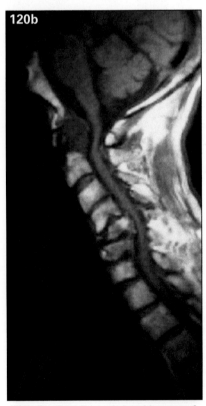

120b Sagittal T1 weighted image of the cervical spine showing erosion of the odontoid peg and subsequent atlantoaxial subluxation.

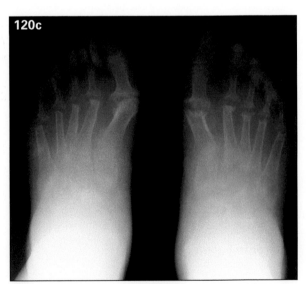

120c Radiograph of both feet of a rheumatoid patient.

CASE 121

History
A young Afro-Caribbean patient presented with left knee pain.

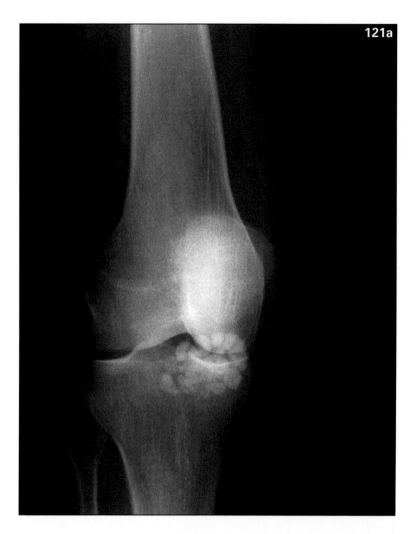

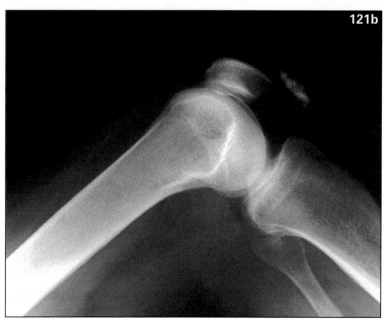

ANSWER 121

Observations (121a, 121b)
AP and lateral radiographs of the left knee show lobulated calcified masses in the soft tissues anterior to the left knee. Taking into consideration the age and ethnicity of the patient, tumoral calcinosis is the most likely diagnosis.

Diagnosis
Tumoral calcinosis.

Differential diagnosis
Of periarticular soft tissue calcification:
- Haematoma.
- Myositis ossificans.
- Crystal arthropathy.
- Scleroderma (121c – note the characteristic distal tuft resorption in the index finger).
- Dermatomyositis.
- Synovial osteochondromatosis.
- Tumoral calcinosis.
- Synovial sarcoma (121d, 121e, 121f, 121g).

Discussion
Tumoral calcinosis is a rare, benign condition characterized by the presence of progressively enlarging periarticular calcified soft tissue masses. It usually affects young black patients and there is a familial tendency. The masses may cause pain and limitation of movement, with overlying skin ulceration and the development of a sinus tract draining chalky fluid. In fact, the masses may contain fluid-fluid levels on imaging that have a milk of calcium consistency. The periarticular region of the hip is the most commonly affected site. The masses can grow to a very large size and there is a tendency for recurrence if the lesions are not completely excised.

Practical tips
The radiological appearances of the varying causes of periarticular calcification can be quite different:
- Tumoral calcinosis – lobulated dense masses, fluid-fluid levels.
- Myositis ossificans and synovial sarcoma may look similar but without fluid levels.
- Dermatomyositis – sheets of calcification.
- Synovial osteochondromatosis – several foci of calcification with lucent centres that are essentially loose bodies within the joint.

Further management
Patients with tumoral calcinosis are usually treated with phosphate depletion. Surgical excision is also a treatment option but needs to be meticulous as recurrence often occurs with incomplete excision.

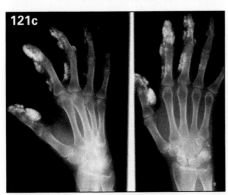

121c Radiograph of the hand in a female adult with scleroderma shows the typical soft tissue calcification. Note the distal tuft resorption affecting the index finger, which is characteristically seen in this condition.

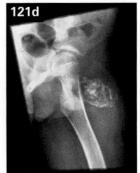

121d Radiograph of the left hip of a child with periarticular calcification arising from a synovial sarcoma.

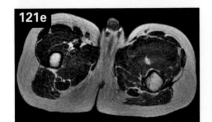
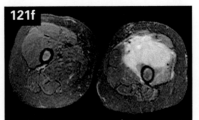
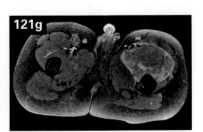

121e, 121f, 121g Axial T1, T2 and fat saturated images of the synovial sarcoma shows a fairly well defined soft tissue lesion which is of low signal on T1 and inhomogeneously high signal on T2.

CASE 122

History
A 40-year-old presented with knee discomfort.

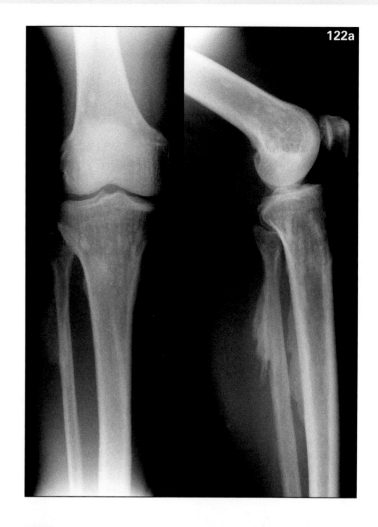

CASE 123

History
Male patient presented with rigidity and kyphosis.

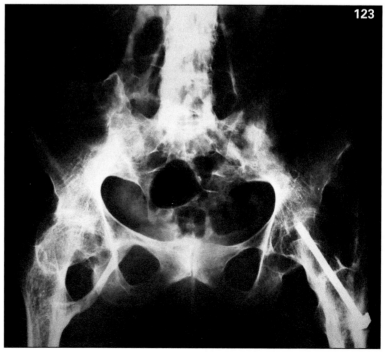

ANSWER 122

Observations (122a)
AP and lateral radiographs of the right knee and upper tibia and fibula demonstrate marked cortical thickening of the diaphyses of the tibia and fibula, which has the appearance of 'dripping candle wax'. This is typical of melorheostosis. There are also multiple small sclerotic foci within the metadiaphysis of the distal femur and the proximal tibia, which have the appearance of osteopoikilosis.

Diagnosis
Melorheostosis and osteopoikilosis.

Differential diagnosis
Sclerotic metastases in a patient with melorheostosis; this is much less likely. However in patients with multiple sclerotic foci alone, sclerotic metastases must always be considered.

Discussion
Melorheostosis is a nonhereditary disease of unknown aetiology that often presents as an incidental finding. It is usually discovered in childhood where it has a rapid progression, but it occasionally presents in adults where it has a slow chronic course. The limb involved often demonstrates joint pain, swelling and limitation of movement. Males and females are equally affected.

Radiological signs of melorheostosis are as follows:
- Cortical hyperostosis in one or multiple tubular bones with streaks of sclerosis beginning at the proximal end of the bone and extending distally. This produces the characteristic 'dripping candle wax' appearance. This is shown particularly well in Figure **122b**, where the right humerus and scapula are affected in another patient.
- Predominantly affects the diaphysis of the bone.
- The lower extremities are more commonly affected than the upper.
- Although a single bone may be involved, contiguous bones of an extremity are more often affected.
- Bilateral signs are extremely rare and should prompt consideration of other causes of sclerosis.
- Limb length discrepancy is also a feature and the sclerosis may cross the joint and result in joint fusion.

The skull, spine and ribs are rarely involved. Melorheostosis is associated with osteopoikilosis, osteopathia striata (asymptomatic disease consisting of longitudinal striations along the metaphyses of long bones) and arteriovenous malformations.

Osteopoikilosis is an autosomal dominant disorder that is more common in males. It is asymptomatic and consists of multiple ovoid bone islands parallel to the long axis of the bone. These bone islands normally measure 2–10 mm and are found at the metaphysis and epiphysis, rarely extending into the midshaft. It usually affects the pelvis, wrist and ankle and rarely affects the skull, ribs and mandible. The differential diagnosis of this condition, which often leads to clinical confusion and concern, is disseminated sclerotic metastases.

Practical tips
Osteopoikilosis tends to be distributed around joints, whereas multiple sclerotic metastases will not be so confined.

Further management
No further management is normally necessary. Both these conditions are usually found incidentally. The main thing is to ensure that a patient with multiple sclerotic lesions has osteopoikilosis and not sclerotic metastases.

Further reading
Levine S, Lambiase R, Petchprapa C (2003). Cortical lesions of the tibia: characteristic appearances at conventional radiography. *RadioGraphics* **23**: 157–177.

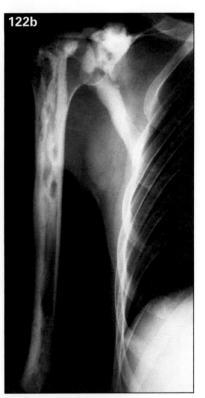

122b AP radiograph of melorheostosis affecting the humerus and scapula demonstrating the typical 'dripping candle wax' appearance.

ANSWER 123

Observations (123)
This AP radiograph of the pelvis reveals thick linear columns of calcification and ossification around both hips and in the paravertebral regions bilaterally. The hip joints, sacroiliac joints and spine are fused. The patient has had previous internal fixation of the left hip. The appearances are in keeping with myositis ossificans progressiva.

Diagnosis
Myositis ossificans progressiva.

Discussion
This is an 'Aunt Minnie'. Myositis ossificans progressiva is also known as fibrodysplasia ossificans progressiva. It is a rare slowly progressive disease characterized by exacerbations and remissions of fibroblastic proliferation leading to ossification and calcification of skeletal muscle, subcutaneous fat, tendons and ligaments.
Radiological features are:
- Linear columns of ossification and calcification.
- Ossified bridges between different bones.
- Ankylosis.
- Kyphosis – due to rigidity of the muscles of the spine and upper limbs.

Half of patients present by the age of 2 years. Initially subcutaneous painful masses develop in the neck and upper limbs, which may ulcerate and bleed. Eventually there is progressive involvement of the remaining musculature, including that of the pelvis and lower extremities. Torticollis also occurs due to restriction of the sternocleidomastoid muscles.

Ankylosis and limitation of movement progress and the patient gradually becomes a 'stone person'. Eventually, respiratory failure develops due to calcification of the thoracic muscles. Skeletal anomalies are associated with this condition including microdactyly of the big toes and thumbs and shortening of the first metatarsal with hallux valgus deformity. Some patients may have a shallow acetabulum with shortening and widening of the femoral necks. Fusion of the middle ear ossicles may lead to conductive hearing loss.

Practical tips
Ossified bars and bridges between bones are the hallmark of this rare condition.

Further management
Treatment is supportive. Attempts at surgery to relieve rigidity have led to accelerated ossification at the surgical site.

CASE 124

History
A child presented with retarded growth.

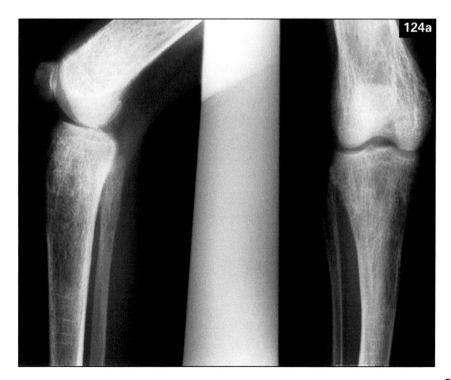

ANSWER 124

Observations (124a)
There is diffuse, coarse trabeculation of the visible bones causing a 'cobweb-like' appearance. Erlenmeyer flask deformity of the distal femurs is present. The features are in keeping with thalassaemia major.

Diagnosis
Thalassaemia major.

Discussion
Thalassaemia is an inherited disorder of haemoglobin synthesis characteristically seen in Mediterranean patients. The homozygous form, thalassaemia major, is more severe. The radiological signs result from marrow hyperplasia and expansion due to extramedullary haematopoiesis. Every part of the skeleton may be affected in patients with untreated disease. Radiological features of the complications of treatment such as recurrent transfusions and iron chelation therapy may also be seen. In fact, abnormalities secondary to iron chelation therapy are now more common than those due to marrow hyperplasia.

The radiological signs to look for depend on the site of the body imaged:
- Peripheral skeleton:
  - Coarse trabeculation causing 'cobweb' appearance (**124a**).
  - Loss of concavity of tubular bones (**124a**).
  - Erlenmeyer flask deformity of metaphyses of long bones (**124a**).
  - Arthropathy and chondrocalcinosis as a result of haemochromatosis secondary to hypertransfusion.
  - Fraying of metaphyses and dense metaphyseal bands secondary to iron chelation therapy.

- Skull:
  - 'Hair on end' appearance.
  - Frontal bossing (**124b**) due to diploic expansion.
  - Obliteration of paranasal sinuses (except for ethmoid sinuses) due to marrow hyperplasia (**124b**).

- Axial skeleton:
  - Coarse trabeculation causing 'cobweb' appearance (**124c**).
  - Biconcave vertebrae.
  - 'Bone within bone' appearance of spine and ribs.
  - Paraspinal masses (due to extramedullary haematopoiesis).
  - Expansion of the ribs posteriorly, particularly at the costochondral junctions, due to marrow hyperplasia (**124c**).

Practical tips
- The only sign may be a diffuse but subtle coarsening of the bony trabeculae.
- On an AXR look for evidence of hepatosplenomegaly (a result of extramedullary haematopoiesis) and gallstones.
- On a CXR look for cardiomegaly secondary to anaemia, as well as a paraspinal mass due to extramedullary haematopoiesis.

Further management
Death usually occurs within the first decade. Treatment is by multiple transfusions, however as explained in the discussion this too leads to skeletal abnormalities.

Further reading
Tyler P, Madani G, Chaudhuri R, et al. (2006). The radiological appearances of thalassaemia. *Clinical Radiology* **61(1)**: 40–52.

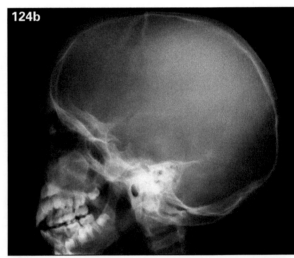

124b Lateral radiograph of a child with thalassaemia; there is frontal bossing with expansion of the diploic space and obliteration of the maxillary sinuses.

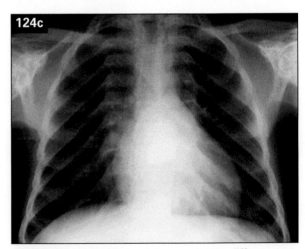

124c Radiograph of chest demonstrates diffuse coarse trabeculation producing a 'cobweb' appearance with expansion of the ribs due to marrow hyperplasia.

CASE 125

History
A 10-year-old child presented with leg pain and fever.

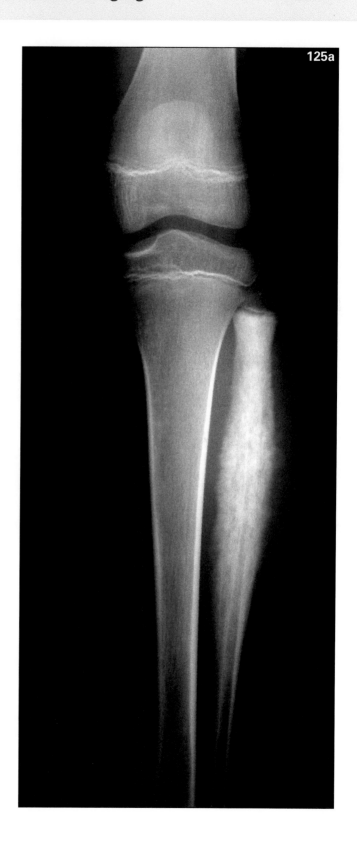

ANSWER 125

Observations (125a)
There is a mostly sclerotic lesion arising in the diaphysis of the proximal fibula in this unfused skeleton. This has a wide zone of transition and demonstrates a florid 'hair on end' periosteal reaction. The features are in keeping with an aggressive lesion. Ewing's sarcoma and osteosarcoma are the two main differential diagnoses and the patient should be referred urgently to a specialist unit.

Diagnosis
Ewing's sarcoma.

Differential diagnosis
Osteosarcoma.

Discussion
Ewing's sarcoma is the most common malignant bone tumour in children, with a peak age of 15 years. Most patients (96%) are Caucasian with a male to female ratio of 1:2. These are round cell tumours and are clinically, radiologically and histologically very similar to primitive neuroectodermal tumours (PNET). Patients present clinically with severe pain that may be associated with a soft tissue mass. Fever and leukocytosis are also features. Long bones are affected in the majority of cases and this usually affects the diaphysis of the bone rather than the metaphysis (which is the more common site of involvement for osteosarcoma). Flat bones such as the pelvis and ribs are affected in 40% of cases and this is predominantly seen in older patients, whereas younger patients tend to present with long bone lesions. In most cases the lesion is lytic rather than dense and there is often a permeative 'moth eaten' appearance. Invasion into local soft tissues is seen in up to a half of cases and there is usually an aggressive periosteal reaction causing a 'sunburst' or 'hair on end' appearance. A Codman's triangle may also be seen.

These features can all be seen in osteosarcoma and sometimes it can be difficult to differentiate the two conditions radiologically. A radiograph of the right femur and knee in a 12-year-old boy with osteosarcoma is shown (**125b**). This can be seen as a sclerotic density with a wide zone of transition in the metadiaphysis of the distal femur, with aggressive periosteal reaction. Overall, the appearances are quite similar to those seen in Figure **125a** and both diseases have a similar 60–80% 5 year survival rate. The practical tips section below lists some features that may help differentiate the two.

Practical tips
- In assessing focal bone lesions, the first concern is whether the lesion is benign or aggressive (note that aggressive lesions are not necessarily malignant – infection, for example, can cause aggressive appearances). One of the most important factors is the clarity and extent of the margin between the lesion and adjacent normal bone, the so-called 'zone of transition'. A wide zone of transition indicates an indistinct and extended junction between lesion and normal bone, and is a hallmark of the aggressive lesion. Conversely, benign lesions show a narrow zone of transition. The presence and type of periosteal reaction are other important features to assess. Aggressive lesions more commonly show periosteal reaction, which may be irregular, lamellated or spiculated. Codman's triangle is the term applied to the elevated corner of periosteum at the margins of the periosteal reaction, and is frequently seen in malignancy. Cortical destruction is another sign of the aggressive lesion, though one can see cortical thinning and pathological fracture through benign bone lesions.
- The other two important factors in establishing a diagnosis in the focal bone lesion are the patient's age and the location of the lesion. Location includes not only which bone, but whether the lesion is epiphyseal, metaphyseal or diaphyseal. A comprehensive discussion of the distribution of benign and aggressive lesions by age and location is beyond the scope of this case discussion, but an appreciation is vital in establishing a meaningful differential diagnosis.

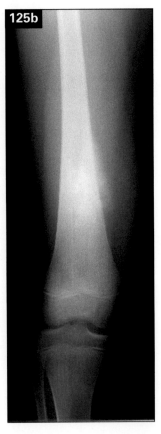

125b AP knee radiograph in a 12-year-old child demonstrates a sclerotic lesion of the femoral metaphysis that has a wide zone of transition and aggressive periosteal reaction. This proved to be an osteosarcoma.

- To summarize the approach to the focal bone lesion, ask yourself:
    - Is it benign or aggressive?
    - Diaphysis, metaphysis or epiphysis?
    - How old is the patient?

- In the young patient with an aggressive lesion such as those illustrated, the two main primary tumours to consider are Ewing's and osteosarcoma. The two can be difficult to differentiate radiologically, and can also cause similar clinical features such as fever and leukocytosis. The features shown in *Table 2* may help, though none are pathognomonic.

Further management
MRI is helpful in assessing local spread and aids planning of surgical resection.

Further reading
Murphey M, Robbin M, McRae G, *et al.* (1997). The many faces of osteosarcoma. *RadioGraphics* **17**: 1205–1231.

Table 2 *Differentiating features of Ewing's sarcoma and osteosarcoma*

	Ewing's sarcoma	Osteosarcoma
Age	Children	Older children and young adults
Location	More common in diaphysis	More common in metaphysis
Appearance	More commonly lucent or permeative	More commonly sclerotic
Metastases	To bone	To lung

CASE 126

History
A 35-year-old male presented with shoulder pain.

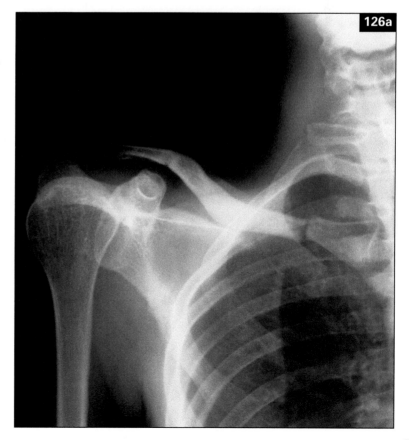

ANSWER 126

Observations (126a)
There is a transverse fracture at the medial third of the clavicle, which is likely to be an insufficiency fracture as there are Looser zones at the lateral aspect of the clavicle and the lateral border of the body of the scapula. The bones are generally osteopenic with marked thinning of the cortices. The findings are consistent with a diagnosis of osteomalacia.

Diagnosis
Osteomalacia.

Discussion
Osteomalacia is a disorder of insufficient osteoid mineralization causing bone softening. Aetiology can be due to dietary deficiency, decreased absorption or deficient metabolism of vitamin D.

Radiological features of osteomalacia include:
- Generalized osteopenia.
- Cortical thinning.
- Bowing of long bones.
- Protrusio acetabuli.
- Coarse trabecular pattern (**126b**).
- Looser zones:
  - Pseudofractures that consist of transverse lucent clefts with sclerotic margins.
  - These are mostly seen in the pelvis, femoral necks (**126c**) and scapula.
- Insufficiency fractures.

Practical tips
Osteomalacia is related to renal failure and secondary hyperparathyroidism therefore:
- On an abdominal radiograph look for a peritoneal dialysis catheter or a tunnelled femoral haemodialysis line.
- On a chest radiograph look for a central haemodialysis line and eroded lateral clavicles.
- Prominent vascular and soft tissue calcification may be seen.
- Brown tumours may be present and appear as lytic lesions, which may also be associated with pathological fracture.

Further management
Treatment involves reversing the cause of vitamin D deficiency.

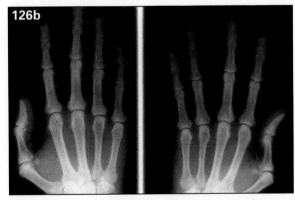

126b Radiograph of both hands in a patient with osteomalacia demonstrates diffusely coarsened trabecular pattern.

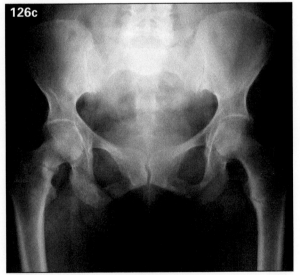

126c AP pelvic radiograph with Looser zones in both proximal femora.

CASE 127

History
A 5-year-old child presented with marked bowing deformity of right leg.

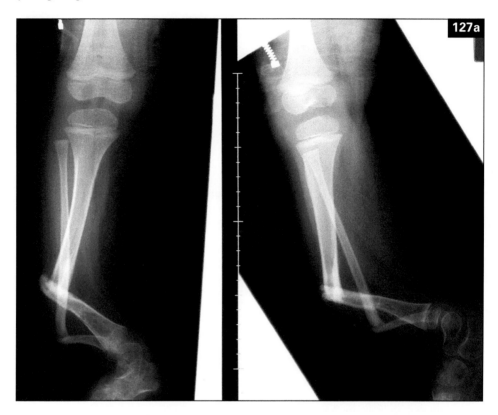

CASE 128

History
A young adult with nail abnormalities.

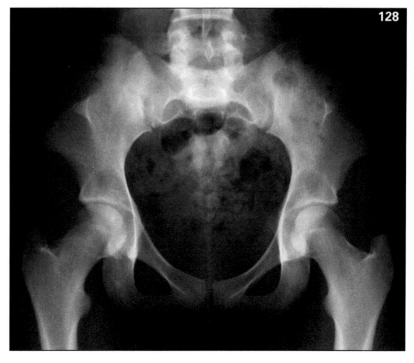

ANSWER 127

Observations (127a)
There is marked angulation deformity of the diaphyses of the lower tibia and fibula with the formation of pseudarthroses. The bones are also generally osteopenic. The most likely diagnoses are nonunion of previous fractures, neurofibromatosis or osteogenesis imperfecta.

Diagnosis
Neurofibromatosis.

Differential diagnosis
- Nonunion of a fracture.
- Osteogenesis imperfecta.
- Fibrous dysplasia.
- Congenital.

Discussion
Congenital – affects the middle to lower third of the tibia and fibula. Half of congenital pseudarthroses present in the first year of life and later on there may be cupping of the proximal bone end and pointing of the distal bone end.

Neurofibromatosis type 1 (NF1) is a common genetic disorder and in addition to cutaneous and neurological abnormalities, osseous lesions are also seen. There may be anterolateral bowing of the tibia with or without a hypoplastic fibula. Focal narrowing and intramedullary sclerosis or cystic change at the apex of the angulation is due to hamartomatous fibrous tissue, typically at the junction of the middle and distal third of tibia. Pathological fracture with nonunion often results in pseudarthrosis of the tibia and fibula, with 'pencil pointing' of the bone fragments. Prophylactic bracing of limbs with bowing deformity may prevent the development of pseudarthrosis. Osteotomy with bone grafting and pinning (127b) is the treatment of choice if the pseudarthrosis has already occurred.

Osteogenesis imperfecta – all four types can result in bowing of the long bones due to bone softening and multiple fractures. Bowing typically involves all the long bones and can result in pseudarthroses. Again osteotomies and pinning are the preferred treatment although bisphosphonates have been shown to produce some success.

Cleidocranial dysplasia is associated with congenital pseudarthrosis of the femur.

Ankylosing spondylitis can lead to pseudarthrosis in the spine.

Practical tips
- Severe osteopenia and multiple fractures of differing ages that have exuberant callus formation suggest osteogenesis imperfecta. Remember that some osteopenia may result from disuse, however, e.g. in fracture nonunion.
- Look for soft tissue nodules indicative of neurofibromatosis.
- A 'ground glass' density lesion associated with the pseudarthrosis is suggestive of fibrous dysplasia.

Further management
As in this case, osteotomy with bone grafting and pinning is the treatment of choice.

Further reading
Cheema J, Grissom L, Harcke H (2003). Radiographic characteristics of lower-extremity bowing in children. *RadioGraphics* **23**: 871–880.

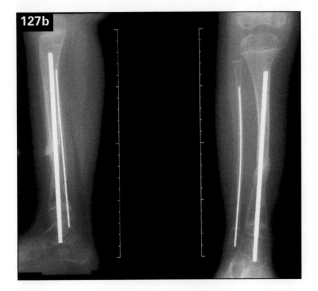

127b Radiograph of the same patient postfixation with pins.

ANSWER 128

Observations (128)
There are bilateral posterior iliac horns consistent with Fong's disease.

Diagnosis
Fong's disease.

Discussion
This case is an 'Aunt Minnie'. Fong's disease, also known as nail–patella syndrome and osteo-onychodysplasia, is a rare autosomal dominant disorder characterized by symmetrical ectodermal and mesodermal anomalies. Patients tend to present with abnormalities of nail dysplasia that can manifest as spooning and splitting of the fingernails or even hypoplasia or aplasia. This particularly affects the thumb and index fingernails. Patients may also have abnormal pigmentation of the iris.

The presence of bilateral posterior iliac horns is seen in 80% of cases and is diagnostic of the condition. Hypoplasia of the anterior half of the ilia can result in drooping of the iliac crests. The other major finding is aplasia or hypoplasia of the patellae, which frequently results in recurrent lateral dislocations. Hypoplasia of the capitellum and radial head may also be present and this can lead to an increase in the carrying angle at the elbow. Similarly, genu valgus can occur due to asymmetrical development of the femoral condyles. Some patients may have a short 5th metacarpal.

Practical tips
- Look for a peritoneal dialysis catheter or femoral tunnelled dialysis line on the pelvic radiograph, as these patients may have renal failure.
- If the knees are included on the radiograph, look for hypoplastic or absent patellae and genu valgus deformity.

Further management
The most serious association of this condition is renal dysfunction, which occurs secondary to abnormality of the glomerular basement membrane leading to proteinuria, haematuria and renal failure. The exact mechanism for this is unknown, but renal failure tends to occur in later life. This is an important point to note when diagnosis of this condition is made, often incidentally.

CASE 129

History
A patient presented with head injury.

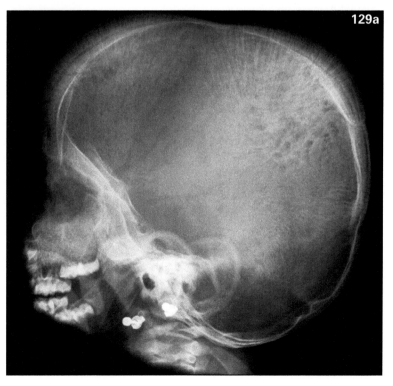

ANSWER 129

Observations (129a)
There is a 'hair on end' appearance to the skull vault and the diploic space is widened. This does not affect the calvaria below the level of the internal occipital protuberance. The maxillary sinuses are obliterated. The most likely cause is thalassaemia major.

Diagnosis
Thalassaemia major.

Differential diagnosis
Of 'hair on end' appearance of skull:
The mnemonic is 'STAN' and is easy to remember when you think of Stan Laurel's hair!
- Sickle cell disease.
- Thalassaemia major.
- Anaemia (other anaemias):
  - Hereditary spherocytosis.
  - Glucose-6-phosphate dehydrogenase deficiency.
  - Severe iron deficiency anaemia.

- Neoplastic:
  - Haemangioma (**129b**).
  - Neuroblastoma metastases in children.

Discussion
The 'hair on end' sign is a finding that can be seen in the diploic space of the skull on radiographs, CT and MRI, and has the appearance of long, thin, vertical striations. On plain radiographs and CT the appearance is caused by alternating thickened trabeculae and radiolucent marrow hyperplasia. On MRI, the alternating bands of hypointense trabeculae and hyperintense marrow produce the distinct striated pattern. Essentially the effect is due to marrow hyperplasia. The diploic space widens and the outer table thins and can become obliterated. With regard to anaemic causes, the marrow hyperplasia begins in the frontal region and can affect the entire calvaria excluding that which is below the internal occipital protuberance, since there is no marrow in this area. Marrow hyperplasia in thalassaemia major is more marked than in any other anaemia and may cause hyperplasia of the facial bones resulting in obliteration of the paranasal sinuses. However the ethmoid sinuses are spared as they do not contain marrow. The 'hair on end' appearance can also be seen in severe childhood cases of iron deficiency anaemia.

The medical literature is split as to whether the 'hair on end' appearance may be reversed following treatment of the anaemia. Some authors have reported that resolution of the appearance occurs with treatment, although the diploic space may remain wider than normal. However others have reported that the appearances persist without regression even over a follow-up period of approximately 20 years.

Practical tips
- Thalassaemia major and sickle cell disease are the most common causes of 'hair on end' skull. To differentiate the two look at the maxillary sinuses – if they are obliterated this suggests thalassaemia. This does not occur in sickle cell disease.
- Is the appearance diffuse or localized? If localized consider neoplastic causes such as haemangioma (**129b**).
- Haemangioma tends to have a 'corduroy' appearance, i.e. thickened and coarsened rather than thin vertical trabeculation due to vascular channels. This is well demonstrated in Figure **129b**.

Further management
Thalassaemia major has a poor prognosis with most affected children not surviving past the first decade. Treatment is by repeated transfusions.

Further reading
Hollar M (2001). The hair-on-end sign. *Radiology* **221**: 347–348.

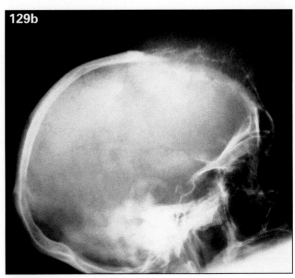

129b The trabeculations here are thickened and coarsened rather than thin, vertical trabeculations. Haemangioma tends to have this appearance.

CASE 130

History
A 45-year-old male presented with left sided chest pain for several weeks. He had suffered minor trauma to the arm.

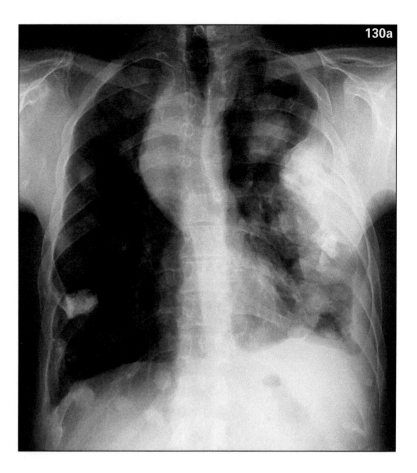

CASE 131

History
A 20-year-old male presented with knee pain.

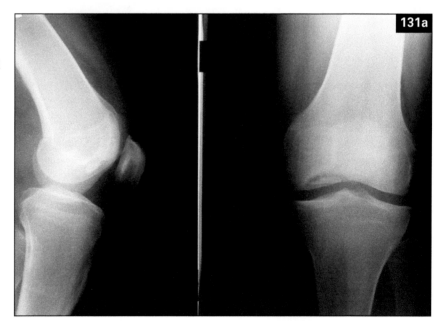

ANSWER 130

Observations (130a)
Multiple bony exostoses are seen arising from the ribs on both sides of the chest. On the left, there is a large associated soft tissue mass projected over the lateral thorax. Given the history of chest pain, sarcomatous transformation must be suspected. Moreover, there is a small left pleural reaction, a large pulmonary nodule in the left upper zone and possible pulmonary nodules in the left lower zone and right costophrenic recess.

The combination of findings suggests sarcomatous transformation in diaphyseal aclasis with pulmonary metastases.

Diagnosis
Diaphyseal aclasis with sarcomatous transformation.

Discussion
Diaphyseal aclasis is an autosomal dominant condition characterized by multiple exostoses (osteochondromas). Osteochondromas are benign cartilaginous tumours. Diaphyseal aclasis is usually discovered in childhood and short stature may occur due to the development of exostoses at the expense of normal bone growth. The exostoses are usually multiple and bilateral and mostly affect the limbs though ribs can be affected, as in this case. The exostoses point away from the nearest joint, as illustrated in image **130b**. A pseudo-Madelung deformity may develop (**130b**), where there is ulnar shortening with bowing of the radius, and ulnar tilt of the distal radial articular surface.

In fewer than 5% of patients, malignant transformation into chondrosarcoma or osteosarcoma can occur. A further example is shown (**130c**) where a patient with diaphyseal aclasis developed a chondrosarcoma affecting the femur. The exostoses may also cause neurological compromise due to nerve compression or entrapment.

Practical tips
- 'Diaphyseal' aclasis is a misnomer as the exostoses arise from the metaphyses.
- They are often multiple and bilateral and point away from the nearest joint.
- The cartilage cap of the exostosis may be calcified.

Further management
In cases of nerve entrapment, surgical excision may be possible. The crucial factor is to identify malignant degeneration when it occurs; suspicious signs include pain and growth of an exostosis after physeal closure and thickening of the cartilaginous cap by greater than 1.5 cm. This is best delineated on MRI.

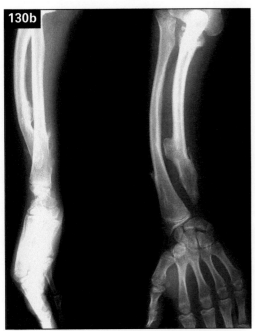

130b AP and lateral radiographs of the ulna demonstrate multiple exostoses. Note how they point away from the joint.

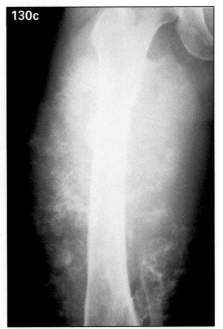

130c AP of right femur demonstrates extensive flocculent calcification in a huge chondrosarcoma, which arose from the exostosis at the medial femoral condyle.

ANSWER 131

Observations (131a)
AP and lateral radiographs of the left knee reveal a well defined defect in the lateral aspect of the medial femoral condyle. A separate bony fragment lies within the defect. Findings are those of osteochondritis dissecans.

Diagnosis
Osteochondritis dissecans.

Differential diagnosis
Spontaneous osteonecrosis.

Discussion
Osteochondritis dissecans is synonymous with osteochondrosis dissecans and osteochondral fracture (**131b**). The cardinal feature is fragmentation of a portion of the articular cartilage and underlying bone, which may separate to form a loose body within the joint. It is thought to occur due to subchondral fatigue fracture as a result of shearing from rotatory impaction forces. Though sometimes asymptomatic, presentation is often with pain aggravated by movement and/or limited movement.

Patients are most commonly affected in adolescence with males affected more than females. The typical location of osteochondritis dissecans at the knee is the **L**ateral **A**spect of **M**edial femoral **E**picondyle (usefully remembered by the 'LAME' mnemonic). The condition can be bilateral in up to 30% of cases. Other commonly affected sites include the humeral head, capitellum and talus. MRI is useful in determining whether the osteochondral fragment is loose as evidenced by a rim of fluid around it on T2 weighted images or a rim of contrast around it on MRI arthrography.

Practical tips
- In the adolescent knee with symptoms but no obvious abnormality on first inspection, check for the subtle osteochondral defect. The 'LAME' mnemonic identifies the classical location.
- When identified, check for radiological evidence of joint effusion and loose bodies.
- Suggest MRI for further evaluation.

Further management
Identification and treatment are important to prevent the development of osteoarthritis. Arthroscopy and removal or pinning of the detached fragment is the treatment of choice when conservative management with rest and NSAIDs fails.

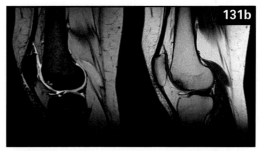

131b T1 and T2 weighted sagittal MRI images of the knee show a traumatic osteochondral fracture in the anterior aspect of the lateral femoral condyle

---

CASE 132

History
A middle aged female presented with painful hands.

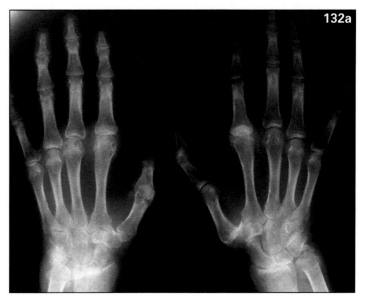

ANSWER 132

Observations (132a)
This radiograph of both hands reveals soft tissue swelling at the metacarpophalangeal joints bilaterally and to a lesser extent at the proximal interphalangeal joints. This is not associated with any erosions, however there is subluxation of several joints including the metacarpophalangeal joint of the right index finger and the right first carpometacarpal joint. Degenerative changes are also noted at both wrists. In summary, there is a bilateral nonerosive arthropathy with evidence of joint subluxation. The differential diagnosis includes collagen vascular disease. Early rheumatoid arthritis should also be considered.

Diagnosis
Systemic lupus erythematosus (SLE).

Differential diagnosis
Of nonerosive deforming arthropathy:
- Collagen vascular disease.
  - SLE.
  - Ehlers–Danlos syndrome.
  - Scleroderma.
- Jaccoud's arthropathy.
- Hypogammaglobulinaemia.

Discussion
Over 90% of patients with SLE develop arthralgia. Nonerosive arthropathy is characteristically present, the main features of which are soft tissue swelling and joint subluxation. In particular, the subluxation affects the first carpometacarpal joints and also the metacarpophalangeal joints leading to ulnar deviation of the fingers. The distribution is often bilateral and symmetrical but the main factor excluding rheumatoid arthritis is of course the absence of erosions. Several different diseases may cause similar appearances as outlined in the differential diagnosis. Soft tissue calcification may be seen with scleroderma and Ehlers–Danlos syndrome. Jaccoud's arthritis is a rare, nonerosive arthropathy affecting the hands and feet of patients following rheumatic valve disease. Figure **132b** shows an example of this demonstrating characteristic subluxation at the metacarpophalangeal joints producing ulnar deviation of the digits. There is also subluxation at the first carpometacarpal joint. Note the absence of erosions.

Practical tips
- The only finding with the nonerosive arthropathies may be periarticular soft tissue swelling in the early stages.
- Subluxation of joints is the major finding and this mostly affects the metacarpophalangeal and first carpometacarpal joints bilaterally.
- The appearances tend to be bilateral and symmetrical.
- Scleroderma (**132c**) and Ehlers–Danlos syndrome may be associated with soft tissue calcification on the hand radiograph.

Further management
SLE is, as its name suggests, a systemic disease and although patients can expect a long life death eventually occurs from renal failure or cardiomyopathy. Treatment is supportive with the aim of suppressing the autoimmune element of the disease.

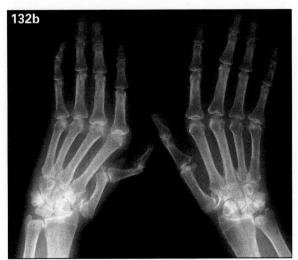

132b Radiograph of both hands in a patient with Jaccoud's arthropathy demonstrating bilateral metacarpophalangeal joint subluxation.

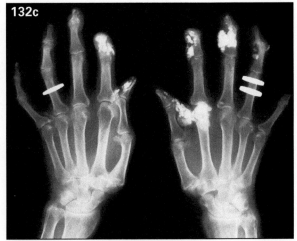

132c Radiograph of both hands in a patient with scleroderma demonstrating florid soft tissue calcification.

CASE 133

History
A 15-year-old male presented with left shoulder pain.

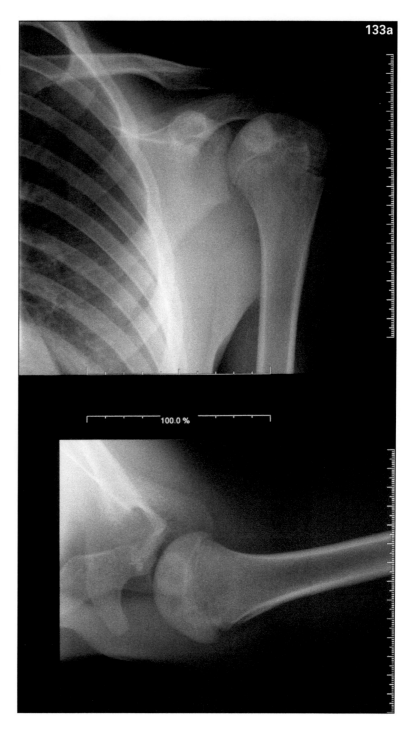

ANSWER 133

Observations (133a)
AP and axial radiographs of the left shoulder demonstrate a well defined lesion in the upper humeral epiphysis. This has a thick sclerotic border and central lucency. The lesion has nonaggressive features including a narrow zone of transition and the likely diagnosis considering the age of the patient and the location of the lesion is chondroblastoma.

Diagnosis
Chondroblastoma.

Differential diagnosis
Of epiphyseal lesions:
- Chondroblastoma – well defined sclerotic border, calcification in 50%, may have periosteal reaction.
- Giant cell tumour (GCT) – closed epiphyses, abuts articular surface, eccentric, no marginal sclerosis. No periosteal reaction unless fracture present.
- Geode – will be other signs of arthropathy; older patients.
- Metastases and myeloma.
- Infection – usually metaphyseal rather than epiphyseal.

Discussion
Chondroblastoma is a rare, cartilage containing tumour that almost always occurs in the epiphyses of long bones. Patients affected are under 30 years of age and tend to present with localized pain. The lesion is usually well defined with a sclerotic border and occurs most commonly about the knee joint. Calcification within the lesion is seen in approximately 50%. The tumour rarely metastasizes but may be locally aggressive (133b, 133c).

As with all focal bone lesions, an assessment of benign vs aggressive features, the patient's age and the location of the lesion within the bone are critical in forming a meaningful differential diagnosis. Fortunately, the differential for epiphyseal lesions is fairly short! One condition that deserves brief discussion is GCT as this can sometimes look similar. The vast majority occur in long bones, most commonly at the knee. Age at presentation is 20–40 years, often with pain. Classical features of GCT are presence in a fused skeleton, epiphyseal subarticular location, eccentric position and absence of marginal sclerosis. Only when all these features are present can one confidently predict GCT from the plain radiograph. What is impossible to say, however, is whether the lesion is benign or malignant.

Figure 133d is a radiograph of the knee in a patient with a GCT. Note how the lesion abuts the articular surface but has no marginal sclerosis unlike the chondroblastoma illustrated (133a). The distinction may not always be this clear however, and further advice is offered in the practical tips section.

Practical tips
- With regard to epiphyseal lesions in young patients, the two main possibilities are chondroblastoma and GCT. However, many chondroblastomas will not have the prominent internal calcifications and sclerotic border seen in Figure 133a. In such cases it is important to check whether the patient has unfused epiphyses as GCT will not normally be seen in this group.
- If doubt still exists as to the nature of an epiphyseal lesion, MRI may help. There is typically marked bony oedema seen surrounding a chondroblastoma but rarely around a GCT.

Further management
Chondroblastoma is a benign tumour that may become locally aggressive. Treatment is by curettage and bone chip grafting.

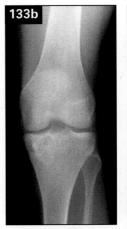
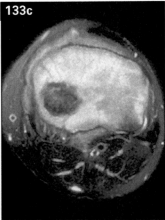

133b, 133c Plain radiograph of a lucent tibial epiphyseal lesion and axial T2 weighted MRI image of the same case, which shows a well defined hypointense lesion in the tibial epiphysis consistent with a chondroblastoma. The high signal thoughout the tibial plateau is in keeping with marrow oedema. This reactive oedema is a common feature of chondroblastoma and can lead to overestimation of the aggressiveness of the lesion.

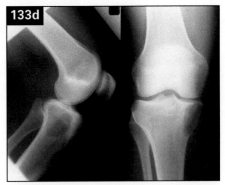

133d Radiograph of knee demonstrating a lucent subarticular lesion typical of a GCT.

CASE 134

History
A 25-year-old male presented with knee pain and fever.

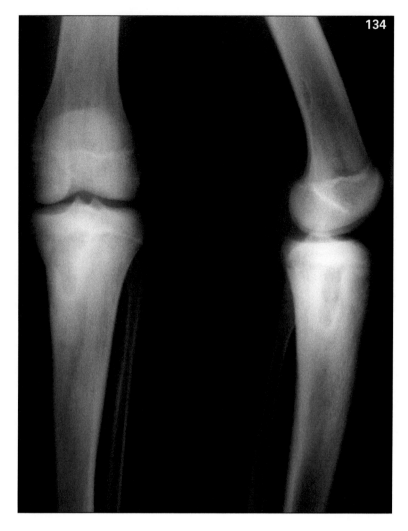

CASE 135

History
A 28-year-old male with bilateral hip pain.

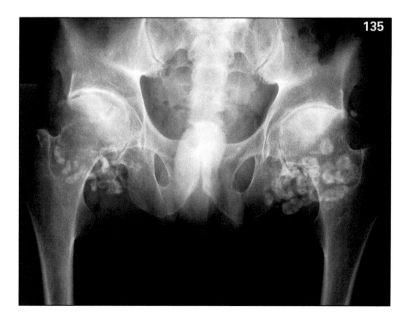

ANSWER 134

Observations (134)
AP and lateral radiographs of the right knee reveal a well demarcated area of lucency in the metaphysis of the proximal tibia. This is surrounded by sclerosis and there is no evidence of extension through the growth plate into the epiphysis. A small amount of smooth periosteal reaction is seen medially. Together with the history of pyrexia, the findings best fit with the diagnosis of Brodie's abscess.

Diagnosis
Brodie's abscess.

Differential diagnosis
- Osteosarcoma.
- Giant cell tumour (GCT) (in child).

Discussion
Brodie's abscess is the term used to describe a subacute pyogenic osteomyelitis. It is a smouldering, indolent infection that is most commonly caused by *Staphylococcus aureus*. Children and males are more commonly affected. It has a predilection for the ends of tubular bones and is characteristically located in the metaphysis. The proximal and distal metaphyses of the tibia are the most common sites involved. The carpal and tarsal bones are other commonly affected sites. The characteristic appearance is of a central area of lucency surrounded by a dense rim of reactive sclerosis. A lucent, tortuous channel extending towards the growth plate is pathognomonic when seen. Periosteal reaction and new bone formation are features and there may be adjacent soft tissue swelling. On MRI, a 'double line' effect may be seen on T2 weighted images. This refers to the high signal intensity of granulation tissue surrounded by low signal intensity of bone sclerosis. The abscess may also be more conspicuous on MRI after IV gadolinium injection. The disease is generally indolent and may persist for several months.

Practical tips
- Giant cell tumour in children is often located in the metaphysis rather than its characteristic epiphyseal location in adults. Therefore GCT in children may look like a Brodie's abscess when marginal sclerosis is limited.
- In more subtle cases where the abscess is present near the cortex of a bone, the lesion may mimic an osteoid osteoma.
- In difficult cases where the abscess is not well defined, the appearances may look like those of a malignant process and when considering the metaphyseal location of the disease the findings may look suspicious of an osteosarcoma. This is where local periosteal reaction is important and if smooth rather than aggressive, will suggest benign disease.

Further management
Treatment is surgical drainage.

Further reading
Rosenberg Z, Beltran J, Bencardino J (2000). MR imaging of the ankle and foot. *RadioGraphics* 20: S153–S179.

ANSWER 135

Observations (135)
Pelvic radiograph shows bilateral irregularity of the femoral heads with decreased joint space, sclerosis and large subchondral cysts. This is associated with multiple calcified foci adjacent to both hips. These foci have lucent centres and appearances are consistent with synovial osteochondromatosis.

In summary, there is irregularity of the femoral heads from an underlying condition that has led to premature osteoarthritis and secondary synovial osteochondromatosis. The main possibilities are epiphyseal dysplasia (including Meyer's dysplasia) and previous avascular necrosis.

Diagnosis
Meyer's dysplasia with secondary synovial osteochondromatosis.

Differential diagnosis
Of irregular epiphyses:
- Avascular necrosis.
- Multiple epiphyseal dysplasia.
- Meyer's dysplasia.
- Morquio's syndrome.
- Congenital hypothyroidism.
- Chondrodysplasia punctata.

Discussion
Meyer's dysplasia, also known as congenital multicentric ossification of the femoral heads, is an epiphyseal dysplasia that is confined to the upper femoral epiphyses. The femoral heads become irregular, fragmented and collapsed, leading to premature degenerative joint disease. It can be an incidental finding in asymptomatic hips of young

Answer 135

children. The differential diagnoses for irregular (or stippled) epiphyses are listed and all may lead to premature osteoarthritis (OA).

The radiological features are:
- Irregularity of contour.
- Sclerosis.
- Collapse.
- Irregular epiphyseal calcifications.
- Secondary degenerative changes.

Multiple epiphyseal dysplasia normally arises in childhood and resembles Meyer's dysplasia, although unlike the latter it is not confined to the femoral heads and may affect the tarsal bones, knees and ankles.

Synovial osteochondromatosis is due to metaplasia of subsynovial connective tissue to form cartilage nodules that go on to calcify and eventually migrate into the joint to form loose bodies. In this case, secondary synovial osteochondromatosis has developed. Compared to primary synovial osteochondromatosis, the intra-articular loose bodies tend to be larger and more varied in size.

Practical tips
- Multiple epiphyseal dysplasia will be seen in other joints and there may be a family history. Meyer's is confined to the hips.
- When irregular/stippled epiphyses identified:
  - Look for ancillary signs of avascular necrosis:
    - Signs of sickle cell anaemia, e.g. endplate infarctions of the vertebral bodies, and gallstones on an AXR.
    - Associations with steroid therapy on a pelvic x-ray/AXR, e.g. thumb-printing in colon, stoma bag or sacroiliitis.
    - Associations with condition of immunosuppression on a pelvic x-ray, e.g. pelvic transplant kidney.
  - Look for ancillary signs of Morquio's syndrome:
    - Posterior vertebral scalloping.
    - Anterior vertebral body beaks.

Further management
Treatment is supportive. Joint replacement may be needed in the long term.

CASE 136

History
A 32-year-old male presented with thigh pain.

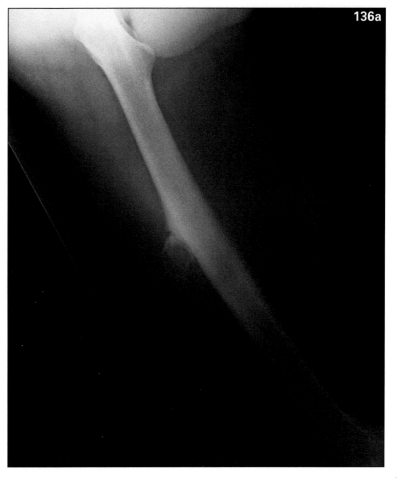

ANSWER 136

Observations (136a)
At the midshaft of the femur there is an ossific mass with mixed sclerosis and lysis lying lateral to the femoral shaft. A radiolucent line separates the mass from the cortex except at its attachment superiorly. Periosteal reaction is also noted. The features are characteristic for a parosteal osteosarcoma.

Diagnosis
Parosteal osteosarcoma.

Differential diagnosis
- Osteochondroma.
- Extraosseous osteosarcoma.
- Juxtacortical haematoma.
- Myositis ossificans.

Discussion
Parosteal osteosarcoma accounts for 4% of all osteosarcomas. The tumour originates in the outer layer of periosteum and is slow growing. Eventually, invasion of the medullary canal may occur. Fifty per cent of patients are more than 30 years of age when affected, with the peak at 38 years. This contrasts with conventional osteosarcoma, where 75% are younger than 30 years of age. Females are more commonly afflicted at a ratio of 3:2. The lesion most commonly affects the posterior aspect of the distal femur. It also affects either end of the tibia, the proximal humerus and the fibula, but is rare in other long bones. The metaphysis is the most common part of the long bone that is affected and the patient may present with a palpable mass. The typical radiological appearances are of a lobulated 'cauliflower-like' ossific mass extending away from the cortex. In over a third of cases a fine radiolucent line separates the tumour mass from the cortex and this is known as the 'string sign'. The attachment to the cortex is described as the tumour stalk, and when considering differential diagnoses this will not be seen with myositis ossificans. Non-aggressive periosteal reaction is also a feature. Another example is shown in a child in Figure **136b**.

A medullary canal mass with aggressive periosteal reaction (e.g. 'sunburst' or 'hair on end') points to conventional osteosarcoma. These features are demonstrated in the typical metaphyseal location in a knee radiograph of a child with osteosarcoma (**136c**). Conventional osteosarcoma affects males more commonly than females and there is a bimodal age distribution with elderly patients being affected due to malignant transformation in Paget's disease. Parosteal osteosarcoma has the best prognosis of all osteosarcomas with an 80–90% 10 year survival rate (60–80% for conventional osteosarcoma).

Practical tips
The 'give away' appearance of this tumour is that it looks like a cauliflower on a stalk attached to the cortex.

Further management
Surgical resection can result in an 80–90% 10 year survival rate, the best prognosis of all types of osteosarcoma.

Further reading
Murphey M, Robbin M, McRae G, *et al.* (1997). The many faces of osteosarcoma. *RadioGraphics* **17**: 1205–1231.

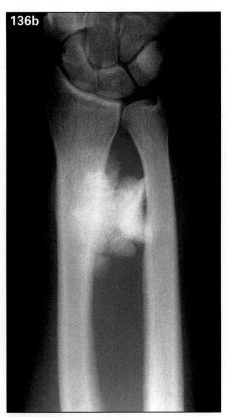

136b Parosteal osteosarcoma of the distal radius of a child.

136c Conventional osteosarcoma affecting the metaphysis of the femur in a child.

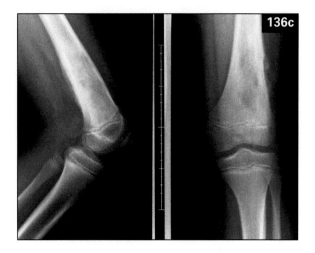

CASE 137

History
A 58-year-old female presented with back pain.

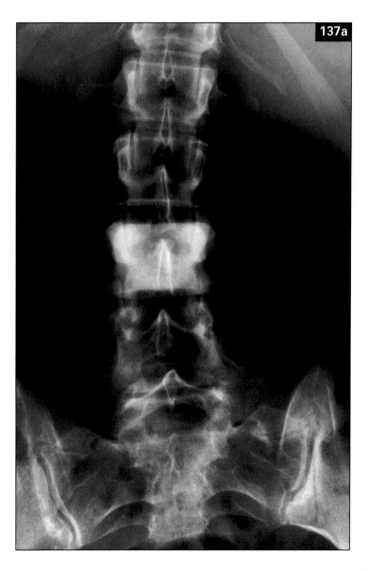

ANSWER 137

Observations (137a)
There is homogeneous sclerosis of the L4 vertebral body producing the appearance of an ivory vertebra. No significant expansion or trabeculation of the vertebral body is seen. The remaining vertebrae and bony skeleton are normal in appearance. The most likely diagnosis in a female patient is sclerotic metastases from a breast carcinoma primary. The differential diagnosis includes lymphoma.

Diagnosis
Sclerotic metastases from breast carcinoma.

Differential diagnosis
(Mnemonic – 'Mets…LP HIM'):
- Lymphoma.
- Paget's disease.
- Haemangioma.
- Infection.
- Mastocytosis.

Discussion
The ivory vertebra sign refers to an increase in opacity of a vertebral body that retains its size and contours.
In adults:
- Osteoblastic metastases elicit a sclerotic response that results in patchy replacement of the vertebral body spongiosa with dense new bone that may be confluent (137b, 137c). Sclerotic metastases from prostate carcinoma in men and breast carcinoma in women are the most common primaries. Occasionally osteosarcoma and carcinoid are responsible.
- Lymphomatous deposits can also elicit a marked osteoblastic response resulting in diffuse sclerosis. When considering lymphoma as a cause, Hodgkin's disease is more frequent than the other reticuloses. However lymphoma is generally more likely to result in destructive lytic lesions than osteosclerosis.
- Paget's disease tends to cause expansion of the vertebral body with coarsening of the vertical trabeculae. In fact, the sclerosis of Paget's tends to be mostly at the periphery with relative lucency of the centre owing to atrophy of the spongiosa. This can produce a 'picture frame' or windowed double contour appearance.
- As with Paget's disease, haemangioma causes increased vertebral trabeculations and expansion in a sclerotic vertebral body. The younger age group will help to differentiate it from Paget's.
- Infection in the healing phase may cause sclerosis in a vertebra, however this rarely involves a single vertebra and endplate destruction with decrease in disc space height will point to the correct diagnosis.
- Mastocytosis is a systemic disease characterized by mast cell proliferation in skin and the reticuloendothelial system. Release of histamine by mast cells in bone promotes osteoblastic activity leading to sclerotic skeletal foci particularly in the spine.
- Vertebroplasty, the introduction of cement into a collapsed vertebral body under imaging guidance, results in high density within the vertebra mimicking an ivory vertebra. This procedure is performed in patients with vertebral collapse who have severe pain unresponsive to medication, and is highly effective. An example is shown (137d) of an elderly patient who had painful osteoporotic collapse at two lumbar levels and was successfully treated with resolution of pain.

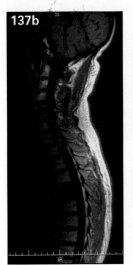

137b Sagittal fat saturated MRI image shows a sclerotic metastasis in the T5 vertebral body.

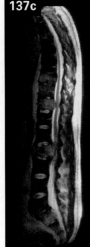

137c Sagittal fat saturated MRI image shows multiple sclerotic and lytic metastases throughout the visuallized spine.

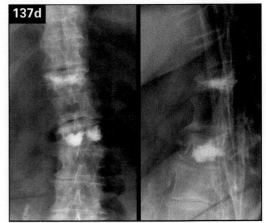

137d AP and lateral radiographs of the thoracolumbar spine following vertebroplasty in a patient with osteoporotic collapse.

Answer 137

In children:
- The ivory vertebra sign is less common in children and frequently the result of lymphoma.
- Less commonly, osteoblastoma, neuroblastoma, osteosarcoma or medulloblastoma deposits can cause the appearance.

Practical tips
- Increased vertical trabeculation and expansion suggest Paget's or haemangioma. The latter affects a younger age group, whereas the former is seen in the elderly and may be polyostotic.
- A paraspinal mass may be seen with lymphoma due to adenopathy, which may also cause anterior scalloping of the vertebral bodies.
- With mastocytosis, look for involvement of several vertebrae and background small bowel thickening/dilatation and hepatosplenomegaly, which may be seen on the spine radiograph.
- Decreased disc space height and endplate changes point to infection.

Further management
The underlying cause can be determined from the age of the patient, ancillary signs on the radiograph (as described above) and the history and examination. An isotope bone scan may be required to locate further deposits in a patient with metastases.

Further reading
Graham TS (2005). The ivory vertebra sign. *Radiology* 235: 614–615.

CASE 138

History
A 67-year-old male presented with a swollen foot.

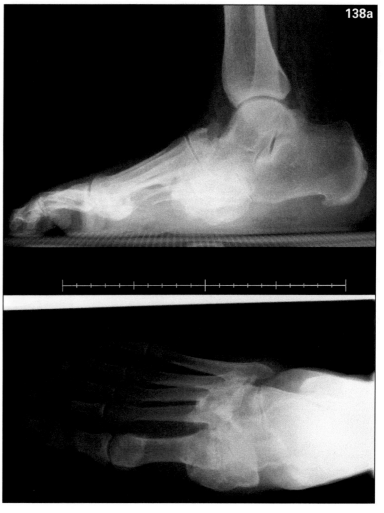

ANSWER 138

Observations (138a)
There is marked abnormality at the midtarsal joint with dislocation, sclerosis and debris formation. Prominent vascular calcification is noted. The appearances are those of a Charcot joint and the most likely cause in view of the vascular calcification is diabetes mellitus.

Diagnosis
Diabetic neuropathic foot.

Differential diagnosis
Of causes of neuropathic joint:
- Shoulder and upper limb joints:
  - Syringomyelia.
  - Congenital insensitivity to pain.
  - Leprosy.
  - Syphilis.

- Spine:
  - Trauma.
  - Tabes dorsalis.

- Hip and knee:
  - Tabes dorsalis.
  - Steroids.

- Ankle and foot:
  - Diabetes mellitus.
  - Alcoholism.
  - Myelomeningocele.
  - Congenital insensitivity to pain.

Discussion
Neuropathic arthropathy is a traumatic arthritis associated with loss of sensation and proprioception of an affected limb. When encountered clinically it is also known as a Charcot joint. The decreased pain sensation produces repetitive trauma leading to eventual destruction of the joint. There is often no history of trauma and the patient may present with a swollen warm joint with normal inflammatory markers. A third have pain at presentation although there is usually a decreased response to deep pain and proprioception at this stage. Because the patient is still using the limb there is no juxta-articular osteoporosis, in fact the bones are sclerotic. The exception to this rule is in patients with superadded infection, which is not uncommon in diabetics. Repetitive trauma leads to destruction, dislocation and deformity with multiple loose bodies within the joint. The likely underlying pathology depends upon the site of the joint and the age of the patient. When considering the ankle and foot, the most common causes in adults are diabetes mellitus and alcoholism, whereas in children the most common causes are myelomeningocele and congenital insensitivity to pain. Examples are shown of a Charcot joint secondary to diabetes mellitus (**138b**) and a Charcot elbow in a patient with syringomyelia (**138c**).

Radiological features of a Charcot joint include:
- Dense (i.e. sclerotic) bones.
- Destruction and fragmentation of articular surfaces.
- Degeneration.
- Debris (loose bodies).
- Dislocation.
- Deformity.
- Joint effusion.
- Excessive callus formation.

Practical tips
Look for vascular calcification on the radiograph as this will often be present in patients with diabetes mellitus and hence point to the underlying cause.

Further management
Treatment is supportive. Amputation may be necessary in severe progression.

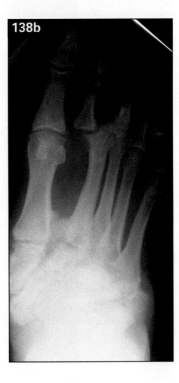

138b Charcot foot in a diabetic showing sclerosis and loose body formation at the midtarsal joint with subluxation and destruction of the 2nd metatarsophalangeal joint.

138c Charcot elbow showing destruction, sclerosis and loose body formation.

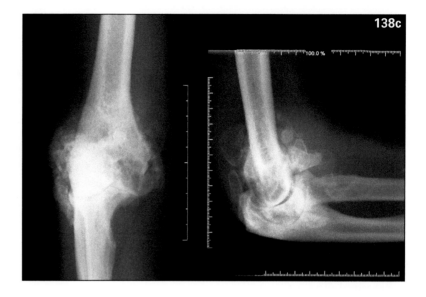

CASE 139

History
A 30-year-old male patient presented with right hip pain and limitation of movement.

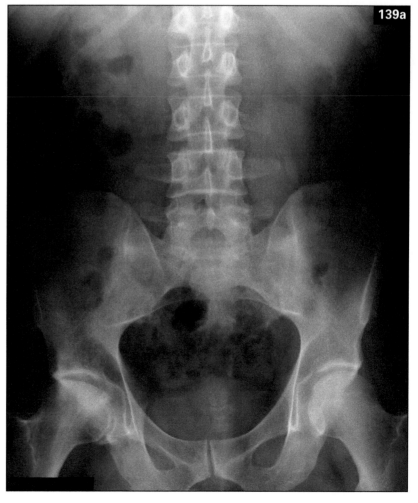

ANSWER 139

Observations (139a)
Irregularity, sclerosis and loss of height of the right femoral head are seen on the pelvic radiograph. There is no significant abnormality of the acetabulum and the left hip is unremarkable. The findings are consistent with avascular necrosis of the right hip. Bilateral sacroiliac joint fusion is also present, though more prominent on the right side. This suggests a background seronegative arthropathy. It is therefore likely that the avascular necrosis is drug induced by treatment for the seronegative arthropathy, or perhaps associated inflammatory bowel disease. No bowel abnormality is seen on this plain film to confirm the latter hypothesis.

Diagnosis
Avascular necrosis (AVN) in a patient on steroids for seronegative arthropathy.

Differential diagnosis
For causes of avascular necrosis (mnemonic – 'DRIED HIP'):
- Diabetes and other metabolic conditions, e.g. hyperlipidaemia, gout, pancreatitis.
- Radiotherapy.
- Inflammatory disorders, e.g. rheumatoid, SLE, scleroderma.
- Endocrine disorders, e.g. Cushing's.
- Drugs, e.g. steroids, anti-inflammatory and immunosuppressive drugs, alcohol.
- Haematological disorders, e.g. sickle cell, haemophilia, polycythaemia, Gaucher's.
- Infection and injury, e.g. fractures, burns and fat embolism.
- Perthe's disease (idiopathic AVN in children).

Discussion
Avascular necrosis is a consequence of interrupted blood supply to bone with death of cellular elements. The many causes are listed in the differential diagnosis and follow the mnemonic 'DRIED HIP'. The femoral head is the most common site affected. Other common locations include the humeral head and femoral condyles. The earliest radiological sign is subtle relative sclerosis secondary to resorption of surrounding bone. A radiolucent crescent parallel to the articular surface may appear. Flattening, fragmentation and sclerosis then ensue. Subchondral cysts and collapse lead to early osteoarthritis of the affected joint. An AP of the pelvis (**139b**) shows the subtle crescent sign in the left hip of a child with early avascular necrosis. This is more clearly seen on the frog lateral view of the same patient (**139c**).

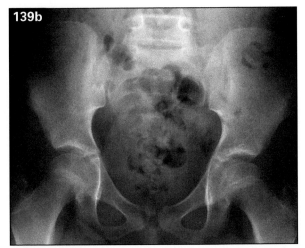

139b AP pelvis in a child. A subtle lucent crescent is present in the subchondral surface of the left femoral head indicating early AVN.

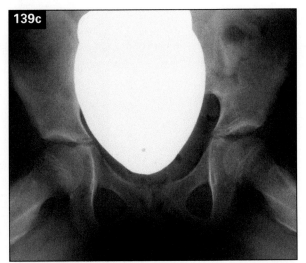

139c The lucent crescent is more clearly visible on this frog lateral view of the same patient as in Figure **139b**.

Answer 139

Practical tips
The list of potential causes for AVN is long and, of course, it may just be idiopathic Perthe's disease in children. The following radiological features are worth checking for in the search for a cause, but clinical history may be required thereafter. For example, the child with AVN shown in Figure **139b** had leukaemia, and steroid treatment was the cause.
Check for:
- Signs of sickle cell anaemia, e.g. vertebral endplate infarctions producing H-shaped vertebrae, altered bony trabecular pattern, gallstones and splenic calcification.
- Associations with steroid therapy, e.g. thumb-printing in colon, presence of a stoma or sacroiliitis.
- Rheumatoid-type arthropathy or changes of scleroderma.
- Vascular calcification, which may point to underlying diabetes.
- Associations with immunosuppressives, e.g. pelvic transplant kidney.

Further management
The underlying cause should be sought and treated. Many patients will develop debilitating secondary arthritis and go on to require replacement of the affected joint.

CASE 140

History
A 64-year-old patient presented with abdominal pain.

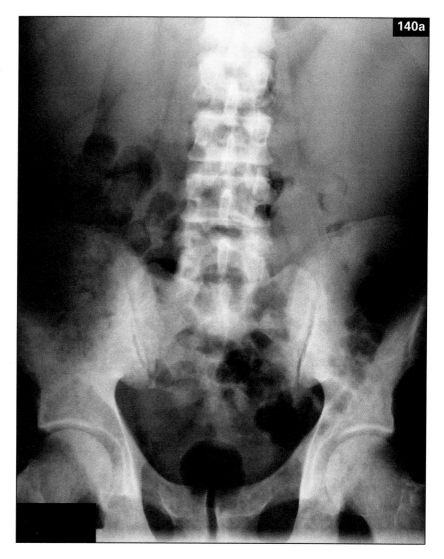

ANSWER 140

Observations (140a)
There is diffuse osteosclerosis affecting the visible skeleton. There is also massive splenomegaly making the likely diagnosis that of myelofibrosis. Lymphoma is another possibility and less likely, mastocytosis.

Diagnosis
Myelofibrosis.

Differential diagnosis
Of diffuse bony sclerosis and splenomegaly:
- Lymphoma.
- Mastocytosis.

Of generalized osteosclerosis in adults:
- Sclerotic metastases (especially breast or prostate carcinoma).
- Lymphoma.
- Myelofibrosis.
- Paget's disease (**140b**).
- Renal osteodystrophy.
- Sickle cell disease.
- Mastocytosis.
- Osteopetrosis.
- Pyknodysostosis.
- Fluorosis.

Osteopetrosis and pyknodysostosis have onset in the paediatric age group.

Discussion
This myeloproliferative disorder results in progressive marrow replacement by fibrosis and consequent anaemia, extramedullary haematopoiesis and splenomegaly (often massive). Typical age of onset is over 50 years.

Practical tips
- Osteosclerosis is often missed when the appearance is blamed on the quality of the film, i.e. when it is thought to be due to the radiograph being underpenetrated. Assessment of the intervertebral discs should be made – if they are visible then the appearance is likely to be real. This is well demonstrated in Figure **140c**: there is diffuse osteosclerosis affecting all the bones on this CXR of a patient with osteopetrosis. Note how the intervertebral discs are clearly seen, reinforcing the fact that the radiograph is not underpenetrated.
- Patients with renal osteodystrophy may have a haemodialysis line on CXR or peritoneal dialysis line on AXR. There may be evidence of subperiosteal bone resorption, soft tissue and vascular calcification, and 'rugger jersey' spine.
- When sclerotic metastases are suspected on a CXR, check the breast shadows: in female patients there may be a mastectomy, while in males enlargement of breast tissue may be seen due to hormone therapy for prostatic carcinoma. Figure **140d** shows such features – sclerotic prostate metastases and gynaecomastia.

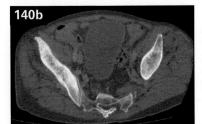

140b Axial CT image of the pelvis shows sclerosis of the right hemipelvis with cortical thickening and thickened internal trabeculations typical for Paget's disease.

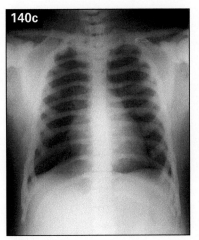

140c CXR of an adult with osteopetrosis demonstrates diffuse dense osteosclerosis.

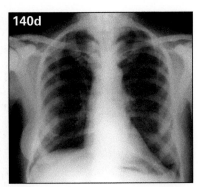

140d CXR of a male patient with diffuse osteosclerotic metastases from prostatic carcinoma. Note the gynaecomastia secondary to hormone therapy.

Answer 140

- Massive splenomegaly on the AXR suggests myelofibrosis.
- Splenic atrophy (possibly with calcification) suggests sickle cell disease, and there may be other signs of this such as gallstones, avascular necrosis of the femoral heads and endplate infarctions causing H-shaped vertebral bodies.
- Splenomegaly and small bowel thickening suggest mastocytosis.
- On the AXR of a patient with osteopetrosis a generalized 'bone within bone' appearance may be seen and the vertebral bodies may have densely sclerotic endplates producing 'sandwich vertebrae'. Erlenmeyer flask deformity of the femurs should also be looked for. Figure **140e** is an orthopantomogram in an adult patient with osteopetrosis demonstrating diffuse osteosclerosis and supernumerary teeth.
- Paget's disease can also produce a 'bone within bone' appearance, however coarse trabeculation and cortical thickening normally differentiate this from other causes.
- Fluorosis is associated with ligamentous insertion calcification.

Further management
There is no specific treatment for myelofibrosis. Splenectomy is not routinely performed, but is indicated for splenic enlargement that causes recurrent painful episodes, severe thrombocytopenia or an unacceptably high red blood cell transfusion requirement. Median survival from time of diagnosis is approximately 5 years. End stage myelofibrosis is a wasting illness characterized by general disability, liver failure and bleeding from thrombocytopenia.

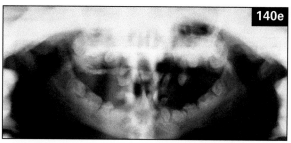

140e OPG of an adult with osteopetrosis; this demonstrates diffuse osteosclerosis and supernumerary teeth, which is an associated finding.

CASE 141

History
A 34-year-old male presented with right hip pain.

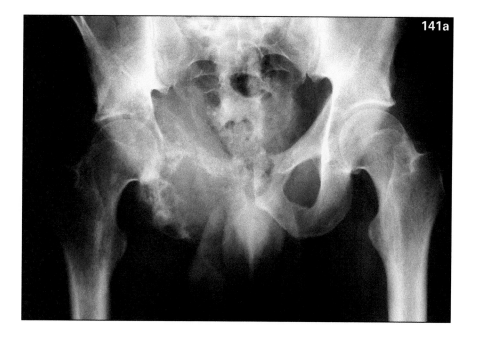

ANSWER 141

Observations (141a)
There is a large, expansile, mixed lytic/sclerotic destructive lesion involving the right anterior hemipelvis. There is marked cortical destruction with a soft tissue component. The lesion has a wide zone of transition. This is an aggressive lesion and the most likely diagnosis in a patient of this age is a primary malignancy such as lymphoma or chondrosarcoma. Metastasis should also be considered.

Diagnosis
Chondrosarcoma.

Differential diagnosis
- Lymphoma.
- Metastasis.

Discussion
Chondrosarcoma is the third most common primary bone malignancy with multiple myeloma being the most common and osteosarcoma following second. Chondrosarcoma can be primary, or secondary following malignant transformation in a pre-existing skeletal lesion such as an osteochondroma, enchondroma or a parosteal chondroma. Chondrosarcoma most commonly presents in the 4th or 5th decade of life with a male predilection of 2:1. Radiographs typically reveal a mixed lytic and sclerotic appearance. The sclerotic areas represent chondroid matrix mineralization and are seen in 60–78% of lesions. The characteristic appearance of mineralized chondroid matrix is a 'ring and arc' pattern of calcification that can coalesce to form 'snowflake-type' calcification. This characteristic chondroid calcification usually allows confident radiological diagnosis of a cartilaginous lesion.

Radiological signs:
- Mixed lytic/sclerotic lesion.
- Wide zone of transition.
- 'Ring and arc' and 'snowflake' calcification.
- Cortical destruction.
- Soft tissue mass.

Chondrosarcomas are also characterized as central or peripheral. Central chondrosarcomas make up the majority and are intramedullary in origin, although they may erode through the cortex into the soft tissues. Central chondrosarcomas usually arise in the pelvis or femur and are often expansile with the characteristic calcification described. Endosteal scalloping is often seen and can help differentiate low-grade chondrosarcomas from enchondromas. Clinical symptoms are nonspecific, with pain being the most frequent symptom. Peripheral chondrosarcoma is also termed exostotic chondrosarcoma and refers to malignant degeneration in an exostosis (i.e. is a secondary chondrosarcoma). An example is shown in Figure **141b** – note the flocculent calcification of the chondrosarcoma, which had arisen from the exostosis at the lateral femoral condyle. This should always be suspected when there is growth of an exostosis after skeletal maturity or if an exostosis becomes painful. The cartilage cap of a suspicious exostosis can be measured on MRI, and if the thickness is greater than 1.5 cm then malignant transformation should be suspected. Again, flocculent chondroid calcification is characteristic for malignant degeneration.

Practical tips
It can often be difficult to differentiate an enchondroma from an intramedullary chondrosarcoma, however the latter is more likely to present with pain and unlike enchondroma will often demonstrate periosteal reaction and cortical breakthrough.

Further management
As with most primary bone tumours, a suspected chondrosarcoma should only be biopsied in a specialist bone tumour centre so as not to seed tumour or contaminate the surgical field.

Further reading
Murphey M, Walker E, Wilson A, *et al.* (2003). Imaging of primary chondrosarcoma: radiologic-pathologic correlation. *RadioGraphics* **23**: 1245–1278.

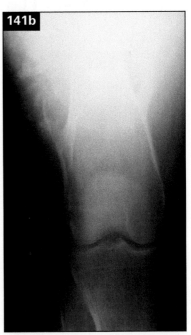

141b Flocculent calcification from a chondrosarcoma that has arisen from the exostosis at the lateral femoral condyle.

CASE 142

History
A 45-year-old male presented with severe back pain for several weeks.

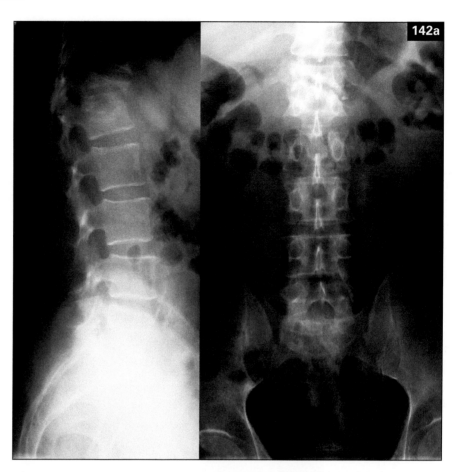

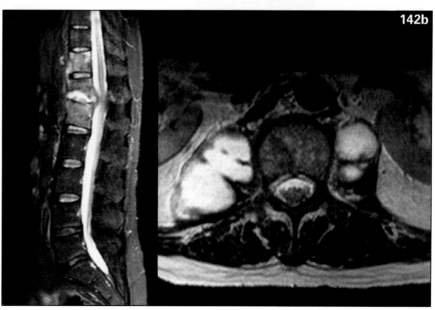

ANSWER 142

Observations (142a, 142b)
AP and lateral images (**142a**) of the thoracolumbar spine show marked deformity at the T12/L1 level with erosive destruction of the opposing vertebral endplates. There is anterior slip at this level with anterior angulation (gibbus deformity). Appearances are in keeping with a discitis.

Axial and coronal T2 weighted MR images (**142b**) demonstrate high signal in the T12/L1 intervertebral disc. Signal change extends throughout the adjacent vertebrae, and there is endplate destruction and partial vertebral collapse at T12. T11 vertebra has increased marrow signal suggesting it is also involved. The axial image demonstrates high-signal fluid collections in both psoas muscles consistent with bilateral psoas abscesses.

Diagnosis
Tuberculous spondylitis (Pott's disease) with associated psoas abscess.

Discussion
The spine is the most common bony location to be involved in TB. Presentation is often late since initial symptoms are of vague back pain and stiffness. The most common location is the upper lumbar/lower thoracic region, particularly around L1 level. The anterior aspect of the vertebral body is most typically affected. The disk space then becomes involved via extension along the anterior or posterior longitudinal ligament or directly through the endplate.

Radiological features of discitis include:
- Reduction in height of the intervertebral disc, which is usually the first sign of a discitis.
- Erosion of the vertebral endplates.
- Involvement of the vertebral bodies leads to collapse and resulting gibbus deformity.
- Spread of infection into adjacent soft tissues resulting in psoas/paraspinal abscesses.
- Neurological involvement arises due to intraspinal spread of infection and vertebral body collapse. This occurs much more commonly when the infective organism is TB.

Practical tips
- Discitis will cause bony abnormality of the superior and inferior endplates of the adjacent vertebral bodies, i.e. abnormality will be centred at the level of the disc.
- The vertebral disc space is maintained longer in TB spondylitis than in pyogenic discitis.
- Look at the paraspinal regions to look for spread of infection. Infection can present as leg pain/swelling due to tracking of collections down the iliopsoas muscle.
- Look at, and around the spinal cord for extradural collections and spinal involvement.

Further management
Treatment is with antituberculous medication. Drainage of associated psoas or epidural abscesses may be required.

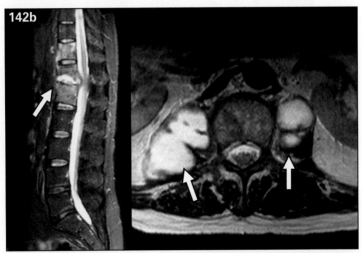

142b (left) Vertebral body collapse with abnormal marrow signal in the vertebral bodies above and below it. Bilateral psoas abscesses (right).

CASE 143

History
A 40-year-old male patient presented with painful fingers.

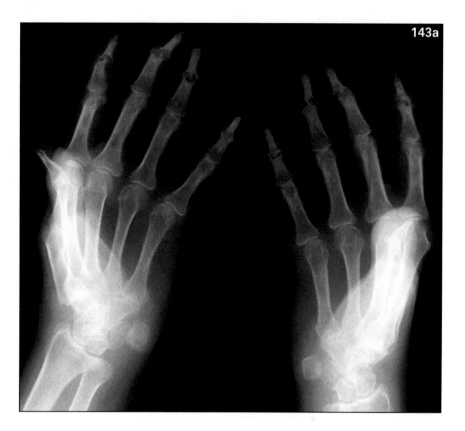

CASE 144

History
A young male presented with pain in left hand following a fight.

(see page 258 for case answer)

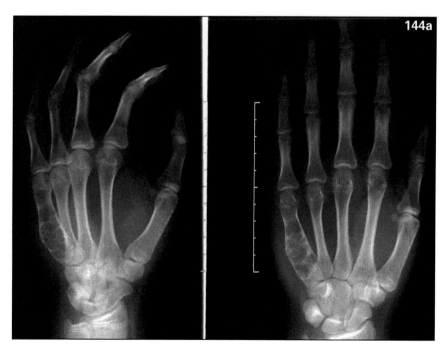

ANSWER 143

Observations (143a)
There is a bilateral symmetrical erosive arthropathy affecting the distal interphalangeal joints. Bone density is preserved and there is 'pencil in cup' deformity with bony proliferation. At the left little finger there are signs of ankylosis of the distal interphalangeal joint. The appearances are consistent with psoriatic arthropathy.

Diagnosis
Psoriatic arthropathy.

Differential diagnosis
- Ankylosing spondylitis.
- Rheumatoid arthritis (RA).

Discussion
This is a seronegative arthropathy affecting synovium and ligamentous attachments, and affects fewer than 5% of psoriasis patients. In approximately 15%, the arthropathy can predate development of skin changes by several years. The pattern of disease is variable, though the case illustrated is classical, i.e. asymmetric erosive oligoarthritis affecting the distal joints of hands and feet. New bone formation is characteristic, and may result in ankylosis of interphalangeal joints, as in this case. Resorption of the distal phalangeal tufts may be seen with accompanying nail changes.

Spondyloarthropathy is another pattern of disease, often with sacroiliitis and paravertebral ossifications. Other disease patterns include symmetrical polyarthritis mimicking rheumatoid, monoarthritis and arthritis mutilans, a grossly destructive pattern that may progress to form 'opera glass hand'.

Practical tips
- When presented with a hand radiograph with evidence of erosive arthropathy, certain differentiating features can help identify the most likely aetiology. The radiological differentiating features of the more common erosive arthropathies are as follows:
- Psoriatic arthropathy:
  - Usually *asymmetrical* erosive.
  - Interphalangeal joints, particularly the distal interphalangeal joints, are affected.
  - *Bony proliferation/periosteal reaction and preserved bone density* characteristic.
  - 'Pencil in cup' deformity.
  - Ankylosis.

- RA:
  - Bilateral *symmetrical erosive* arthropathy.
  - Metacarpophalangeal and proximal interphalangeal joints affected, i.e. *proximal small joints of digits*.
  - *Marginal* erosions.
  - Subluxation with ulnar deviation of digits.
  - *Decreased bone density*.
  - Ankylosis.
  - Figure **143b** is a radiograph of both hands in a patient with rheumatoid arthritis demonstrating bilateral symmetrical erosive destruction of the metacarpophalangeal joints. There is also generalized decreased bone density and arthropathy at the carpal joints and radiocarpal joints. Figure **143c** shows similar changes in the feet of a rheumatoid patient with marginal erosions and symmetrical subluxation at the metatarsophalangeal joints bilaterally.

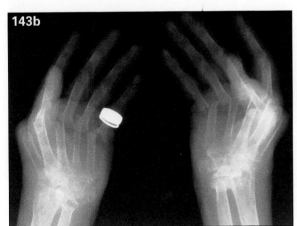

143b Radiograph of both hands of a patient with rheumatoid arthritis. Bilateral symmetrical erosive destruction is present affecting the metacarpophalangeal joints and the wrists. Note the telescoping of bone ends and the periarticular osteoporosis.

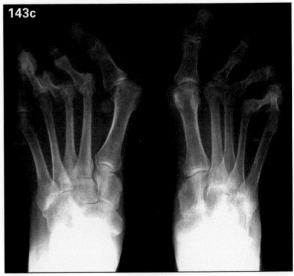

143c Rheumatoid arthritis of the feet with marginal erosions and lateral subluxation of the digits.

- Gouty arthropathy:
  - Asymmetrical erosive arthropathy.
  - Erosions are *juxta-articular with overhanging edges*.
  - Preserved bone density and joint space.
  - Bony proliferation/periosteal reaction.
  - *Gouty tophi* causing soft tissue masses in 50%.
  - Figures **143d** and **143e** are radiographs of gout demonstrating an asymmetrical erosive arthropathy with 'punched out' erosions. These erosions have overhanging edges, which are best seen at the proximal interphalangeal joints of the index fingers bilaterally and the metacarpophalangeal joint of the right thumb. Further large 'punched out' juxta-articular erosions with associated tophi are seen around the base of the right big toe in particular. Note the preservation of bone density.

- It is impossible to distinguish the spondyloarthropathy of psoriasis from Reiter's syndrome though it is notable that in psoriasis the hand is most affected and in Reiter's, the foot.
- Spondyloarthropathy of psoriasis is different radiographically from ankylosing spondylitis – the paravertebral ossification is asymmetrical and not due to true syndesmophytes.

Further management
Given the inflammatory nature of the disease, treatment consists of anti-inflammatory and immunosuppressive drugs as for other inflammatory arthropathies.

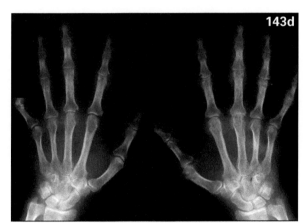

143d Radiograph of both hands demonstrates several 'punched out' erosions with overhanging edges and associated soft tissue swelling in a patient with gout.

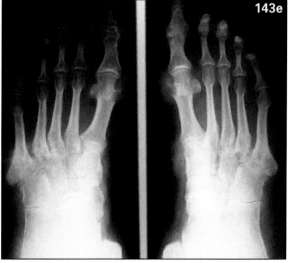

143e Radiograph of both feet in a patient with gout with characteristic 'punched out' erosions affecting the big toes.

ANSWER 144

Observations (144a)
Radiographs of the left hand reveal a lucent expansile lesion of the diaphysis of the 5th metacarpal. There is thinning of the cortex but no cortical breakthrough or periosteal reaction. No pathological fracture has occurred and no fracture is seen elsewhere. The lesion has a narrow zone of transition and nonaggressive features and is consistent with an enchondroma.

Diagnosis
Enchondroma.

Differential diagnosis
For lytic lesion in the digits (mnemonic – 'SEGA GAME F'):
- Simple bone cyst – rare in the hand.
- Enchondroma is by far the most likely lesion with this appearance at this site.
- Giant cell tumour of tendon sheath.
- Aneurysmal bone cyst – rare in the hand.
- Glomus tumour – painful.
- Abscess/osteomyelitis.
- Metastases and myeloma.
- Epidermal inclusion cyst (intraosseous) – distal phalanx; history of trauma, erythema and swelling may be present.
- Fibrous dysplasia – rare in the hand.

Discussion
Enchondroma is a common benign cartilaginous tumour most commonly seen in the tubular bones (50% in hands and feet) of patients under the age of 30 years.
The cardinal radiological features are listed below:
- Central lesion within the medullary canal.
- Lucent expansion of bone.
- Narrow zone of transition.
- Thinning of the cortex but no cortical breakthrough.
- No periosteal reaction unless pathological fracture.
- Stippled calcification may be present.
- Cortical endosteal scalloping.
- Affects small tubular bones.

Ollier's disease occurs when multiple enchondromas are present (144b). The enchondromas are most commonly seen in the femur, tibia and hands in an asymmetrical distribution. In the long bones, presentation is with asymmetric limb shortening due to impairment of epiphyseal fusion. The lesions do not increase in size after cessation of normal growth. Malignant transformation to chondrosarcoma can occur in up to 25% of patients with Ollier's disease by the age of 40. Malignant change is more common in central lesions and should be suspected when there is abnormal continued growth with pain and swelling and/or imaging findings of growth in a previously stable lesion, bony erosion and new or increasing calcification.

Maffucci's syndrome describes multiple enchondromas with multiple soft tissue haemangiomas, which present on imaging as multiple phleboliths in the soft tissues. It presents later, usually after puberty, and has a much higher incidence of malignant transformation.

Practical tips
- Chondroid pattern calcification, often seen in enchondroma, is however frequently absent in lesions of the tubular bones of the hands and feet.
- A painful enchondroma without pathological fracture should be suspected of having undergone malignant transformation until proven otherwise.

Further management
There is no specific treatment for enchondroma as it is a benign bony lesion that is often picked up incidentally or when a pathological fracture occurs.

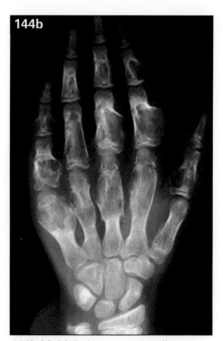

144b Multiple lucent expansile lesions of the tubular bones of the hand represent enchondromas in this patient with Ollier's disease. Note that the absence of phleboliths excludes the main differential diagnosis, Maffucci's syndrome.

CASE 145

History
Follow-up hand x-ray in an older child.

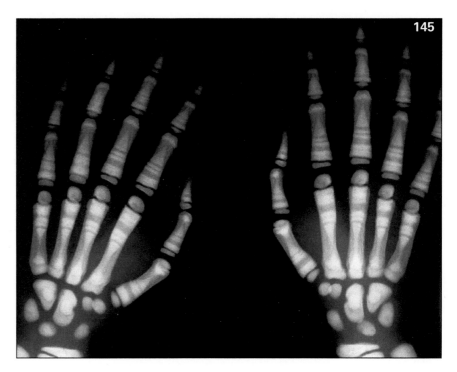

CASE 146

History
Adult patient presented with heel pain.

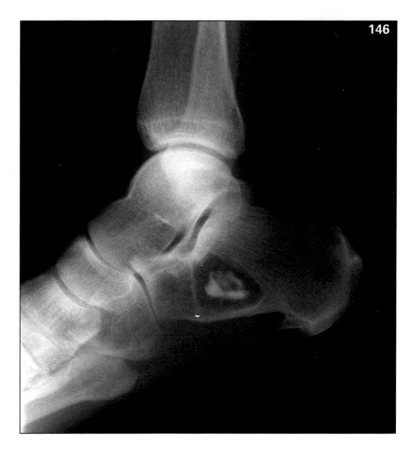

ANSWER 145

Observations (145)
There is diffuse osteosclerosis with a 'bone within bone' appearance. The most likely diagnosis is osteopetrosis.

Diagnosis
Osteopetrosis causing a 'bone within bone' appearance.

Differential diagnosis
Of 'bone within bone' appearance (mnemonic – 'SHARPS POOL'):
- Sickle cell disease.
- Hypervitaminosis D.
- Acromegaly.
- Rickets.
- Paget's disease.
- Scurvy.
- Post-radiation therapy/thorotrast/heavy metal poisoning.
- Osteopetrosis and oxalosis.
- Osteomyelitis.
- Leukaemia.

Discussion
'Bone within bone' describes the radiological appearance where one bone appears to arise within another. It can be seen as part of normal development, especially in the spine. Growth arrest may also cause the appearance but there are several pathological causes as listed. The diffuse osteosclerosis and age of the patient in this case (145) point to the correct diagnosis.

Practical tips
The differential diagnosis of 'bone within bone' appearance is large but there are certain features of the underlying disease process that may point to the specific cause:
- Osteopetrosis may have Erlenmeyer flask deformity of the ends of long bones and sclerotic vertebral endplates producing 'sandwich vertebrae'.
- There may be ancillary signs of sickle cell disease on the radiograph such as avascular necrosis of femoral and humeral heads, gallstones, H-shaped vertebrae due to endplate infarction and splenic atrophy or calcification.
- Acromegaly is associated with rectangular-shaped vertebrae and chondrocalcinosis.
- In children, consider rickets and look for splaying and fraying of the metaphyses.
- If the patient is elderly, consider Paget's and look for increased trabeculation and cortical thickening.

Further management
The only treatment available for osteopetrosis is bone marrow transplantation. Patients are more prone to fractures than the normal population.

Further reading
Williams H, Davies A, Chapman S (2004). Bone within a bone. *Clinical Radiology* 59: 132–144.

ANSWER 146

Observations (146)
Within the body of the calcaneus there is a well-defined lucent lesion with a narrow zone of transition. The lesion has a very thin sclerotic border and centrally within the lesion is a clump of calcification. There is no periosteal reaction or overlying soft tissue mass. The lesion has a nonaggressive appearance and the findings are typical of an intraosseous lipoma.

Diagnosis
Intraosseous lipoma.

Differential diagnosis
- Unicameral bone cyst.
- Post-traumatic cyst.
- Giant cell tumour (GCT).
- Desmoplastic fibroma.

Discussion
The calcaneus is the most common location for an intraosseous lipoma. Other sites of involvement include the proximal femur, tibia, humerus, pelvis, mandible and vertebrae. When involving tubular bones, it is usually located at the metaphysis. Patients of any age may develop an intraosseous lipoma, with no gender predilection. There is an association with hyperlipoproteinaemia. The typical radiological features are an expansile, nonaggressive radiolucent lesion with a thin, well defined sclerotic border. There is no periosteal reaction or cortical destruction. Sometimes the lesion may be septated. A central clump of calcification is virtually diagnostic and represents dystrophic calcification from fat necrosis. Patients may be asymptomatic or have localized bone pain. The radiographic appearances are similar to a unicameral bone cyst. Other differential diagnoses are listed for completeness but the central calcification and characteristic appearances of the lesion (146) make it virtually diagnostic of an intraosseous lipoma.

Practical tips
- Intraosseous lipoma ('lipoma of bone') can occur at any age.
- A central clump of calcification is virtually diagnostic.

Further management
This is a benign bony lesion and no further management is necessary.

CASE 147

History
A 30-year-old female presented after a fall onto outstretched hand.

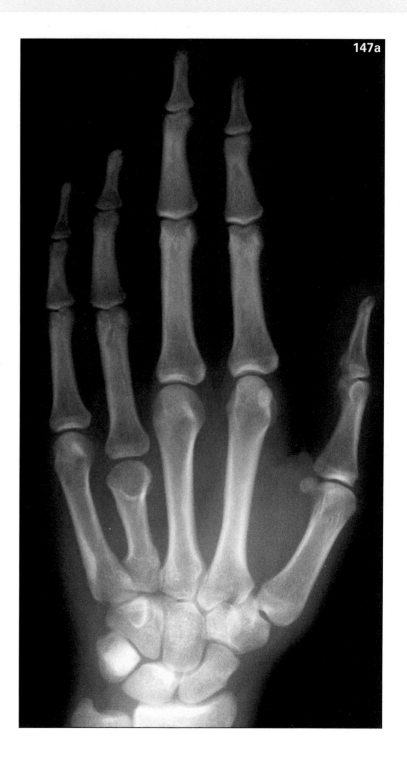

ANSWER 147

Observations (147a)
There is shortening of the 4th metacarpal. No acute bony injury is seen. The findings are most likely to be idiopathic or due to previous trauma. However, less common causes such as Turner's syndrome, pseudohypoparathyroidism and pseudopseudohypoparathyroidism should also be considered.

Diagnosis
Idiopathic shortening of the 4th metacarpal.

Differential diagnosis
For short 4th metacarpal/metatarsal:
- Post-traumatic.
- Postinfarction (e.g. from sickle cell disease).
- Turner's syndrome.
- Pseudohypoparathyroidism.
- Pseudopseudohypoparathyroidism.

Discussion
Shortening of the 4th metacarpal can result from previous trauma, particularly that involving the growth plate during childhood. Pseudohypoparathyroidism is a congenital X-linked dominant abnormality of renal and skeletal resistance to parathyroid hormone due to end-organ resistance and defective hormone. Patients therefore have the same characteristics as those with hypoparathyroidism but also short obese stature, round face, mental retardation, abnormal dentition and hypocalcaemia. Shortening of the 3rd metatarsal occurs along with shortening of the 4th and 5th metacarpals and is seen in up to 75% (**147b**).

Pseudopseudohypoparathyroidism has identical clinical and radiological features but patients have normal calcium.

Turner's syndrome results from nondisjunction of the sex chromosomes, with affected females having 45 XO chromosomes. Patients have absent secondary sexual characteristics with short stature, webbed neck and small iliac wings. Aortic coarctation is seen in 10% of patients and horseshoe kidney is a common finding. Madelung deformity and shortening of the 4th metacarpal are also seen, sometimes also with accompanying shortening of the 3rd and 5th metacarpals.

Practical tips
- The short 4th metacarpal is an 'Aunt Minnie' case but don't be put off by the same finding in the feet! Figure **147c** shows short 3rd–5th metatarsals in the same patient as seen in Figure **147b** with pseudohypoparathyroidism.
- If the wrist is also visualized, check for the presence of Madelung deformity. This would suggest Turner's syndrome is more likely.
- Involvement of multiple metacarpals is not specific to any of the differential diagnoses but involvement of the 4th and 5th metacarpals is particularly characteristic of pseudohypoparathyroidism.

Further management
There is no further treatment. This finding is most commonly idiopathic or related to previous trauma and is often incidental.

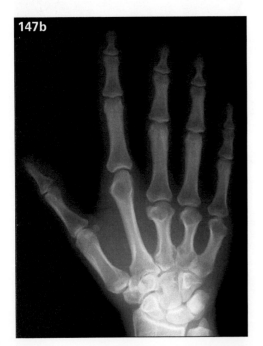

147b Hand radiograph of a patient with pseudohypoparathyroidism demonstrates shortening of the 3rd to 5th metacarpals.

147c Radiograph of the foot in the same patient as in Figure **147b** demonstrates shortening of the 3rd to 5th metatarsals.

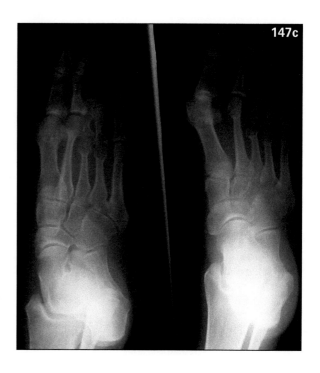

CASE 148

History
A 14-year-old boy presented with thigh pain, which was worse during the night.

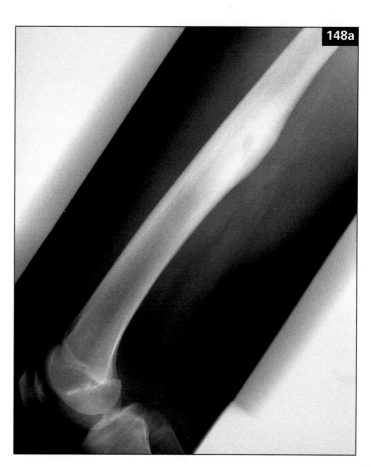

ANSWER 148

Observations (148a)
There is an area of dense sclerosis affecting the shaft of the femur with associated cortical thickening. Within this is an area of central lucency. This likely represents a nidus and the features are therefore consistent with an osteoid osteoma. Depending on other clinical features, infection might be considered as a differential diagnosis.

Diagnosis
Osteoid osteoma.

Differential diagnosis
- Infection.
- Eosinophilic granuloma.

Discussion
Osteoid osteoma is a relatively common, benign skeletal neoplasm composed of woven and osteoid bone, with loose intervening fibrovascular tissue. The lesion itself rarely exceeds 1.5 cm in maximum dimension and there are three main types: cortical, cancellous and subperiosteal.

Cortical lesions are the most common and have characteristic findings. Radiographs show dense reactive sclerosis that affects the shaft of a long bone, especially the tibia and femur. The lesion itself, however, is a radiolucent area within this area of osteosclerosis known as the nidus. This is more clearly seen on the CT images of the same patient (**148b**).

Cancellous osteoid osteomas have a site predilection for the femoral neck, posterior elements of the spine and the small bones of the hands and feet. By comparison, the sclerosis associated with a cancellous lesion is usually mild or moderate and may be distant from the lesion. Unlike the classical cortical osteoid osteoma, the cancellous lesion may not necessarily be situated at the centre of the sclerosis, making treatment more difficult.

The subperiosteal type is rarest, and typically located at the medial aspect of the femoral neck or in the hands and feet. It produces a soft tissue mass immediately adjacent to the affected bone rather than osteosclerosis. Cancellous and subperiosteal osteoid osteomas typically arise in an intra-articular or juxta-articular location.

Osteoid osteomas most commonly occur in the femur and tibia, where they are usually diaphyseal or metadiaphyseal. The most commonly affected area in the spine is the neural arch of the lumbar spine. Atypical locations include the skull, ribs, mandible and patella. Intra-articular lesions are most commonly found in the hip.

The affected population is young, with about half presenting between the ages of 10 and 20 years. Almost all patients are Caucasian with a male predominance. Pain is the usual mode of presentation and is worse at night. It is thought to be related to the vascularity of the lesion. Symptoms may be present before the lesion is radiologically visible and approximately 75% of patients report relief of pain after salicylates. CT can aid plain radiography in identifying the nidus. When the history is atypical, the location unusual or radiographs unexpectedly normal, bone scintigraphy can be very helpful. The characteristic finding is a 'double density' sign, in which there is a small area of intense radionuclide activity corresponding to the nidus, superimposed on a second larger area of increased tracer accumulation due to reactive sclerosis.

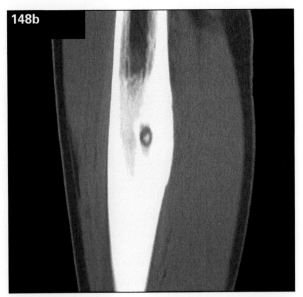

148b CT reconstruction in the same patient clearly shows the lucent lesion with surrounding sclerosis and central nidus.

Answer 148

Practical tips
- In young patients with bony sclerosis in the tibia or femur, look for a radiolucent nidus to confirm this diagnosis.
- When suspected, suggest a CT scan to confirm and accurately localize the nidus.
- When the history and patient's age are strongly suggestive, consider an isotope bone scan if radiographs and CT are unrevealing.

Further management
Treatment consists of complete removal of the nidus. Conventional treatment is surgical, however many cases are now treated radiologically with CT-guided laser photocoagulation. Greater than 90% success rates are reported with this technique.

Further reading
Gangi A, Guth S, Dietemann J, Roy C (2001). Interventional musculoskeletal procedures. *RadioGraphics* 21(3): 1.

Kransdorf M, Stull M, Gilkey F, Moser R (1991). Osteoid osteoma. *RadioGraphics* 11(4): 671–696.

CASE 149

History
A young adult presented after falling onto left arm.

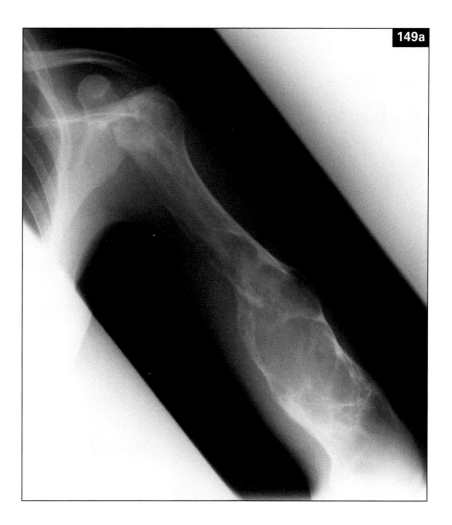

ANSWER 149

Observations (149a)
There is an extensive, expansile lucent lesion involving the length of the left humerus, predominantly the metaphyses and diaphysis. Remodelling of the bone is evident and the lesion has 'ground glass' density in some places. There is, however, no cortical break or periosteal reaction and the lesion has nonaggressive features. The most likely diagnosis is fibrous dysplasia.

Diagnosis
Fibrous dysplasia.

Discussion
Fibrous dysplasia is a benign fibro-osseous developmental anomaly of bone whereby the medullary cavity becomes replaced by an immature matrix of collagen and woven bone. Males and females are equally affected and 75% of patients develop the disease before the age of 30 years. The monostotic form, which most commonly affects the ribs, proximal femur and craniofacial bones, accounts for 80% of cases.

The polyostotic form (i.e. involving more than one site) is seen in the remaining 20% and predominantly affects the femur, tibia, pelvis and facial bones. A subtype of the polyostotic form is McCune–Albright syndrome, where polyostotic unilateral fibrous dysplasia is associated with 'café-au-lait' spots and precocious puberty in young girls. Radiologically, a 'ground glass' density lesion in the medullary cavity is the characteristic feature. The metaphysis is the primary site of involvement with extension into the diaphysis and the lesion may undergo calcification.

The craniofacial form is termed leontiasis ossea and is hemicranial, unlike Paget's disease. The frontal and sphenoid bones are most commonly involved. Sclerotic overgrowth of the facial bones and calvaria results in facial deformity, exophthalmos and visual impairment and obliteration of the sinuses. Sclerosis of the skull base may narrow the neural foramina causing cranial nerve symptoms. Frontal and lateral skull radiographs (**149b**, **149c**) of a patient with leontiasis ossea show these features.

Complications of fibrous dysplasia include pathological fracture, and malignant transformation into osteosarcoma, fibrosarcoma or malignant fibrous histiocytoma in up to 1% of cases.

Osteofibrous dysplasia is an entity that was mistaken in the past for fibrous dysplasia. It is almost exclusively confined to the diaphysis of the tibia and is seen in young children. The appearances are very similar to fibrous dysplasia with a nonaggressive expansile, lucent/ 'ground glass' lesion. Enlargement of the tibia occurs with anterior bowing. As with fibrous dysplasia, pathological fractures commonly occur. The lesion often regresses spontaneously with age. An example is shown (**149d**) that illustrates the typical appearances and mid-diaphyseal location in a young child.

The radiological features of fibrous dysplasia are:
- Lucent/'ground glass' lesion in medullary cavity.
- Expansile.

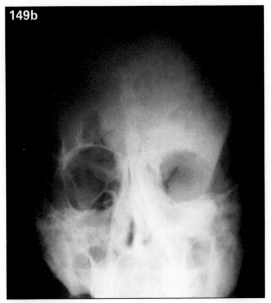

149b Occipitomental radiograph of skull in a patient with leontiasis ossea demonstrating hemicranial sclerosis and expansion.

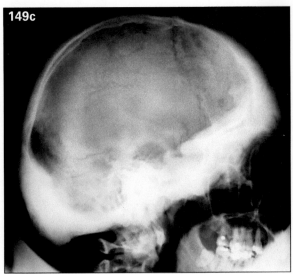

149c Lateral radiograph of the skull in the same patient as in Figure **149b** showing sclerosis and expansion of the calvaria.

Answer 149

- Metadiaphyseal location.
- Remodelling/alteration in bone architecture.
- Endosteal scalloping.
- 'Shepherd's crook' deformity when affecting proximal femur.
- Limb length discrepancy.
- Pathological fracture.
- No cortical destruction.
- Nonaggressive features.

Practical tips
The appearances of fibrous dysplasia overlap with those of many benign bone lesions and it is reasonable to include it on the differential diagnosis list in many cases. As a result, it is often the first differential provided by radiology trainees in a viva even when the lesion in question has characteristic features of something else! Only if a lesion has the characteristic features should fibrous dysplasia be the first diagnosis mentioned – more often, it should be further down the list.

Further management
There is no specific treatment for fibrous dysplasia. Pathological fractures often occur and may necessitate surgical fixation.

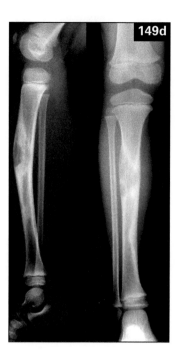

149d Radiographs of the leg in a child demonstrate a lucent/'ground glass' lesion in the diaphysis, which has nonaggressive features and is typical of osteofibrous dysplasia.

CASE 150

History
A 44-year-old female presented with wrist pain.

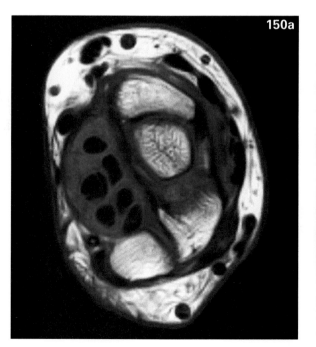
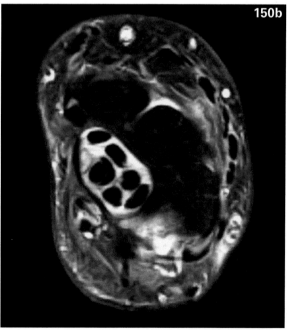

Answer 150

Observations (150a, 150b)
Axial images of the wrist with T1 weighting (**150a**) and T2 fat saturation (**150b**) are shown. Inflamed tendon sheaths are of high signal on T2 fat saturated images and low signal on T1 weighted images. In addition, there is palmar bowing of the flexor retinaculum. The median nerve is of increased signal on the T2 weighted image. This combination of features is consistent with a diagnosis of carpal tunnel syndrome.

Diagnosis
Carpal tunnel syndrome.

Discussion
Carpal tunnel syndrome is a disease that arises due to chronic pressure on the median nerve as it passes within the carpal tunnel, usually associated with repetitive wrist movements. It is more commonly seen in females with a ratio of 4:1 and is bilateral in 50% of cases. Usually diagnosis is made by clinicians with positive findings on clinical examination, electromyelography and nerve conduction studies. Radiological examinations have a role in the few cases where these investigations are inconclusive. Ultrasound is usually the first examination undertaken although MRI has been shown to be more specific and sensitive. US findings are of:
- Median nerve swelling in the proximal tunnel/level of the distal radius.
- Nerve flattening in the distal tunnel.
- Bowing of the flexor retinaculum.

On MRI these same findings can be appreciated:
- Median nerve swelling proximal to the carpal tunnel is termed pseudoneuroma.
- Palmar bowing of the flexor retinaculum.
- Features of tenosynovitis – which appear as high signal on T2 weighted images around the flexor tendons.
- Increased signal in the median nerve on T2 weighted imaging.
- Median nerve enhancement following contrast injection is variable and there can be marked enhancement due to oedema or absence of enhancement due to ischaemia.

Practical tips
Assessment of nerve swelling can be made by comparing the size of the median nerve at the level of the distal radius and at the hamate.

Further management
Methods to decrease oedema and swelling within the carpal tunnel such as treatment of hypothyroidism or restriction of fluid intake can help relieve symptoms. However the gold standard treatment for carpal tunnel syndrome is surgical decompression.

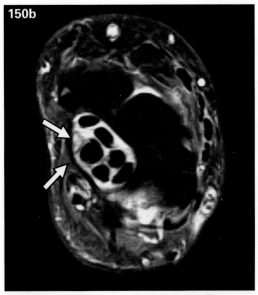

150b High signal of median nerve on T2 weighted image (upper arrow); palmar bowing of flexor retinaculum (lower arrow).

CASE 151

History
An adult female patient with back pain.

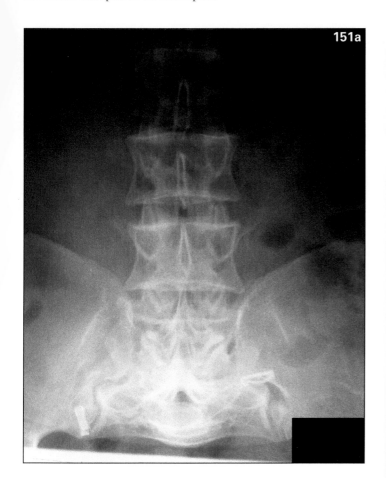
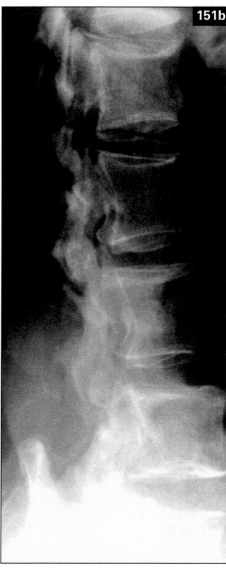

ANSWER 151

Observations (151a, 151b)
AP and lateral radiographs of the lumbar spine show posterior vertebral scalloping of the lower lumbar vertebrae with a narrowed anteroposterior canal diameter. The AP film (**151a**) shows that the interpedicular distance is abnormally narrowed at L5 level and there is squaring of the iliac wings. The features are consistent with achondroplasia.

Diagnosis
Achondroplasia.

Differential diagnosis
Of posterior vertebral scalloping:
- Pressure effect – tumours in spinal canal, syringomyelia and communicating hydrocephalus.
- Dural ectasia. This occurs in neurofibromatosis, Marfan's and Ehlers–Danlos.
- Acromegaly.
- Achondroplasia.
- Congenital disorders such as mucopolysaccharidoses, e.g. Morquio's syndrome.

Discussion
Achondroplasia is an autosomal dominant disease of defective enchondral bone formation related to advanced paternal age. Those with the homozygous form are usually stillborn or die in the neonatal period. Those with heterozygous achondroplasia can have a long life and have normal intelligence.

Radiological features to look for include the following:
- Macrocephaly with bulging forehead (**151c**). A narrow foramen magnum may be associated with hydrocephalus.
- Small J-shaped sella due to flattening of tuberculum sellae.
- Short flared ribs.
- Posterior vertebral scalloping.
- Anterior-inferior vertebral body beaks.
- Short pedicles and caudal narrowing of interpedicular distance (this should normally increase in the caudal direction). These abnormalities can lead to spinal stenosis.
- Squared iliac wings.
- 'Champagne glass' pelvic inlet (**151d**).
- Horizontal sacrum.
- Shortening and bowing of long bones with a 'trumpet' appearance due to disproportionate metaphyseal flaring (**151e**).
- Brachydactyly leading to short stubby fingers (**151f**).

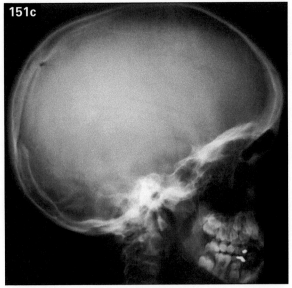

151c Macrocephaly and bulging forehead on lateral skull radiograph.

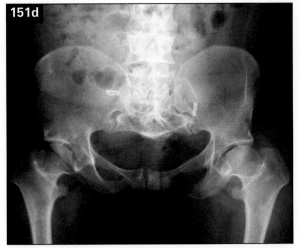

151d AP pelvis in an achondroplastic showing the typical 'champagne glass' pelvis with squaring of the iliac wings. The interpedicular distance is narrowed caudally and the sacrum is horizontal in orientation and difficult to visualize.

Answer 151

Practical tips
- Achondroplasia is an 'Aunt Minnie' – familiarity with the features makes it a straightforward viva case.
- When the sacrum is not seen, possibilities include agenesis, destruction and a horizontal position as in achondroplasia – check for other supporting evidence of the latter, such as narrowing of the interpedicular distance in the lower lumbar spine.
- Posterior vertebral scalloping on plain film – check for:
  - Narrowing of the interpedicular distance caudally in achondroplasia.
  - Cutaneous nodules of neurofibromatosis.
  - Rectangular vertebrae with chondrocalcinosis in acromegaly.

Further management
There is no cure for the condition but affected individuals can normally expect a long life.

Further reading
Cheema J, Grissom L, Harcke H (2003). Radiographic characteristics of lower-extremity bowing in children. *RadioGraphics* **23**: 871–880.

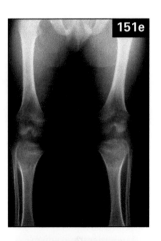

151e Shortening of both legs is seen in this achondroplastic with flaring of the metaphyses producing a 'trumpet' appearance.

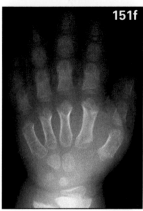

151f Radiograph of the hand demonstrating short, stubby tubular bones.

CASE 152

History
A middle aged female presented with dysphagia.

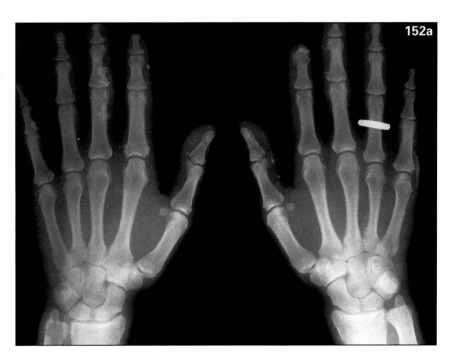

ANSWER 152

Observations (152a)
Destruction of the distal right index finger is seen with almost complete absence of the distal phalanx. Resorption of the distal phalangeal tufts affects several other fingers, most notably the left index finger. There is also widespread soft tissue calcification. The features are characteristic of scleroderma.

Diagnosis
Scleroderma.

Differential diagnosis
Of acro-osteolysis (mnemonic – 'SHARTEN'):
- Scleroderma.
- Hyperparathyroidism.
- Arthropathy – psoriasis, erosive osteoarthritis, rheumatoid, etc.
- Raynaud's.
- Trauma and thermal injury.
- Epidermolysis bullosa.
- Neuropathy, e.g. syringomyelia and diabetes.

Of fingertip calcification:
- Scleroderma.
- Raynaud's.
- Hyperparathyroidism.
- Dermatomyositis.

Discussion
Acro-osteolysis is the term used to describe resorption or destruction of the distal phalangeal tufts. There are many causes but only the more relevant and common ones are listed. The three main patterns of involvement are: distal tuft, midportion and periarticular (i.e. at the base). Periosteal reaction is not usually seen at the site of resorption.

Practical tips
- Soft tissue calcification is characteristic in scleroderma but can also be seen in other causes of acro-osteolysis such as hyperparathyroidism and Raynaud's. When present, check for erosive arthritis, tapered fingers (sclerodactyly) or swollen fingers (sausage fingers) in scleroderma. Hyperparathyroidism may also show classical subperiosteal resorption along the radial aspect of the middle phalanges.
- With regard to the three different patterns of acro-osteolysis:
  - Hyperparathyroidism can cause any of the three patterns but is the only commonly occurring condition that causes resorption of the midportion of the phalanx.
  - Scleroderma can cause erosion of the distal tuft (by pressure erosion from tight skin) or at the base of the phalanx (by virtue of erosive arthropathy).
  - Resorption of the proximal phalanx is, not surprisingly, caused by the erosive arthropathies, in particular psoriatic arthropathy – look for erosive arthropathy of the interphalangeal joints with ankylosis and 'pencil in cup' deformity.
- Most of the other conditions listed affect the distal tuft.
- Scleroderma is a multisystem disease so look for other changes e.g. lung fibrosis, oesophageal dilatation (**152b**) – see Case 17.

Further management
There is no cure for scleroderma. Treatment is supportive.

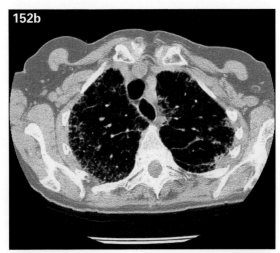

152b Single axial CT image of the same patient with scleroderma showing lung parenchymal changes of fibrosis with subpleural reticulation. There is also a dilated oesophagus.

CASE 153

History
A child presented having had a fall on outstretched hand.

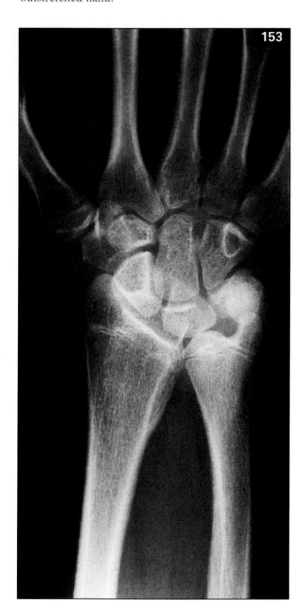

CASE 154

History
An 15-year-old male presented with back pain.

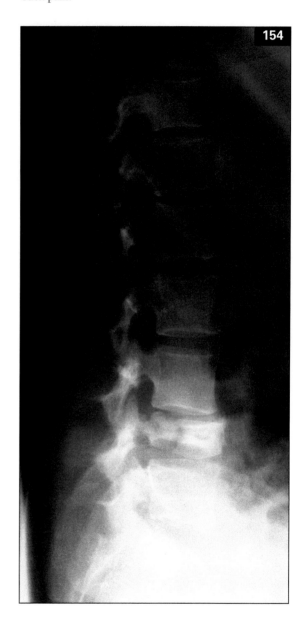

ANSWER 153

Observations (153)
There is relative shortening and ulnar curve of the distal radius with wedging of the carpus between the distal radius and ulna. The features are consistent with Madelung deformity. There are no exostoses to indicate diaphyseal aclasis, and a more specific cause cannot be established from this film.

Diagnosis
Madelung deformity.

Differential diagnosis
Of causes of Madelung deformity (mnemonic – 'TILDti'):
- Turner's syndrome.
- Idiopathic.
- Leri–Weil disease (dyschondrosteosis).
- Diaphyseal aclasis.
- Trauma and Infection can lead to pseudo-Madelung deformity.

Discussion
Madelung deformity comprises a short distal radius which has abnormal dorsal and ulnar curvature resulting in ulnar tilt of the distal radial articular surface. The distal ulnar is also subluxed dorsally, and the triangular-shaped carpus is wedged into the reduced carpal angle created at the wrist. There are several conditions associated with Madelung deformity, shown in the differential diagnosis list below. When idiopathic, Madelung deformity is seen mostly in adolescent or young adult women and tends to be bilateral and asymmetrical. Leri–Weil disease is an autosomal dominant condition where sufferers have bilateral Madelung deformity and mesomelic long-bone shortening with limited motion of the elbow and wrist.

Turner's syndrome is associated with Madelung deformity as well as short stature, webbed neck, horseshoe kidney, aortic coarctation and shortening of the 4th metacarpal.

Trauma and infection may lead to premature fusion of the distal radial growth plate and if this occurs only on the ulnar aspect, there will be resulting ulnar tilt of the distal radius as the radial aspect of the physis allows continued growth on this side. This results in a reduced carpal angle and a pseudo-Madelung deformity.

Practical tips
- Look for metaphyseal exostoses pointing away from the joints indicating diaphyseal aclasis.
- Look for shortening of the 4th metacarpal, which is associated with Turner's syndrome.

Further management
There is no specific treatment for this condition.

ANSWER 154

Observations (154)
There is uniform collapse of the L4 vertebral body causing the appearance of a vertebra plana. The most likely cause in a child for a solitary collapsed vertebra is eosinophilic granuloma.

Diagnosis
Eosinophilic granuloma causing vertebra plana.

Differential diagnosis
For vertebra plana:
- Idiopathic.
- Infection.
- Neoplastic (metastasis, leukaemia).
- Trauma.
- Steroids.
- Haemangioma.

For platyspondyly:
- Thanatophoric dwarfism.
- Osteogenesis imperfecta.
- Morquio's disease.
- Spondyloepiphyseal dysplasia congenital.
- Kniest syndrome.

Discussion
Vertebra plana is the term used to describe uniform collapse of a vertebral body into a thin, flat disk. The most common cause in children is eosinophilic granuloma, with the thoracic vertebrae most frequently affected. The vertebral body is described as having a 'coin on edge' appearance. The disc spaces are preserved and can in fact appear slightly widened. Usually there is no kyphotic deformity associated. The posterior elements of the vertebra are normally spared. Early on, the vertebra will appear lytic and preserved in height before gradually uniform collapse develops. Soft tissue oedema or a paraspinal soft tissue mass are sometimes seen. With healing there is reconstitution of the vertebra to its original height, although some residual compression deformity normally persists. There are many other causes of vertebra plana as outlined in the differential diagnosis. One of these is avascular necrosis, which when idiopathic is termed vertebral osteochondrosis or Calvé–Kummel–Verneuil disease.

Answer 154

Practical tips
- The vertebral body affected has a uniformly flat 'coin on edge' appearance.
- Intervertebral discs are typically spared with normal disc spaces.
- The posterior elements are spared.
- Marked generalized osteopenia suggests osteogenesis imperfecta.
- Malignant causes may affect more than one vertebral body.

Whereas vertebra plana is the term used to describe flattening of a previously normal vertebral body, platyspondyly refers to flattening of the vertebral bodies from birth. Platyspondyly may be generalized, affecting all the vertebral bodies, multiple, affecting some but not all the vertebral bodies, or localized, involving just one vertebral body.

Further management
The underlying cause should be determined if possible. Eosinophilic granuloma is the most common cause in children and usually resolves spontaneously with age.

CASE 155

History
A young adult presented with abdominal pains.

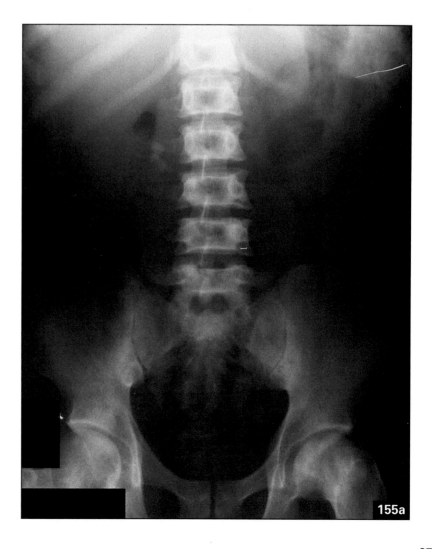

ANSWER 155

Observations (155a)
Three well defined densities in the right upper quadrant are projected outside the contour of the right kidney and are likely to represent gallstones. There is mild, diffuse osteosclerosis and increased trabeculation of the bony skeleton with vertebral endplate infarctions causing H-shaped lumbar vertebrae. Sclerosis and flattening of the left femoral head suggest avascular necrosis. The spleen is noted to be atrophic and calcified. Overall the features are consistent with a diagnosis of sickle cell disease.

Diagnosis
Sickle cell disease.

Discussion
Sickle cell disease is an inherited disorder mostly seen in Afro-Caribbeans. The sickling of the red blood cells leads to increased blood viscosity, occlusion of small vessels and bone infarction leading to necrosis. Chronic haemolytic anaemia also ensues. Marrow hyperplasia leads to coarsening of the trabeculae and may cause diffuse osteosclerosis. A CXR in a 17-year-old female with sickle cell disease is shown (**155b**). This demonstrates diffuse osteosclerosis with H-shaped thoracic vertebrae (due to endplate infarctions) and cardiomegaly (secondary to chronic anaemia).

Practical tips
Ancillary signs of sickle cell disease on the radiograph depend on the area of the body imaged:
- Abdominal radiograph:
  - H-shaped vertebrae due to endplate infarctions.
  - Avascular necrosis of the femoral heads causing flattening and fragmentation.
  - Gallstones (secondary to haemolytic anaemia).
  - Splenic atrophy and calcification.
  - Renal papillary necrosis may be caused by sickle cell disease due to sloughing of papillae from infarction; a sloughed papilla may be seen within the renal calyx (on an IVU) (**155c**).

- Chest radiograph:
  - H-shaped vertebrae due to endplate infarctions.
  - Avascular necrosis of the humeral heads.
  - Cardiomegaly (due to chronic anaemia).

- Skull radiograph:
  - 'Hair on end' appearance of skull vault due to marrow hyperplasia.
  - Widening of diploic space.

Further management
Treatment is generally supportive with multiple transfusions being necessary. There is a high incidence of infection of bone and lung. Skeletal pain can occur not only from osteomyelitis but also from bone marrow infarction.

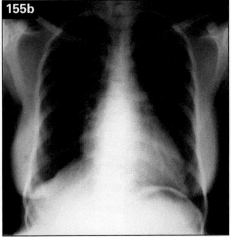

155b CXR in a patient with sickle cell disease demonstrating diffuse osteosclerosis with cardiomegaly and H-shaped thoracic vertebrae.

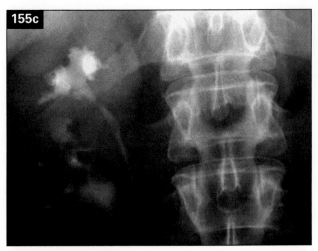

155c Sloughed papilla.

CASE 156

History
An 80-year-old woman presented with left arm and right leg pain.

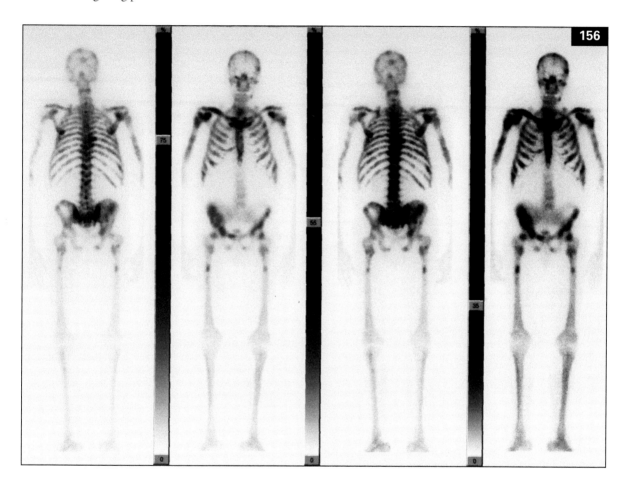

ANSWER 156

Observations (156)
A full body bone scan is presented. There is widespread, diffuse increased skeletal uptake with more focal areas of increased uptake located in the skull, spine, ribs, pelvis and limbs. No renal uptake of isotope is seen, however there is some uptake in the bladder. The findings are therefore consistent with a 'superscan' and the most likely cause is widespread metastases.

Diagnosis
'Superscan' due to widespread metastases.

Differential diagnosis
Of causes of a 'superscan':
- Diffuse skeletal metastases.
- Renal osteodystrophy.
- Osteomalacia.
- Hyperparathyroidism.
- Hyperthyroidism.
- Myelofibrosis.
- Leukaemia.
- Aplastic anaemia.
- Widespread Paget's disease.

Discussion
Diffusely increased activity in the bones on an isotope bone scan can result in an 'absent kidney sign' where there is little or no activity in the kidneys but good visualization of the urinary bladder. This is termed a 'superscan'. The key finding is the absence of activity in the kidneys, which can be easily missed when the diffuse increase in skeletal activity is overlooked. In fact many such scans were reported as normal in the past until the importance of absent renal activity secondary to diffuse skeletal uptake was realized.

The most common cause is skeletal metastases, most of the other causes being metabolic. In this particular case, there are multiple foci of increased uptake on a background of increased activity, however more difficult cases of 'superscan' might show homogeneous activity that would be more easily overlooked. The diffuse increase in activity is usually more prominent in the axial skeleton, calvaria, mandible, sternum, costochondral junctions and long bones. The femoral cortices become visible and there is also increased metaphyseal activity.

Radiological signs in 'superscan' are:
- Diffuse increased skeletal activity.
- Prominent uptake in axial skeleton, long bones and sternum.
- Absent/little uptake in the kidneys.
- Visualization of bladder.
- Increased bone to soft tissue ratio.
- Increased metaphyseal and periarticular uptake.
- Visible femoral cortices.

Practical tips
- Diffusely increased activity in the bones on a 'superscan' is particular prominent in the sternum producing a 'tie sternum'.
- Metabolic causes tend to cause more diffuse uptake whereas metastatic causes may produce more focal areas of increased uptake.

Further management
When a 'superscan' is seen, the most important factor is to determine whether the cause is due to metabolic or malignant disease. This may be evident from the history and clinical examination.

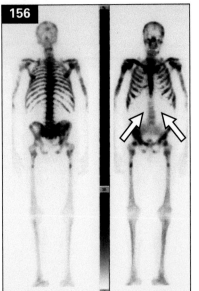

156 No renal uptake.

CASE 157

History
An elderly patient presented with leg pains.

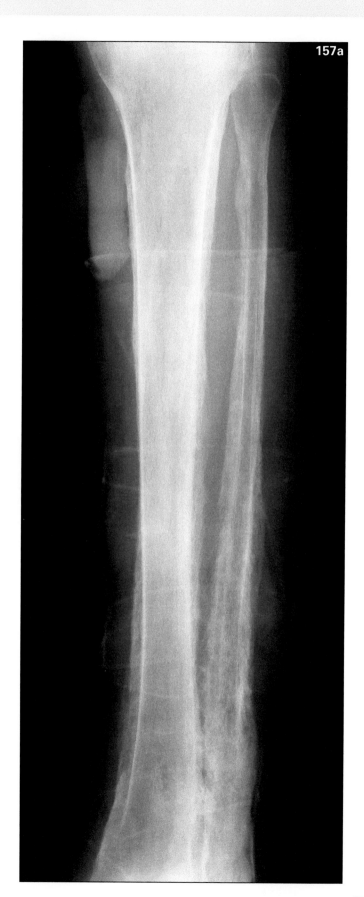

ANSWER 157

Observations (157a)
There is diffuse, thick periosteal reaction along the metadiaphyses of the left tibia and fibula. Bandages are also noted around the leg and an elongated soft tissue opacity in the upper medial leg may well indicate a varix. There is no arterial calcification of note. The most likely cause of the periosteal reaction is chronic venous insufficiency, though it is still advisable to obtain a chest radiograph to exclude hypertrophic pulmonary osteoarthropathy from an occult lung tumour.

Diagnosis
Venous insufficiency.

Differential diagnosis
Of diffuse bilateral periosteal reaction in adults:
- Hypertrophic pulmonary osteoarthropathy (HPOA).
- Vascular insufficiency.
- Pachydermoperiostosis.
- Thyroid acropachy.
- Fluorosis.

Discussion
Focal periosteal reaction demands careful assessment for an underlying bone lesion including tumour, infection, fracture, etc. However, diffuse reaction that is bilateral and may well affect multiple bones is a different scenario requiring this brief differential diagnosis:
- HPOA is the most likely cause for such an appearance in adults. The condition presents with painful swelling and clubbing may occur. The periosteal reaction is of variable thickness and typically affects the lower half of the arm and leg. Soft tissue swelling and periarticular osteoporosis may be appreciable radiologically. A chest radiograph should be requested to exclude a lung tumour. Other causes of hypertrophic osteoarthropathy include fibrotic lung disease, suppurative lung disease, liver cirrhosis and inflammatory bowel disease.
- Vascular insufficiency (arterial or venous) is almost always seen in the lower limbs.
- Thyroid acropachy – periosteal reaction typically affects the radial side of the thumb and index fingers. Clubbing of the fingers may be present. An example is shown (157b), although the thumb and index fingers are affected, periosteal reaction is also seen along most of the phalanges and the 5th metacarpal.
- Pachydermoperiostosis is an autosomal dominant condition, typically seen in young black males. It is relatively pain free and self-limiting but causes skin thickening and clubbing. Enlarged paranasal sinuses are also seen. Periosteal reaction most commonly affects the lower half of the arm and leg, though hands can also be affected. Periosteal reaction looks very similar to HPOA but begins around ligament and tendon insertions, i.e. close to the epiphysis.
- Fluorosis – ligamentous calcification present.

Practical tips
- On identifying diffuse periosteal reaction on radiographs of the limbs always ask for a CXR as this can be the first manifestation of a primary lung tumour.
- Bandages and phleboliths point to chronic venous insufficiency and arterial calcification to arterial disease.
- Though all five causes can affect the hands, remember thyroid acropachy in particular with this distribution.
- Fluorosis is something that is unlikely to be seen outside of exam vivas but remember ligamentous calcification is characteristic!

Further management
This depends on the cause. HPOA is the most common cause and the most important management aspect is to exclude the presence of an underlying lung tumour.

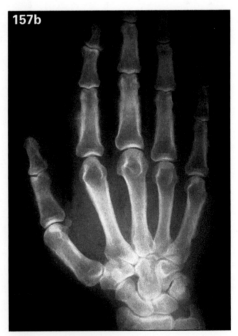

157b Hand radiograph of a patient with thyroid acropachy demonstrating periosteal reaction along the diaphyses of most of the phalanges and the 1st and 5th metacarpals.

CASE 158

History
A 14-year-old male presented with arm pain.

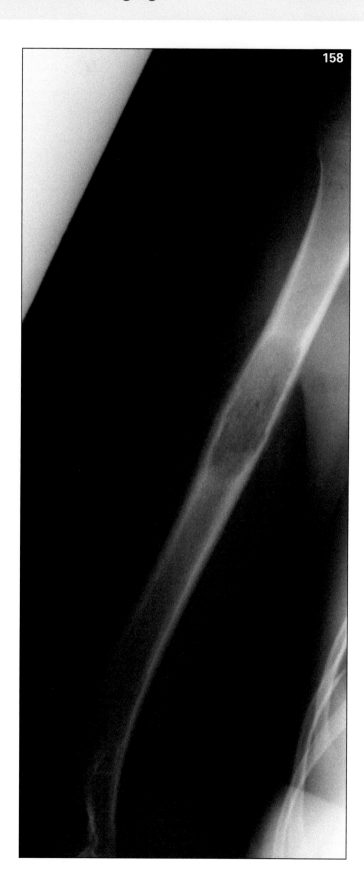

ANSWER 158

Observations (158)
Within the midshaft of the diaphysis of the humerus there is a relatively well defined lytic lesion that has a narrow zone of transition. There is endosteal scalloping and smooth lamellated periosteal reaction. The lesion has nonaggressive features and in this age group eosinophilic granuloma or infection is the most likely diagnosis.

Diagnosis
Eosinophilic granuloma.

Differential diagnosis
- Osteomyelitis.
- Fibrous dysplasia.
- Leukaemia.
- Lymphoma.

Discussion
Langerhans cell histiocytosis is a spectrum of disease characterized by idiopathic proliferation of histiocytes producing focal or systemic manifestations. Eosinophilic granuloma is the term used to describe the disease when limited to bone and is mostly seen in patients aged between 5 and 30 years. The clinical and radiological features may mimic infection as well as other benign and malignant diseases. The cause and pathogenesis of the condition are unknown. Clinical manifestations relate to the affected bone with local pain, tenderness and masses commonly observed. Patients may have low-grade fever or elevated inflammatory markers, which confuses the clinical picture with infection. The disease may occur in any bone, although there is a predilection for the flat bones with more than half occurring in the skull, mandible, ribs and pelvis. Lesions are solitary in 50–75% of cases. Approximately one-third of lesions occur in the long bones, most commonly the femur followed by the humerus and tibia. Most lesions occur in the diaphysis, and in general the growth plate acts as a barrier to extension.

Radiographic appearances are varied. Lesions typically appear lytic but may have reactive sclerosis. Margins can be well demarcated or poorly defined and they may even have a permeative appearance. A lamellated periosteal reaction is often seen. Invasion of overlying soft tissue may result if the lesion penetrates through the cortex. In the skull, the lesion is often round with a punched out appearance and uneven destruction of the inner and outer skull tables results in a 'double contour' or 'bevelled edge' appearance. If there is more than one lesion, these may coalesce producing 'geographical skull'. In the spine, the vertebral body is the most common site of involvement. Lung involvement occurs in 10%. Treatment of the bone lesions consists of conservative therapy or surgical treatment such as curettage or excision.

Practical tips
Always keep this condition in mind when forming differential diagnoses for lytic bone lesions in the young patient – the appearances are varied and the clinical picture may be confusing.

Further management
The prognosis of eosinophilic granuloma is excellent with spontaneous resolution of bony lesions occurring in 6–18 months.

Further reading
Levine S, Lambiase R, Petchprapa C (2003). Cortical lesions of the tibia: characteristic appearances at conventional radiography. *RadioGraphics* 23: 157–177.

Stull M, Kransdorf M, Devaney K (1992). Langerhans cell histiocytosis of bone. *RadioGraphics* 12(4): 801–823.

CASE 159

History
A 24-year-old male presents with knee instability following a football injury 2 months previously.

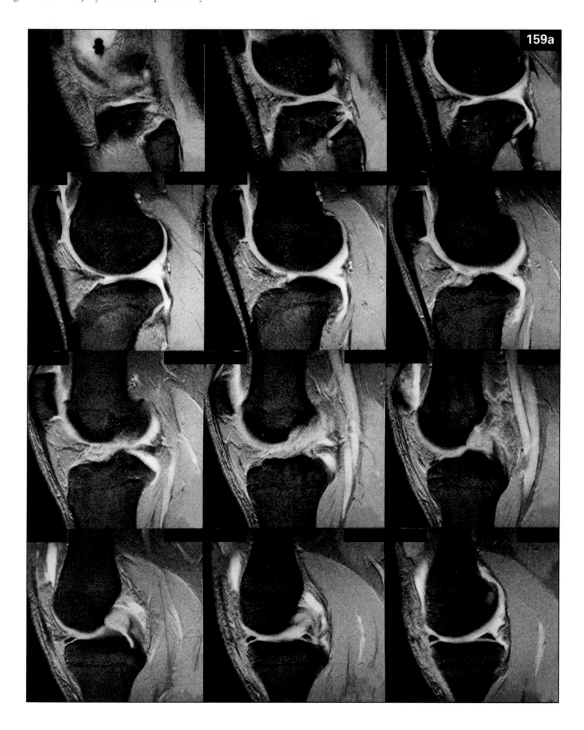

ANSWER 159

Observations (159a)
Sagittal T2 weighted images of the knee demonstrate a rupture of the anterior cruciate ligament, no intact fibres being demonstrated. In keeping with this, there is mild anterior tibial translocation. The posterior cruciate ligament (PCL) is intact.

There is loss of the normal 'bow tie' appearance of the lateral meniscus with non-visualization of the body and much of the posterior horn. Furthermore, abnormal low signal tissue is present in the intercondylar region just lateral to the PCL. These findings are indicative of a 'bucket handle' tear of the lateral meniscus with a fragment of meniscus displaced medially. A joint effusion is also present.

Diagnosis
Anterior cruciate ligament (ACL) rupture with 'bucket handle' tear of the lateral meniscus.

Differential diagnosis
None.

Discussion
The ACL is best evaluated on T1 weighted images and fibres should run parallel to the roof of the intercondylar notch (159b). ACL tears most commonly leave no normal residual fibres visible on MRI. Sometimes, residual fibres of the ACL are seen, but following a more horizontal than normal course.

Sagittal images of normal menisci show a 'bow tie' appearance on at least two contiguous slices (159c). This is because the normal meniscus is approximately 9 mm in width and the sagittal images are 3–4 mm in thickness. Thus, at least two sagittal slices should pass through a contiguous section of meniscus.

'Bucket handle' tears constitute about 10% of meniscal tears. The vertical tear through the inner edge produces a mobile fragment that flips through approximately 180°, much like a handle flipping from one side of a bucket to the other. In such circumstances, the residual part of meniscus will be reduced in thickness and will not be seen on the usual number of sagittal scans. If the 'bow tie' is seen on less than two contiguous sagittal images, a 'bucket handle' tear must be excluded. The mobile fragment should then be sought elsewhere in the joint, e.g. medially in the intercondylar region; anterior to the posterior cruciate ligament (PCL) producing the 'double PCL' sign (159d); in the anterior joint, in front of the anterior horn of the meniscus.

Other types of meniscal tear include:
- Oblique and horizontal – linear signal change within the meniscus that extends to the inferior or superior surface.
- Radial (also known as 'parrot beak' tear) – a vertical tear through the free edge will produce an absent 'bow tie' sign similar to a 'bucket handle' tear. However, the defect is only small and so the defect in the 'bow tie' is much smaller.

As an aside, if the 'bow tie' appearance of the meniscus is seen on more than two sagittal images this can be indicative of a discoid meniscus. This is probably a congenital abnormality where the meniscus has a more disc-like shape than the normal 'C-shape' due to a wider than normal body. They are more prone to tearing and can be symptomatic even without being torn.

Further management
- A complete ACL tear causes instability that is treated by surgical repair with a prosthetic or tendon graft.
- Meniscal tears often require arthroscopic debridement.

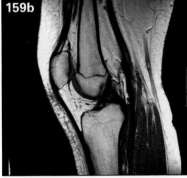

159b Sagittal T1 weighted image shows an intact anterior cruciate ligament.

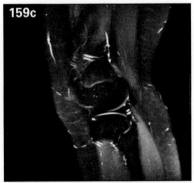

159c Sagittal T2 weighted image shows a normal lateral meniscus.

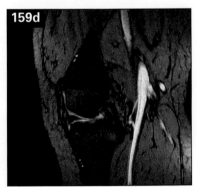

159d Sagittal T2 weighted image shows the 'double PCL' sign of a 'bucket handle' tear of the medial meniscus

CASE 160

History
A female patient presented with joint pains.

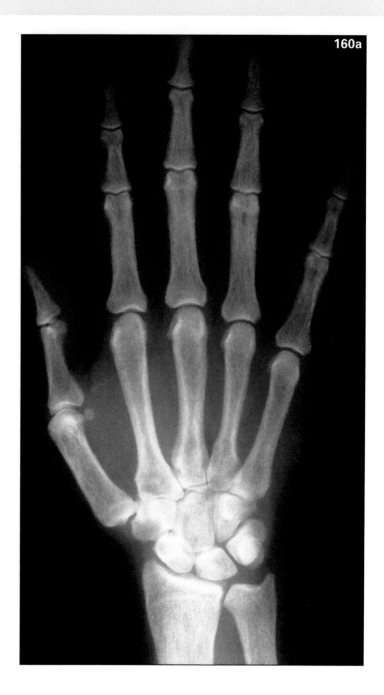

ANSWER 160

Observations (160a)
There is subperiosteal resorption of the radial aspect of the middle phalanges of the index and middle fingers. No evidence of marginal erosions or brown tumours is seen though the trabecular pattern is coarsened. The findings are consistent with hyperparathyroidism.

Diagnosis
Hyperparathyroidism.

Discussion
The uncontrolled production of parathyroid hormone in hyperparathyroidism is primary, secondary or tertiary. Primary hyperparathyroidism is caused by a parathyroid adenoma. The raised parathyroid hormone levels lead to resorption of bone and hypercalcaemia. Secondary hyperparathyroidism is usually a consequence of renal insufficiency, where chronic hypocalcaemia leads to parathyroid hyperplasia. Some patients with secondary hyperparathyroidism then go on to develop the tertiary form, whereby a parathyroid adenoma arises within a chronically overstimulated hyperplastic parathyroid gland.

The cardinal radiological feature is subperiosteal bone resorption. The different sites affected are shown below, the classical location being the radial aspect of the middle phalanx of the index and middle fingers. Figure **160b** shows another pattern of erosion – band-like zones in the middle of the terminal tufts. Bone softening may result in wedged vertebrae, kyphoscoliosis and bowing of long bones. Parathyroid-hormone-stimulated focal osteoclastic activity can cause brown tumours, which are characteristically expansile, lytic, well demarcated lesions. These can be the solitary sign of hyperparathyroidism in 3% of cases. Figure **160e** shows a pathological fracture through a brown tumour.

Radiological features of hyperparathyroidism are as follows:
- Bone resorption:
  - Radial aspect middle phalanx of 2nd and 3rd fingers (**160a**).
  - Terminal phalangeal tufts (**160b**).
  - Distal end of clavicles and superior aspect of ribs on CXR.
  - Medial aspect proximal tibia (**160c**).
  - Medial femoral and humeral necks.
  - Lamina dura of skull and teeth producing 'floating teeth'.
  - 'Pepper-pot' skull due to trabecular resorption (**160d**).
  - Pseudo-widening of joints, e.g. sacroiliac joints.
  - Marginal erosions of the hands.

- Bone softening:
  - Wedged vertebrae.
  - Kyphoscoliosis.
  - Bowing of long bones.

- Brown tumour (**160e**).
- Osteosclerosis (more common in secondary hyperparathyroidism).
  - 'Rugger jersey' spine.

- Soft tissue calcification:
  - Periarticular.
  - Chondrocalcinosis.
  - Arterial.

- Renal calculi.
- Medullary nephrocalcinosis.

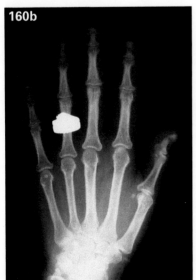

160b Left hand radiograph demonstrating lucent bands of resorption across the mid-portions of the distal phalanges of the first three digits.

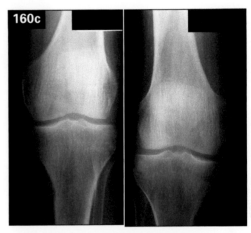

160c AP radiograph of both knees demonstrates subperiosteal resorption at the medial aspect of both tibial metaphyses.

Answer 160 — Musculoskeletal Imaging

Practical tips
- On CXR look for subperiosteal resorption at the superior aspects of the ribs – Figure **160f** demonstrates very subtle resorption at the superior aspects of the posterior left 7th and 8th ribs. Also look for erosion of the lateral ends of the clavicles (**160g**). Hyperparathyroidism is associated with renal failure so there may be a haemodialysis line on the film and prominent soft tissue calcification. Lucent bone lesions may be due to brown tumours.
- On AXR look for a peritoneal dialysis catheter. There may be renal calculi or medullary nephrocalcinosis. A 'rugger jersey' spine may be seen along with widening of the sacroiliac joints due to resorption.

Further management
Primary hyperparathyroidism is treated by surgical resection of the parathyroid gland. After clinical and serological diagnosis of hyperparathyroidism, US and/or sestamibi scintigraphy of the neck is often performed to locate the adenoma pre-operatively (**160h**). In suspected ectopic parathyroid adenoma, MRI or scintigraphy may be required to locate the tumour.

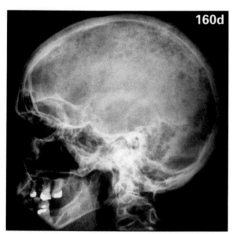

160d Diffuse bone resorption of the calvaria producing a 'pepper-pot' skull appearance.

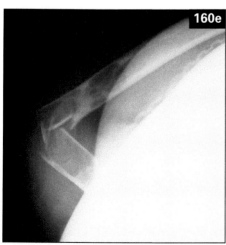

160e Radiograph of the humerus in a patient with brown tumours; there are lytic lesions with an associated pathological fracture.

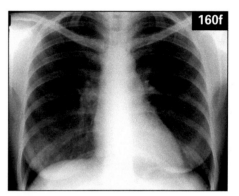

160f CXR in a patient with hyperparathyroidism with subtle erosions of the superior aspects of the left posterior 7th and 8th ribs.

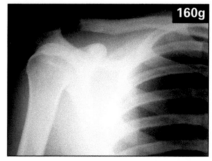

160g AP radiograph of right shoulder demonstrating erosion of the lateral end of the right clavicle.

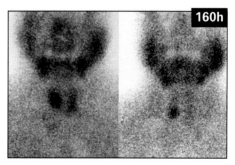

160h Sestamibi scan with images at 10 min and 90 min post injection show retained tracer in a right parathyroid adenoma.

Chapter 5

PAEDIATRIC IMAGING

The approach to paediatric imaging is essentially a composite of the suggested approaches in the other chapters. The approach with paediatric films is as for adult films but the differential diagnosis list will be completely different in many cases. Some additional points when approaching paediatric films are:

- It is very useful to know whether the child has had a premature birth as conditions such as hyaline membrane disease and necrotizing enterocolitis are essentially diseases of the premature neonate. In addition, patterns of disease can vary between infants born prematurely and those born at term. For example, hypoxic/ischaemic brain injury in the premature infant leads to periventricular leukomalacia, a pattern of injury rather different to that otherwise seen.
- Particularly in the child under 2 years, always consider the possibility of 'non accidental injury' (NAI) in suspected trauma. However, while it is important to be vigilant for NAI, a false assumption can have severe consequences for the family and must not be declared likely without due consideration. Although certain injuries such as metaphyseal fractures and depressed skull fractures may be highly suspicious for NAI, a multidisciplinary approach should be used with involvement of a specialist paediatric radiologist and appropriate clinical correlation.
- The distribution of categories of disease is very different in children and adults. For example, degenerative disease is largely a feature of adult medicine, and while malignancy is certainly seen in children, it is far less common than in adults. Conversely, congenital disorders are a much bigger consideration in children and there are many such rare conditions that remain outside the realm of the general radiologist's experience. For example, there are many varieties of skeletal dysplasia causing widespread abnormalities of the skeleton. In the examination viva for general radiological training, it is unlikely that you will be expected to know specific details of the less common varieties. However, it is reasonable to expect you to recognize that a skeletal dysplasia is likely and suggest specialist review by a paediatric radiologist with an interest in such disorders.
- Imaging that utilizes ionizing radiation has an associated risk that must always be balanced against the potential benefit of diagnosis. This is even more important in the child, where the risk of ionizing radiation is greater. As such, while CT imaging is now commonplace in the early work-up of adult illness, greater reliance may be placed on modalities such as ultrasound and MRI in the paediatric population.

CASE 161

History
Stillborn fetus.

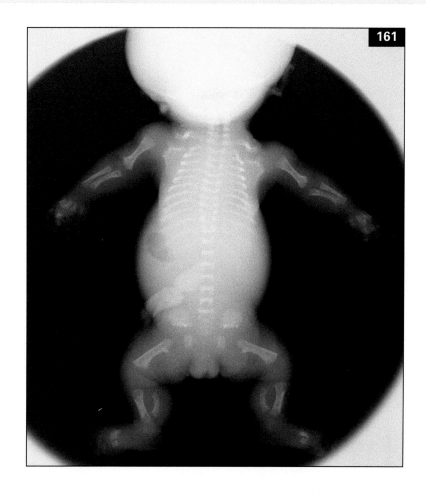

CASE 162

History
An 8-year-old child presented with headaches.

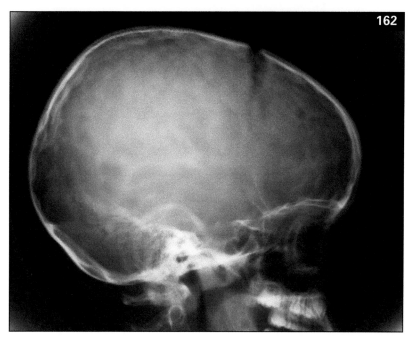

ANSWER 161

Observations (161)
This radiograph is of a stillborn baby as there is no air seen within the lungs. The cut umbilical cord is seen, confirming that this is a newborn. The thoracic cage is narrow and there is squaring of the iliac wings. There is bowing of the long bones with flaring of the metaphyses producing a characteristic 'telephone handle' shape. There is no evidence of fractures to suggest osteogenesis imperfecta. The most likely diagnosis is thanatophoric dysplasia.

Diagnosis
Thanatophoric dysplasia.

Differential diagnosis
Of lethal neonatal dysplasia:
- Osteogenesis imperfecta.
- Thanatophoric dysplasia.
- Jeune's syndrome (asphyxiating thoracic dysplasia). The narrow elongated thorax contains a normal size heart but leaves little room for the lungs. There is an 80% mortality rate from respiratory failure.

Discussion
Thanatophoric dysplasia, which is also known as thanatophoric dwarfism, is one of the more common causes of lethal neonatal dysplasia. The most common is osteogenesis imperfecta.

Practical tips
It may be possible to identify the specific cause of the lethal neonatal dysplasia from certain features on the babygram:
- Osteogenesis imperfecta will cause generalized osteopenia with bowing of long bones and multiple fractures. Multiple wormian bones may also be seen in the skull.
- Thanatophoric dysplasia is associated with a narrow thoracic cage and 'telephone handle' long bones. The iliac wings may be small and squared.
- Narrowing of the thoracic cage and small squared iliac wings are also seen in Jeune's syndrome. The ribs may also be small and horizontal in this condition.

Further management
No further management options.

ANSWER 162

Observations (162)
There is significant widening of the coronal suture. The skull vault also has a 'copper beaten' appearance. The combination of findings suggests raised intracranial pressure and urgent CT or MRI should be advised.

Diagnosis
Suture diastasis due to raised intracranial pressure.

Differential diagnosis
Of the causes of suture diastasis follows the mnemonic 'TRIM':
- Traumatic diastasis.
- Raised intracranial pressure:
  - Intracerebral tumour.
  - Hydrocephalus.
  - Subdural collection.

- Infiltration (of the sutures):
  - Leukaemia.
  - Lymphoma.
  - Neuroblastoma.

- Metabolic:
  - Hypoparathyroidism.
  - Rickets.
  - Hypophosphatasia.

Discussion
Abnormal widening of the cranial sutures is suggested if there is widening of >10 mm at birth, >3 mm at 2 years and >2 mm at 3 years. The appearance of wide sutures may just be a normal variant but there are several pathological causes, as listed Suture widening due to elevated intracranial pressure is unlikely after 10 years of age.

Practical tips
- Suture diastasis, copper beaten skull appearance and erosion of the dorsum sella are classical plain film signs of raised intracranial pressure.
- A tense fontanelle is a useful clinical sign to confirm raised intracranial pressure.

Further management
In most cases, clinical suspicion of elevated intracranial pressure will lead directly to CT or MRI evaluation, but this is clearly the next step should such findings be encountered on plain films with no other explanation.

CASE 163

History
Emergency plain CT of the brain in a 4-year-old child with acute seizures and hypoxia.

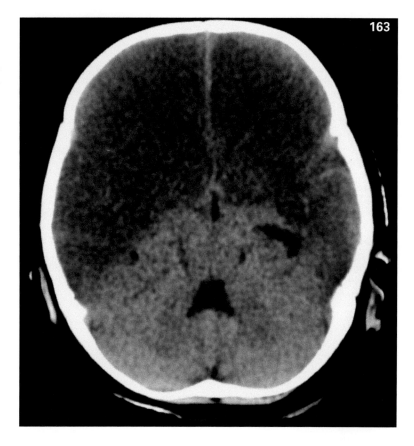

CASE 164

History
A newborn presented with breathing difficulties at birth.

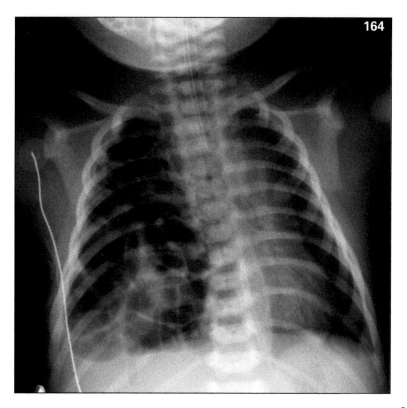

ANSWER 163

Observations (163)
The CT scan image shows diffuse cerebral oedema with effacement of the sulci and gyri. The grey and white matter of the cerebral hemispheres are low in attenuation resulting in loss of the normal corticomedullary differentiation. There is sparing of the cerebellum and brainstem which have an increased density by comparison. The features are typical of the acute 'reversal sign' indicating that there has been severe hypoxic-ischaemic brain injury.

Diagnosis
Severe hypoxic-ischaemic injury producing the 'reversal sign'.

Discussion
When hypoxia, ischaemia or circulatory arrest occur in children, diffuse hypoxic-ischaemic brain injury can ensue. The cerebral circulation redistributes to the most vital areas, i.e. hindbrain so that the cerebrum is first affected. CT in the first 24 hr may show subtle hypoattenuation of the basal ganglia and insular cortex with effacement of the cisterns around the midbrain. Subsequent CT scans (at 24–72 hr) show diffuse cerebral oedema with effacement of the sulci and cisterns, and decreased grey matter – white matter differentiation.

CT features of the so-called 'reversal sign' are hypodensity of the cerebrum with reduced, lost, or even reversed grey matter–white matter differentiation. The thalami, brainstem and cerebellum are relatively spared and retain a more normal density, thus appearing denser than the cerebrum. This finding indicates irreversible brain damage and a universally poor prognosis.

Further reading
Barkovich A (2005). *Paediatric Neuroimaging*, 4th edn. Lippincott, Williams and Wilkins, Baltimore, pp. 240–241.

ANSWER 164

Observations (164)
An endotracheal tube is in place in a satisfactory position. The right hemithorax is filled by a large septated lucent mass, which is causing mediastinal shift to the contralateral side. The hemidiaphragm is not visualized. The most likely cause is a congenital diaphragmatic hernia, however cystic adenomatoid malformation should be considered.

Diagnosis
Congenital diaphragmatic hernia (CDH).

Discussion
Congenital diaphragmatic hernia results from failure of closure of the pleuroperitoneal fold during gestation and presents with respiratory distress soon after birth. It is the most common thoracic fetal anomaly, affecting 1 in 2,500 livebirths. The left side is much more commonly affected than the right. The solid abdominal organs can be herniated as well as bowel. The two main types of hernia are the posterolateral Bochdalek and the anteromedial Morgagni hernias. Survival depends on the size of the hernia, as this determines the degree of pulmonary hypoplasia that will have resulted. There is an association with CNS neural tube defects.

The main differential diagnosis on imaging is cystic adenomatoid malformation (CAM). This congenital cystic abnormality of the lung results from arrest of the normal bronchoalveolar differentiation *in utero*. The imaging features can be almost identical to those of a diaphragmatic hernia, although the cysts may be fluid filled and thus appear solid.

Practical tips
- Bochdalek occurs at the Back of the thorax and accounts for 90% of CDH.
- Morgagni occurs More on the right (heart prevents development on left) and accounts for the other 10%.

Further management
Many cases will be expected from antenatal scans and delivery in an appropriate setting can be arranged. Unexpected cases present a medical emergency and may first be suspected when bowel sounds are heard in the chest of an infant with respiratory distress. If suspected, formal airway intubation should be undertaken as soon as possible as 'bag and mask' ventilation may further distend the upper GI tract with air. Adequate oxygenation often requires ventilation or perhaps extracorporeal membrane oxygenation (ECMO). Ultimately, surgical correction is required.

Cross-sectional imaging can be helpful in better characterizing the anatomy and differentiating a hernia from CAM.

CASE 165

History
A 29-week premature neonate presented with respiratory distress a few hours after birth.

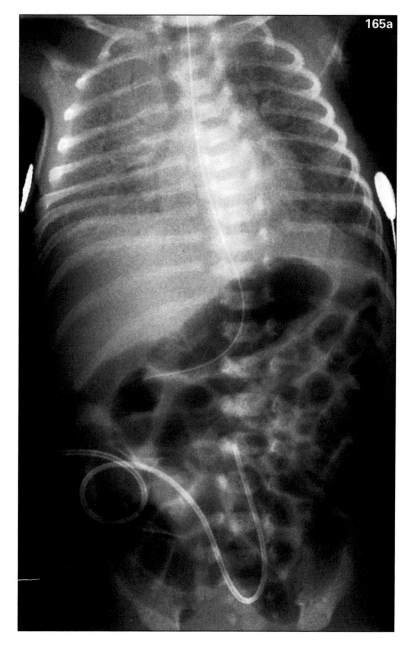

ANSWER 165

Observations (165a)
An NG tube lies in the stomach and there is an umbilical artery catheter in a satisfactory position with the tip at the level of L4 vertebra. The lungs are small in volume with a fine reticulogranular pattern affecting all lung zones with air bronchograms. In view of the history and radiographic findings, the likely diagnosis is hyaline membrane disease.

Diagnosis
Hyaline membrane disease (HMD).

Discussion
Hyaline membrane disease is one of the most common causes of respiratory distress in newborns. It is most common in premature infants but occasionally also occurs in term infants of diabetic mothers. It is due to lack of surfactant, an agent responsible for decreasing the surface tension in alveoli and produced by the type 2 alveolar cells. Without it the alveoli are poorly distensible and remain collapsed causing respiratory distress shortly after birth. Classically the lungs are small in volume with either 'ground glass' opacity or a fine reticulogranular pattern and air bronchograms extending out to the lung periphery.

Treatment consists of surfactant therapy and positive pressure assisted ventilation. However, the elevated airway pressures may lead to air dissecting through into the interstitium (pulmonary interstitial emphysema – PIE). This can lead to a sudden deterioration in the infant's condition due to the interstitial air causing obstruction to the pulmonary veins. This characteristically appears as elongated bubbles extending to the lung periphery in a bilateral, symmetrical pattern. Pneumomediastinum and pneumothorax are other complications of positive pressure ventilation. Figure **165b** demonstrates a left tension pneumothorax in an infant being treated for hyaline membrane disease. Note the shift of the mediastinum to the right and the air bronchograms in the left lung radiating out to the periphery. Figure **165c** is an example of an infant with pulmonary interstitial emphysema and a left sided tension pneumothorax displacing the mediastinum to the right. Elongated lucencies due to air tracking along the interstitium and lymphatics are seen, most clearly in the left lung.

Practical tips
- Signs of prematurity on the film are reduced subcutaneous fat and absence of humeral ossification centres.
- Similar lung opacities are seen with neonatal pneumonia or neonatal retained fluid syndrome, however unlike HMD, the lung volumes in these patients will be normal or increased.

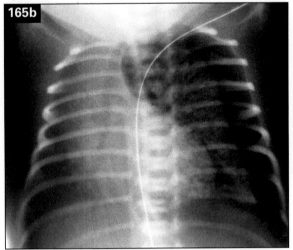

165b Chest radiograph of a child with HMD and left pneumothorax secondary to ventilation therapy. Note the left sided air bronchograms.

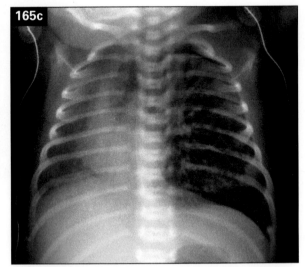

165c Chest radiograph of a child with HMD who developed pulmonary interstitial emphysema and a left pneumothorax secondary to ventilation therapy. Note the bubbly interstitial emphysema radiating to the lung edge.

Answer 165

- Air bronchograms are a characteristic feature of HMD and are not seen in conditions such as meconium aspiration syndrome.
- Check the position of all lines and tubes on the neonatal film:
  - Umbilical artery catheter (**165a**) – has characteristic 'U bend' as it passes inferiorly from the umbilicus in the umbilical artery then ascends in the internal and common iliac arteries and thus into aorta. The tip should lie either above the renal arteries at T8–12 or below them at L3–4.
  - Umbilical vein catheter – straight course cranially from umbilicus passing in umbilical veins, into ductus venosus and IVC to terminate in the right atrium (**165d**).

Further management
- Treatment involves oxygenation, ventilation and administration of surfactant.
- Complications of HMD treatment should always be sought, namely pulmonary interstitial emphysema, pneumothorax and pneumomediastinum.

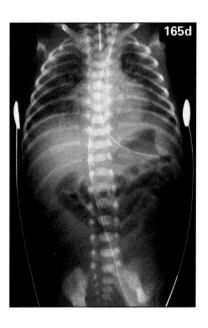

165d Radiograph demonstrating position of an umbilical catheter.

CASE 166

History
Unconscious 1-month-old born at term.

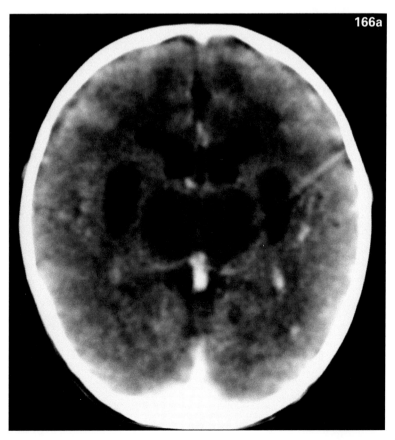

ANSWER 166

Observations (166a)
This axial contrast enhanced CT image shows bilateral and symmetrical low density in the basal ganglia, involving the putamina and thalami. There are several possible causes for this appearance. Hypoxia and hypotension should be self-evident. If not present, levels of glucose and carbon monoxide should be checked urgently.

Diagnosis
Low-density basal ganglia secondary to severe hypoxia/ischaemia.

Differential diagnosis
Of low-density basal ganglia:
- Hypoxia
- Hypotension
- Hypoglycaemia
- Carbon monoxide poisoning
- Wilson's disease

Of basal ganglia calcification (mnemonic 'PIE MAPS'):
- Physiological – the most common cause and increasingly so with age.
- Infection – cytomegalovirus (CMV), toxoplasma, congenital rubella, HIV.
- Endocrine – hypoparathryroidism (and pseudo/pseudopseudohypoparathyroidism), hyperparathyroidism, hypothyroidism.
- Metabolic – Leigh disease, Fahr disease, Wilson's disease.
- Anoxia – at birth, cerebrovascular accident (CVA).
- Poisoning – carbon monoxide, lead.
- Syndromes – Down's, Cockayne's syndrome, neurofibromatosis.

Discussion
Apart from Wilson's disease, the listed differential diagnoses for this appearance are of acute disorders that ultimately result in reduced cerebral oxygenation or glucose provision. The effect of hypoxia/hypotension on the infant brain depends on whether the infant is term or premature, and whether the insult is mild or severe. In the premature infant up to about 34 weeks, it is the deep white matter that is most vulnerable and hypoxic-ischaemic injury results in periventricular leukomalacia (PVL) with sparing of sub-cortical white matter and cortex. Since the corticospinal tract fibres pass through this area, there is usually resulting motor impairment.

In the term infant, the pattern of susceptibility is different. A mild insult results in ischaemia of the 'watershed' areas of the cerebrum where blood supply is most tenuous. These are the boundaries between the areas supplied by the anterior, middle and posterior cerebral arteries. Vital areas of the brain are protected by redistribution of blood flow. After a severe insult, however, vital areas of the brain can no longer be protected, and it the most metabolically active areas at this time of life that are affected. Thus, ischaemic damage occurs in the deep grey matter (thalami, putamina and brainstem nuclei), the peri-rolandic gyri and corticospinal tracts. This case illustrates such a pattern.

In older children, severe hypoxic-ischaemic injury may produce a different pattern, that of global cerebral injury. The resulting cerebral oedema and loss of grey–white matter differentiation with sparing of the brainstem and cerebellum can produce the acute reversal sign on CT described elsewhere (see Case 163).

As a comparative aside, high-density basal ganglia due to calcification are illustrated (**166b**) and the differential diagnosis listed.

Practical tips
- Comparative densities of grey and white matter in the infant brain are variable on CT depending on stage of myelination. Normality of the basal ganglia density can be confirmed by comparison with other grey matter structures.
- MRI is the most sensitive modality for detecting hypoxic-ischaemic injury but may be logistically difficult in the acutely unwell infant. Ultrasound may be practically the easiest imaging option but has reduced sensitivity.

Further management
Urgent correction of hypoxia, hypotension and hypoglycaemia is required followed by exclusion of other causes.

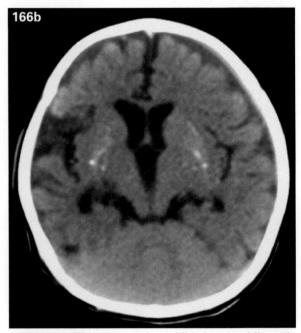

166b Axial CT brain scan in a child showing bilateral basal ganglia calcification.

Paediatric Imaging

CASE 167

History
A premature neonate presented with abdominal distension and sepsis.

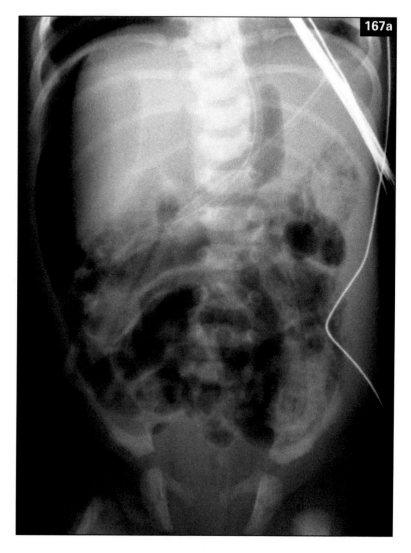

CASE 168

History
An adolescent male presented with a history of trauma.

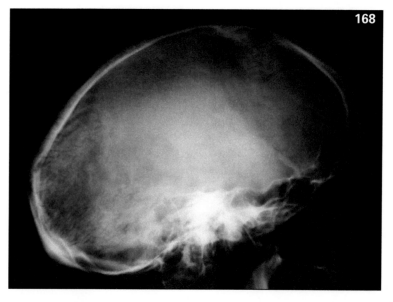

ANSWER 167

Observations (167a)
A cord clamp is noted indicating that the neonate is no more than a few days old. The bowel is abnormal with gaseous distension and a bubbly appearance to the bowel wall indicating mural gas. A large pneumoperitoneum is present with most of the gas adjacent to the liver. The features are consistent with necrotizing enterocolitis and perforation. No gas is seen within the portal veins.

Diagnosis
Necrotizing enterocolitis (NEC).

Discussion
Up to 80% of cases are related to prematurity and NEC is the most common gastrointestinal emergency seen in premature babies, usually occurring in the first 2 weeks of life. Ischaemia of the bowel is thought to occur secondary to perinatal stress, hypoxia or infection. Presentation is with diarrhoea or bloody stools. Radiographic features consist of distended thick walled bowel which has a bubbly appearance due to submucosal gas, i.e. pneumatosis intestinalis. Gas may track from the bowel into the portal venous system and can be seen on plain radiography (branching gas extends towards the periphery of the liver unlike air in the biliary tree, which is central). Such a finding in adults is an ominous and usually premorbid sign, but in NEC, this is not the case at all. Bowel strictures are a potential long term complication.

Pneumoperitoneum should be carefully looked for, as this necessitates immediate surgery. In the supine position, free gas often collects anteriorly as a large rounded lucency in the central abdomen producing the 'football' sign.

When perforation occurs *in utero*, meconium within the peritoneal cavity calcifies and can be seen on plain radiography. An example is shown in a neonate (**167b**) where there is peritoneal calcification (best seen over the inferior tip of liver) with a pneumoperitoneum causing a positive Rigler sign, i.e. visualization of both walls of the bowel.

Practical tips
- The earliest radiological sign on plain film is bowel dilatation (due to ileus).
- If a contrast enema is required to exclude obstruction then water-soluble contrast should be used – barium is contraindicated.

Further management
Mortality rates are dependent on the degree of prematurity, with rates quoted at 5% in term infants and 12% in premature newborns. Initial treatment is supportive with bowel rest but if serial radiographs or clinical features show progression or perforation then surgical resection of necrotic bowel is required.

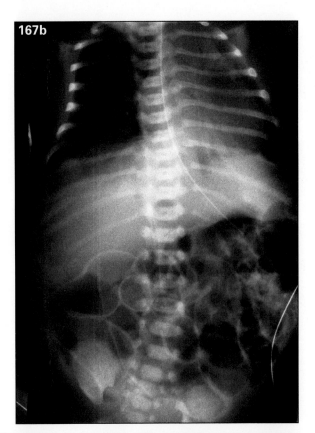

167b Abdominal radiograph in a newborn demonstrates visibility of both sides of the bowel wall, i.e. a positive Rigler sign indicating pneumoperitoneum. Flecks of calcification in the right abdomen confirm the diagnosis of antenatal meconium peritonitis.

ANSWER 168

Observations (168)
No bony injury is seen on this skull radiograph. There are multiple wormian bones, which at this age is abnormal. There is a large differential diagnosis but the most likely cause is idiopathic.

Diagnosis
Multiple wormian bones.

Differential diagnosis
Of wormian bones, with common causes underlined (mnemonic 'PORKCHOPSI'):
- Pyknodysostosis.
- Osteogenesis imperfecta.
- Rickets in healing.
- Kinky hair syndrome (Menkes).
- Cleidocranial dysostosis.
- Hypothyroidism/hypophosphatasia.
- Otopalatodigital syndrome,
- Pachydermoperiostosis.
- Syndrome of Down's.
- Idiopathic – normal in first year of life.

Discussion
Wormian bones are essentially small bones occurring in the sutures of the calvaria. These intrasutural ossicles are usually found in the lambdoid, posterior sagittal and temporosquamosal sutures. They are considered abnormal when seen after 1 year or large and numerous (>10 in number and larger than 6 x 4 mm).

Practical tips
- Because of the wide differential diagnosis, it is difficult to identify a specific cause without the aid of a good clinical history.
- Diffuse osteopenia will be present on the skull radiograph in cases of rickets and osteogenesis imperfecta.
- Pyknodysostosis, on the other hand, will be associated with diffuse osteosclerosis on the film.

Further management
Management is dependent on the underlying cause.

Further reading
Cremin B, Goodman H, Spranger J, Beighton P (1982). Wormian bones in osteogenesis imperfecta and other disorders. *Skeletal Radiology* **8(1)**: 35–38.

CASE 169

History
A child with a history of partial seizures.

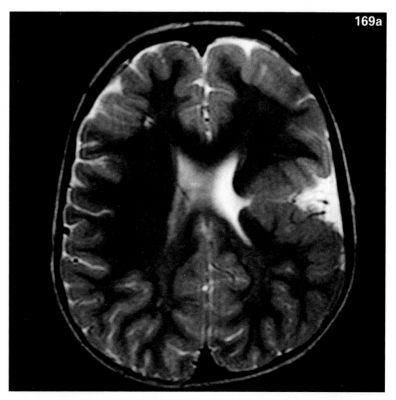

ANSWER 169

Observations (169a)
Axial T2 weighted MR image at the level of the lateral ventricles. This demonstrates a large cleft extending through the full thickness of the left cerebral hemisphere from the surface of the brain to the left lateral ventricle. The cleft is lined by grey matter and is filled with CSF. The findings are consistent with schizencephaly.

Diagnosis
Schizencephaly.

Discussion
During gestation, neurones migrate outwards from the periventricular germinal matrix to form the normal cerebral cortices. This migration can be interfered with by several causes including chromosomal abnormalities, but mostly the reason is unknown. The result is brain tissue lying in the wrong place, typically grey matter.

Schizencephaly is a cleft extending through the full thickness of cerebral hemisphere from the ependyma-lined wall of ventricle to the brain surface. It is lined by pia and grey matter that usually shows polymicrogyria, and is often located around the Sylvian fissure. The lateral end of the cleft may be open and readily apparent (open lip type) but can sometimes be closely opposed and easy to miss (closed lip type). However, even the closed lip type will show a small irregularity in the wall of the ventricle at the site of the cleft. It is not certain whether this condition is due to an ischaemic insult leading to germinal matrix infarction or whether it represents a focal cortical dysplasia.

There are different manifestations of the congenital neuronal migration anomalies which result in varying degrees of mental retardation and/or seizures. The following further patterns are recognized:

- Heterotopic grey matter – when small collections of the neurones arrest on their way to the cortex they can be seen as discrete nodules (most commonly in a subependymal location) or as a subcortical band. Thus there are nodular and band heterotopias. These are isointense to grey matter and show no enhancement. While sometimes asymptomatic, seizures and developmental delay can ensue, especially with band heterotopia. An example of nodular heterotopic grey matter is shown in an axial T2 MR image of the brain (**169b**), where a small area of heterotopic grey matter is seen in a subependymal location adjacent to the occipital horn of the left lateral ventricle.
- Polymicrogyria – sometimes neurones may migrate to the cortex but are abnormally distributed, producing a bumpy appearance to the cortical gyri termed polymicrogyria. An example is shown in a coronal T1 weighted MRI (**169c**), where polymicrogyria affecting the right temporal lobe produces a bumpy

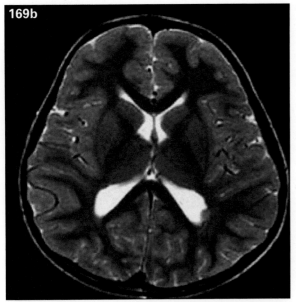

169b Axial T2 MRI of the brain shows a small area of subependymal heterotopic grey matter adjacent to the left occipital horn. Note how it is isointense to the cortical grey matter.

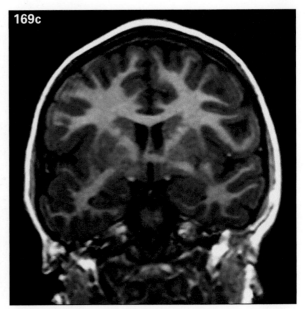

169c Coronal T1 MRI of the brain shows a bumpy appearance to the right temporal lobe gyri due to polymicrogyria.

appearance to the gyri. Note how the normal left temporal lobe gyri are distinct and crisp.
- Pachygyria – in some cases the gyri may be poorly formed (pachygyria). A spectrum exists whereby in the most severe form the surface of the brain appears smooth. This is termed lissencephaly (**169d**). Often these patients have severe mental retardation and limited survival.

Practical tips
Subependymal nodules in tuberous sclerosis can also cause nodularity along the walls of the ventricles. However, the nodules in this condition show a similar signal to white matter rather than the grey matter seen in heterotopia.

Further management
Medical management of epilepsy.

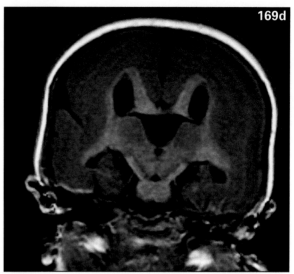

169d Coronal T1 MRI of the brain of a child with lissencephaly; the cortices are smooth with almost no normally formed gyri.

CASE 170

History
A newborn who was born at 41 weeks presented with hypoxia.

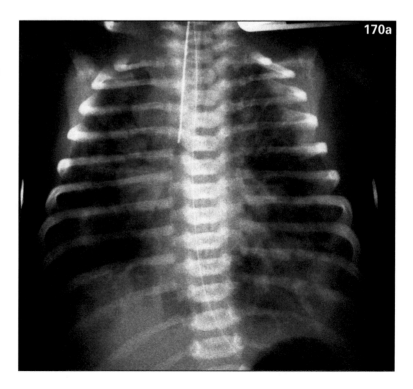

ANSWER 170

Observations (170a)
An endotracheal tube has been placed just above the carina. There is also an NG tube passing into the stomach. There are bilateral diffuse patchy opacities in both lungs indicative of widespread atelectasis and patchy consolidation. However, the lungs appear hyperinflated and there are small pleural effusions. In view of the history, the appearances are likely to be due to meconium aspiration syndrome.

Diagnosis
Meconium aspiration syndrome.

Discussion
Meconium aspiration syndrome is the most common cause of respiratory distress in newborns born at full or post term. The large size of the fetus makes delivery difficult. Perinatal hypoxia and fetal distress lead to meconium defecation *in utero*. Aspiration of the meconium into the tracheobronchial tree then causes obstruction of small peripheral bronchioles (though only a minority of fetuses exposed to meconium stained amniotic fluid develop respiratory symptoms). This results in unevenly distributed areas of subsegmental atelectasis with alternating areas of air trapping. The chest radiograph usually begins clearing within a few days with no long term radiographic sequelae in the lungs.

The radiological features on CXR are:
- Bilateral patchy atelectasis and consolidation.
- No air bronchograms.
- Hyperinflation with areas of air trapping.
- Small pleural effusions.
- Spontaneous pneumothorax and pneumomediastinum may result from the air trapping (**170b**).

Practical tips
- Most common cause of respiratory distress in term babies: meconium aspiration.
- Most common cause of respiratory distress in preterm babies: hyaline membrane disease.

Further management
Almost all neonates with meconium aspiration syndrome make a full recovery of their pulmonary function. Upper airway suction may be employed and ventilatory support may be required in more severe cases of respiratory distress.

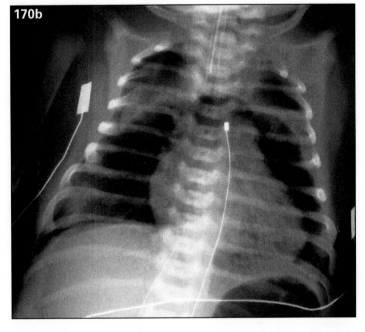

170b CXR in a neonate with a large pneumomediastinum. Air outlines the thymus producing an 'angel's wings' appearance.

CASE 171

History
A newborn presented with regurgitation of feeds.

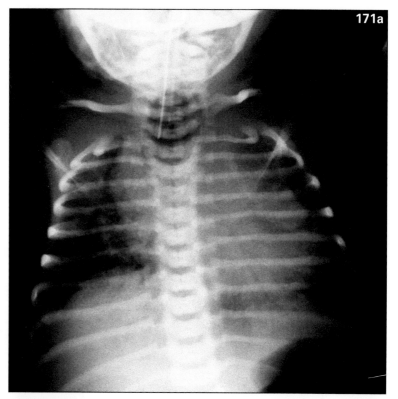

CASE 172

History
Micturating cystourethrogram (MCUG) was taken in a male infant with a previously confirmed urinary tract infection.

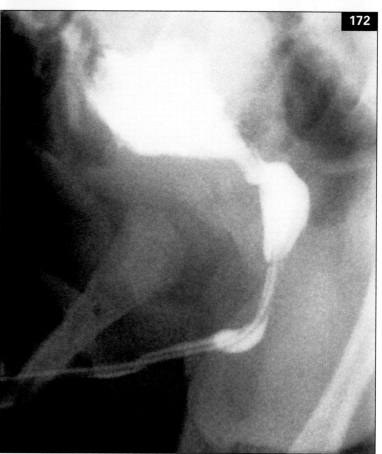

ANSWER 171

Observations (171a)
A feeding tube is seen within a gas-distended blind-ending pouch representing the oesophagus. Air is noted below the diaphragm. There is no convincing evidence of aspiration pneumonia. The features are consistent with oesophageal atresia with a distal tracheoesophageal fistula.

Diagnosis
Congenital oesophageal atresia with tracheoesophageal fistula (TOF).

Discussion
Embryologically the primitive foregut tube separates to form the trachea and oesophagus. Disorders of this separation presenting in infancy result in various combinations of oesophageal atresia and TOF. Presentation is with excessive drooling, regurgitation of feeds or symptoms of aspiration depending on the type of abnormality present.

In 90% of cases there is a component of oesophageal atresia, and the majority of these have an associated tracheoesophageal fistula. Such a fistula can be proximal, distal or both (i.e. between the trachea and the proximal oesophageal segment, the distal segment or both). This case demonstrates the most common subtype (seen in around 80%) where there is oesophageal atresia and a distal TOF. The atresia results in drooling and regurgitation while the distal TOF results in passage of air from trachea into stomach and thus the rest of the bowel.

A minority of cases have TOF without oesophageal atresia and are more likely to present with coughing or choking during feeds and ultimately aspiration pneumonia. An example is shown (**171b**) where water-soluble contrast has been injected via an NG tube in the oesophagus and is seen to pass into the trachea via the fistula.

Practical tips
- Oesophageal atresia – CXR shows a retrotracheal distended pouch of proximal oesophagus and a feeding tube may be coiled within it after attempted passage.
- A gasless abdomen indicates no fistula or a proximal fistula.
- Gas in the abdomen indicates presence of a distal fistula.
- Look for consolidation suggesting associated aspiration pneumonia.
- Oesophageal atresia and TOF can be part of a VACTERL syndrome so check the CXR for abnormalities:
  - Vertebral anomalies.
  - Anorectal anomalies.
  - Cardiovascular anomalies.
  - Tracheo-Esophageal fistula.
  - Renal anomalies.
  - Limb anomalies.

Further management
Surgical repair is required. This can be later complicated by anastomotic leak, oesophageal stricture or abnormal motility resulting in dysphagia and/or aspiration pneumonia.

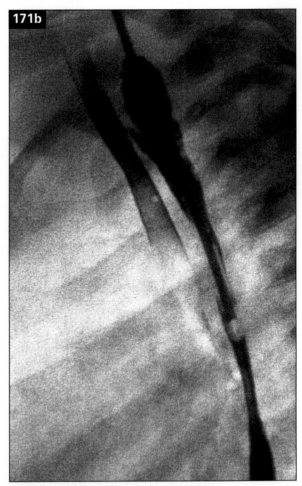

171b Contrast examination via an NG tube demonstrates a tracheoesophageal fistula.

ANSWER 172

Observations (172)
This MCUG study shows a transverse filling defect at the posterior urethra with distension of the proximal posterior urethra. The findings are consistent with posterior urethral valves.

Diagnosis
Posterior urethral valves.

Discussion
Congenital presence of thick folds of mucous membrane in the posterior urethra is the most common cause of urinary tract obstruction in boys. The condition is often suspected on prenatal US where it can lead to oligohydramnios, hydronephrosis, prune belly and urine ascites or urinoma due to leak. If obstruction occurs early *in utero* then multicystic dysplastic kidney may result. After birth, MCUG is the investigation of choice to outline the transverse filling defect caused by the thick mucosal folds. Distension and elongation of the proximal part of the posterior urethra may be seen during voiding and vesicoureteral reflux is present in 50%. Bladder trabeculation and a significant post void residual volume may be noted. Prognosis depends on the duration of obstruction prior to corrective surgery and is worse if associated with vesicoureteral reflux. Approximately three-quarters of cases will have been discovered in the first year of life, though occasionally it can be first noted in adulthood.

Practical tips
Note how diagnosis is still possible when the catheter is *in situ* during the voiding phase of the MCUG (**172**).

Further management
Urological surgical intervention is required with initial treatment aimed at relieving bladder outlet obstruction and ablating the valves. Secondary treatment may be required for vesicoureteral reflux, urinary tract infections, urinary incontinence and renal dysfunction.

CASE 173

History
A newborn presented with abdominal distension and failure to pass meconium.

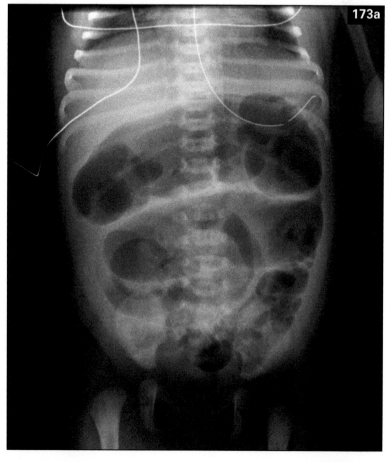

ANSWER 173

Observations (173a)
An NG tube is in the stomach. There are multiple dilated loops of bowel in the abdomen. No fluid levels are seen within the bowel suggesting that the appearances may be due to meconium ileus. However, other pathologies such as Hirschsprung's disease and imperforate anus should be considered.

Diagnosis
Meconium ileus.

Differential diagnosis
- Hirschsprung's disease.
- Imperforate anus.
- Ileal atresia.
- Inguinal hernia.

Discussion
Meconium ileus is the term used to describe small bowel obstruction in neonates secondary to inspissated meconium pellets impacted in the distal ileum. The vast majority prove to have cystic fibrosis and this is the earliest manifestation of the disease. The diagnosis is confirmed by performing a contrast enema, which demonstrates multiple round filling defects (the inspissated meconium) in the distal ileum and proximal colon (**173b**). The colon may be very narrow on the contrast study if it has been unused due to antenatal obstruction, whereby it is termed a microcolon. The enema should be performed using Gastrograffin as this has a therapeutic effect, helping to clear the meconium by drawing water into the gut.

With Hirschsprung's disease, the contrast enema will demonstrate dilated bowel with a transition zone to a distal aganglionic segment.

Practical tips
- On an AXR of a baby it is almost impossible to tell if dilated loops of bowel are large or small bowel. The presence or absence of vomiting/passage of meconium are more helpful to know with regard to assessing if there is high or low bowel obstruction.
- The hernial orifices should be checked for air suggesting an inguinal hernia.
- A 'soap bubble' appearance may be seen on AXR in meconium ileus due to the mixture of gas with meconium.
- Fluid levels are not usually present in meconium ileus because the bowel contents are very viscous.
- Look at the sacrum on the AXR, as imperforate anus is associated with sacral agenesis.

Further management
- Water-soluble contrast enema can be useful for both diagnosis and treatment.
- All patients with meconium ileus should have a 'sweat test' to exclude underlying cystic fibrosis.

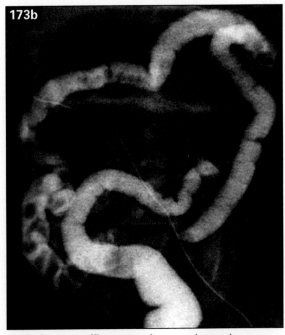

173b Gastrograffin enema in a newborn shows multiple filling defects in the ascending colon and terminal ileum, which represent inspissated meconium. Note the dilated small bowel loops.

CASE 174

History
A 4-year-old child presented with fever and abdominal pain.

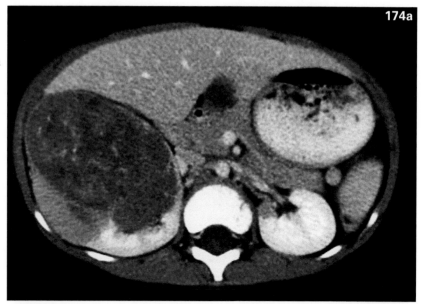

CASE 175

History
A 4-month-old child presented with persistent irritability.

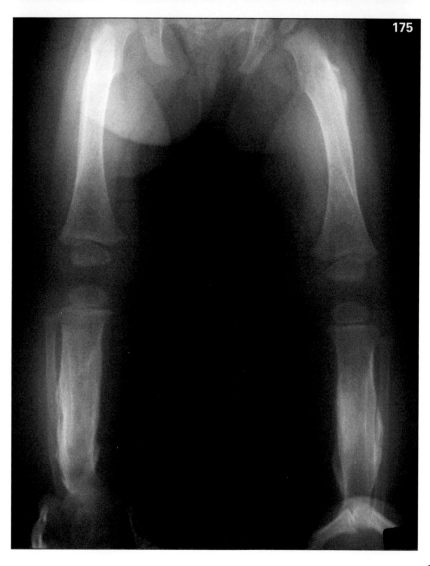

ANSWER 174

Observations (174a)
Axial CT of the abdomen with oral contrast and IV contrast in portal phase. There is a large slightly heterogeneous mass arising from the right kidney. The mass does not enhance as much as the renal parenchyma. There is local mass effect with displacement, but no invasion of the right lobe of liver or encasement of vessels. A small mass of similar density is seen near the hilum of the left kidney. The appearances suggest bilateral Wilms' tumours.

Diagnosis
Bilateral Wilms' tumours.

Differential diagnosis
Neuroblastoma.

Discussion
Wilms' tumour (nephroblastoma) is the most common abdominal malignancy in young children, most commonly presenting at age 3–4 years. The most frequent presentation is with abdominal mass, though hypertension, pain, fever and haematuria also occur. The tumour usually grows to a large size, often measuring over 10 cm. Radiological features include:
- Exophytic mass displacing rather than encasing adjacent structures.
- Less contrast enhancement than normal renal parenchyma.
- Cystic/necrotic areas give it a heterogeneous appearance.
- Invasion of the renal vein and inferior vena cava may occur in up to 10%.

Tumours are bilateral in 10% and this indicates background nephroblastomatosis, a state of persistent nephrogenic blastema that is a precursor to Wilms'. Wilms' tumour is associated with the Beckwith–Wiedemann syndrome (macroglossia, visceromegaly and omphalocele). Other associations include aniridia and hemihypertrophy.

The main differential diagnosis is neuroblastoma, a common malignant tumour of the neural crest that presents in a similar way to Wilms' tumour with a painful abdominal mass and fever. Typical age of presentation is slightly earlier however (under 2 years). Hormone secretion from the tumour (such as catecholamines) may cause other signs, including hypertension and opsoclonus (chaotic jerky eye movements). It can arise anywhere in the sympathetic neural chain including the adrenal gland and the abdominal sympathetic chain.

Practical tips
- Always check for bilateral tumours when Wilms' is suspected.
- Differentiating between neuroblastoma and Wilms' tumour can be difficult radiologically but there are some specific features that can help:
- Almost all neuroblastomas contain calcification whereas only up to 10% of Wilms' tumours calcify.
- Both tumours can cross the midline and look similar on imaging, appearing inseparable from the kidney; however, neuroblastoma tends to encase surrounding vessels such as the aorta while Wilms' tumours tend to displace surrounding tissues and structures. An example of a neuroblastoma is shown (**174b**) encasing the aorta and coeliac axis vessels. Neuroblastoma may also extend into the spinal canal through the neural foramina.
- Look for evidence of metastatic spread; 70% of neuroblastomas have malignant spread at presentation compared to just 10% of Wilms' tumours. Also, Wilms' tumours spread to lung, whereas neuroblastoma spreads to bone.

Further management
Treatment is with radical nephrectomy and chemotherapy. Preoperative chemotherapy is advocated in cases of bilateral Wilms' tumours and when there is IVC extension of tumour (occurs in ~5%).

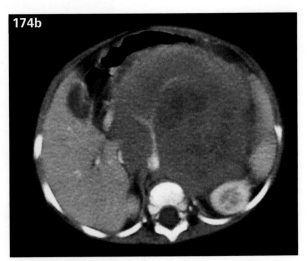

174b CT of a neuroblastoma. The huge mass displaces the spleen and left kidney and shows typical encasement of vessels, in this case the aorta and coeliac axis.

ANSWER 175

Observations (175)
There is bilateral symmetrical thick, smooth periosteal reaction affecting the diaphyses of the long bones. There is no fraying or splaying of the metaphyses to suggest rickets. The most likely diagnosis at this age is Caffey's disease, however other possibilities such as leukaemia need to be considered.

Diagnosis
Caffey's disease.

Differential diagnosis
Of bilateral diffuse periosteal reaction in childhood:
- Normal variant before the age of 4 months.
- Caffey's disease.
- Leukaemia.
- Scurvy.
- Rickets.
- Hypervitaminosis A.
- Non accidental injury (NAI).

Discussion
Infantile cortical hyperostosis (Caffey's disease) is a proliferative bone disease seen in patients under the age of 6 months. Irritability and fever are the presenting symptoms and are associated with soft tissue swelling over the bones. Bilateral symmetrical thick periosteal reaction is the cardinal radiological feature and most commonly affects the mandible, clavicle and the long bones. It usually involves the diaphysis of the bone. In the majority of cases, there is spontaneous complete recovery by the age of 3 years.

Practical tips
- If there is diffuse periosteal reaction with fractures of differing ages, NAI must be considered.
- With rickets, splaying and fraying of the metaphyses will be seen.

Further management
When NAI is considered then a careful analysis of previous radiographs, the clinical presentation and consultation with a specialist paediatric radiologist must be carried out because of the repercussions of a misdiagnosis.

CASE 176

History
None available.

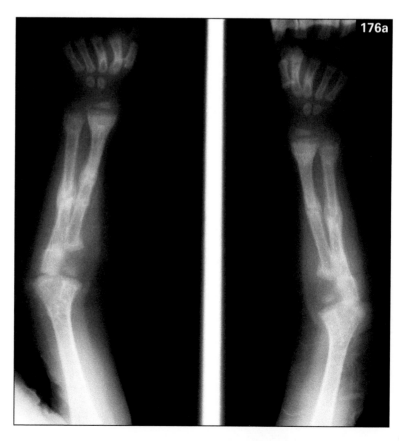

ANSWER 176

Observations (176a)
There is widespread bilateral decreased bone density with healing insufficiency fractures of the radius and ulna bilaterally. These are associated with thick smooth periosteal reaction and there is fraying and splaying of the metaphyses. The features are characteristic of rickets.

Diagnosis
Rickets.

Differential diagnosis
Hypophosphatasia.

Discussion
Rickets is most commonly due to insufficient biologically active vitamin D, though impaired calcium absorption or excessive phosphate excretion can occasionally be to blame. In the western world, pure dietary deficiency of vitamin D is rarely the sole cause; more often it is due to malabsorption or impaired vitamin D metabolism in the liver or kidney.

Rickets is essentially osteomalacia during enchondral bone growth. Portions of the skeleton that have already matured show features of osteomalacia, but loss of normal maturation and mineralization of cartilage cells at the growth plate lead to the additional distinctive radiological features of rickets. Osteomalacia is discussed elsewhere in the book but the radiological features are due to excessive unmineralized osteoid producing Looser's zones, osteopenia, cortical tunnelling, indistinct trabeculae and finally bowing and fractures due to softened bones.

In addition, the following features are seen in rickets:
- Widened growth plate – loss of normal chondrocyte maturation and mineralization result in cell build up here.
- Metaphyses are irregular/frayed, splayed and cupped – impaired mineralization causes the frayed irregular appearance while build up of chondrocytes at the physis indents the metaphysis producing cupping and splaying.
- Epiphysis osteopenic and irregular.
- Periarticular soft tissue swelling.
- Apparent periosteal reaction due to subperiosteal unmineralized osteoid.
- Delayed maturation and growth.

Figure 176b demonstrates rickets of the lower limbs – note the typical changes around the metaphyses in the tibia and also bowing of the fibula. Figure 176c is a CXR of a child with rickets showing splaying of the anterior ends of

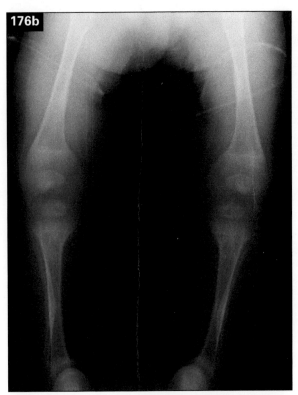

176b AP radiograph of both legs shows typical features of rickets with fraying of the metaphyses.

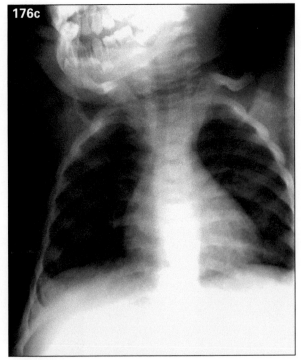

176c Chest radiograph of a child with rickets and splaying of the ribs.

Answer 176 (cont.)

the ribs and the metaphysis of the right humerus. The appearance of the anterior rib ends is due to changes at the costochondral junction growth plates and is termed the 'rachitic rosary'.

Practical tips
- The earliest sign of rickets on the plain film is a widening of the growth plate.
- Looser's zones are rare in rickets compared to osteomalacia in the fused skeleton.

Further management
Rickets is now usually identified early and treated with vitamin D supplements. Significant pelvis deformity and gait disturbances are now rarely seen in the developed world.

CASE 177

History
None available.

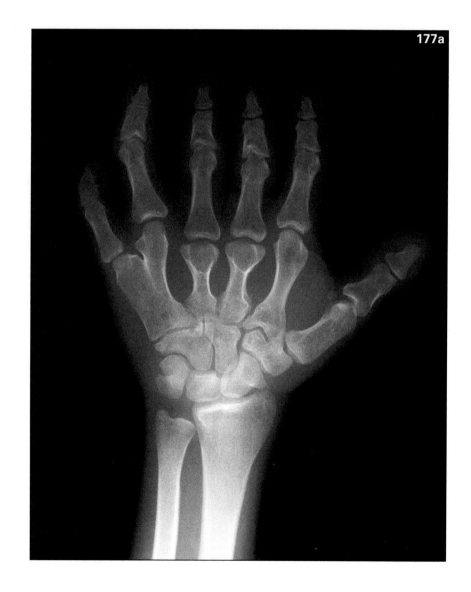

ANSWER 177

Observations (177a)
There is partial fusion of an extra digit with the metacarpal of the little finger. This essentially represents polysyndactyly, the possible causes of which include idiopathic, Ellis–van Creveld syndrome and Carpenter syndrome.

Diagnosis
Ellis–van Creveld syndrome.

Differential diagnosis
Of causes of polydactyly:
- Idiopathic.
- Ellis–van Creveld syndrome.
- Carpenter syndrome.
- Polysyndactyly syndrome.

Of causes of syndactyly:
- Idiopathic.
- Apert's syndrome.
- Carpenter syndrome.
- Down's syndrome.
- Poland's syndrome.
- Neurofibromatosis.

Discussion
There are several causes of syndactyly (fusion of digits) and polydactyly (supernumerary digits), which are both congenital abnormalities. Ellis–van Creveld syndrome is also associated with carpal fusion, as is Apert's syndrome. This is characterized by features in the skull: notably craniosynostosis of the coronal sutures, hypoplastic mid face and enlargement of the sella. All of these features are demonstrated in the lateral skull radiograph in a child with Apert's syndrome (**177b**).

Practical tips
Some exam cases will have an obvious abnormality as part of a syndrome that you don't know – stating that you would seek help from a textbook or specialist colleague is a reasonable answer. You can't know everything!

Further management
Poly/syndactyly will be part of a syndrome with multiple abnormalities.

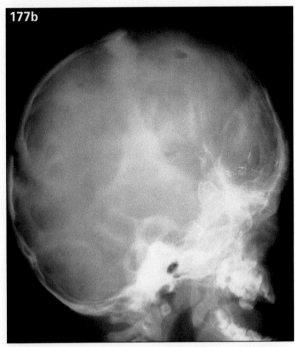

177b Lateral skull radiograph of a child with Apert's syndrome demonstrating craniosynostosis of the coronal sutures, hypoplasia of the midface and enlargement of the sella.

CASE 178

History
None available.

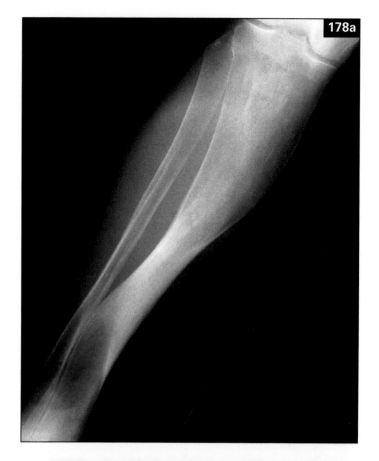

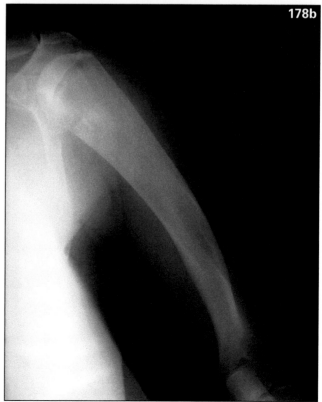

ANSWER 178

Observations (178a, 178b)
There is bowing deformity of the tibia, fibula and humerus. The metaphyses of the bones are widened producing an Erlenmeyer flask deformity. The metaphyses are also relatively lucent when compared with the diaphysis, which is sclerotic. There are no specific features to indicate lead poisoning, osteopetrosis or thalassaemia, so the differential diagnosis lies between Pyle's disease and lipidoses such as Gaucher's or Niemann–Pick disease.

Diagnosis
Pyle's disease.

Differential diagnosis
In this case:
- Craniometaphyseal dysplasia.
- Niemann–Pick disease.
- Gaucher's disease.

Of Erlenmeyer flask deformity (mnemonic – 'Lead GNOME'):
- Lead.
- Gaucher's.
- Niemann–Pick disease – looks like Gaucher's but without avascular necrosis.
- Osteopetrosis.
- Metaphyseal dysplasia (Pyle's) and craniometaphyseal dysplasia (same as Pyle's disease but there is a history of cranial nerve palsies).
- 'E'matological!! – thalassaemia.

Discussion
Pyle's disease is also known as metaphyseal dysplasia. It is a rare autosomal recessive disorder characterized by flaring of the ends of long bones with relative constriction and sclerosis of the central portion of the shafts. Affected patients are usually asymptomatic and genu valgus deformity is often a feature. The expanded metaphyses tend to be lucent and have the appearance of an Erlenmeyer flask (named after the wide necked laboratory flask bearing the name of this German chemist).

Craniometaphyseal dysplasia essentially has the same features but in addition there are cranial nerve palsies due to sclerosis of the skull base.

Gaucher's disease is a hereditary disorder of lipid storage common among Ashkenazi Jews. It is characterized by hepatosplenomegaly with flask-shaped long bones and generalized osteopenia with strikingly thin cortices. Avascular necrosis is also a feature.

Practical tips
Erlenmeyer flask deformity, the metaphyseal expansion of long bones, is also discussed in Chapter 5. Additional differentiating features can be found on the radiograph as to the specific underlying cause of Erlenmeyer flask deformity:
- Diffuse sclerosis and sclerotic vertebral endplates producing 'sandwich vertebrae' indicate osteopetrosis.
- With Pyle's disease, there will be relative sclerosis at the diaphysis and lucency of the metaphysis.
- Gaucher's disease will also be associated with lucency and osteopenia but there may be signs of avascular necrosis of the femoral or humeral heads (loss of height and fragmentation) and on an AXR massive hepatosplenomegaly may be seen.
- Thalassaemia is associated with coarsened trabeculation producing a 'cobweb' appearance.
- Lead poisoning causes dense metaphyseal bands as well as Erlenmeyer flask deformity.

Further management
This condition is usually asymptomatic and requires no direct management.

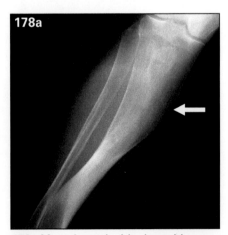

178a Metaphyseal widening with increased lucency.

CASE 179

History
None available.

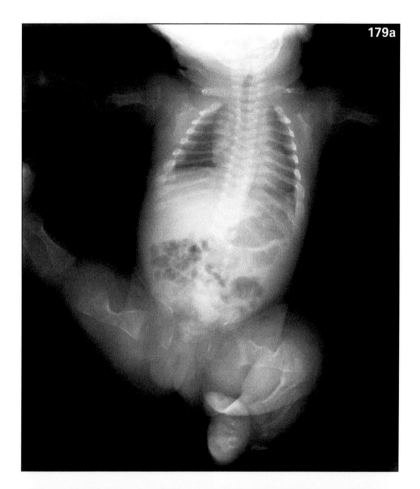

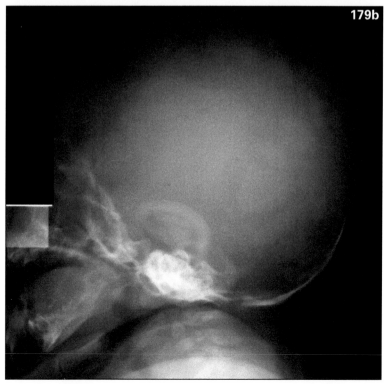

Answer 179 — Paediatric Imaging

ANSWER 179

Observations (179a, 179b)
The lateral skull radiograph (**179b**) demonstrates thinning of the calvaria with multiple wormian bones. Bowing deformities are seen to affect the limbs (**179a**) and there are several fractures of differing ages, mostly seen at the metaphyses of the long bones. There is generalized osteopenia of the skeleton with marked thinning of the cortices. The features are consistent with osteogenesis imperfecta.

Diagnosis
Osteogenesis imperfecta.

Differential diagnosis
Of wormian bones with common causes underlined (mnemonic – 'PORKCHOPSI'):
- Pyknodysostosis.
- Osteogenesis imperfecta.
- Rickets in healing.
- Kinky hair syndrome (Menkes).
- Cleidocranial dysostosis.
- Hypothyroidism/hypophosphatasia.
- Otopalatodigital syndrome.
- Pachydermoperiostosis.
- Syndrome of Down.
- Idiopathic – normal in first year of life.

Discussion
Osteogenesis imperfecta is a connective tissue disorder characterized by fragile bones and blue sclerae. Type 1 is compatible with life. Type 2 is the lethal form associated with perinatal death.

The principal radiological features include:
- Diffuse osteopenia with thinning of cortices.
- Multiple fractures of differing ages with pseudarthroses and bowing deformity.
- Fractures are associated with exuberant callus formation.
- Biconcave vertebral bodies.
- Multiple wormian bones in the skull.
- Poor dentition.

Practical tips
Multiple fractures in children should raise suspicion of non accidental injury (NAI) and sometimes differentiating this from osteogenesis imperfecta can be difficult. Predominantly osteogenesis fractures are diaphyseal compared with metaphyseal NAI fractures but this is not always the case.

Further management
Early medical intervention to increase bone mineral density and surgical intervention to treat/correct scoliosis and treat fractures mean that a multidisciplinary approach to the ongoing treatment is required.

CASE 180

History
A child presented with vomiting and ataxia.

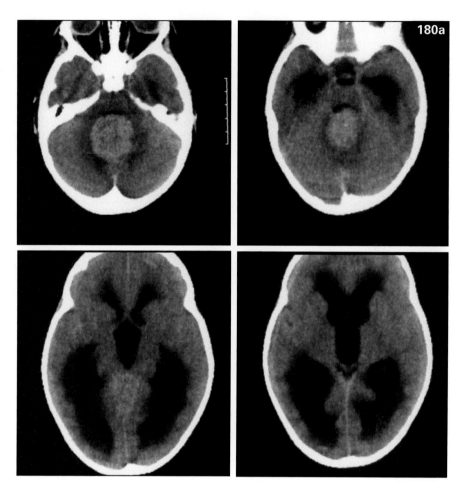

CASE 181

History
A 2-month-old baby presented with cyanosis.

(see page 322 for case answer)

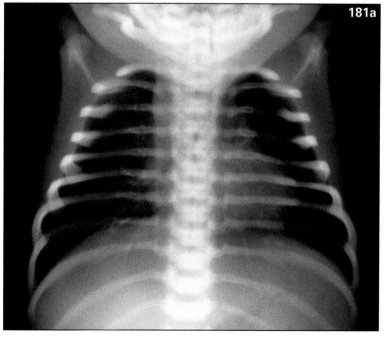

ANSWER 180

Observations (180a)
A series of axial MRI images of skull show a well defined hyperdense mass in the cerebellar vermis causing compression and anterior displacement of the 4th ventricle with obstructive hydrocephalus. A small amount of oedema surrounds the mass. The features are typical of a medulloblastoma.

Diagnosis
Medulloblastoma.

Differential diagnosis
Of posterior fossa tumour in children:
- Medulloblastoma:
  - Predominantly midline posterior to 4th ventricle.
  - Hyperdense on CT with oedema.
  - Avid enhancement.
  - 20% calcify, 50% necrose.

- Juvenile pilocytic astrocytoma:
  - Typically paracentral, posterior to 4th ventricle.
  - Majority are cystic with an enhancing mural nodule, the remainder are solid.
  - 20% calcify; oedema is rare.

- Ependymoma:
  - Arises within 4th ventricle.
  - Heterogeneous appearance and enhancement.
  - 50% calcify.
  - Hydrocephalus is often communicating type due to protein exudate obstructing CSF resorption.
  - Spreads through the exit foramen of fourth ventricle and wraps around brainstem ('plastic growth'). Sagittal and axial T2 weighted MR images (**180b**) demonstrate a high signal lesion arising within the 4th ventricle, wrapping around the brainstem and spreading via the foramina of Luschka and Magendie. Hydrocephalus is present and a syrinx of the upper cervical cord has developed.

- Brainstem glioma:
  - Within pons, possibly causing pontine expansion or 4th ventricle displacement posteriorly.
  - Iso- or hypodense to brain so may be easily missed. Sagittal T1 weighted MRI with contrast (**180c**) demonstrates a large pontine glioma. Note how the lesion is nonenhancing and almost the same signal as surrounding brain. Smaller such lesions can easily be missed due to such imaging characteristics.
  - Enhancement often absent or minimal.
  - Hydrocephalus uncommon (because present with focal neurology before this occurs).

Discussion
Medulloblastoma is the second most common paediatric brain tumour and the most common in the posterior fossa. It is a type of primitive neuroectodermal tumour (PNET)

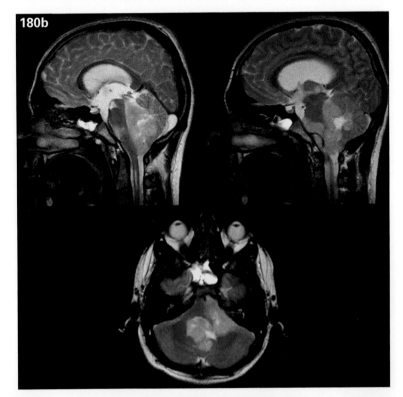

180b Sagittal and axial T2 MRI of the brain demonstrating an ependymoma in the 4th ventricle, which extends into the foramina of Luschka and Magendie and causes obstructive hydrocephalus. A syrinx of the upper cervical cord has developed.

Answer 180 — Paediatric Imaging

arising from the roof of the 4th ventricle. The majority of patients affected are under the age of 15 years, with 80% of lesions arising from the cerebellar vermis, and the rest lying more laterally in the cerebellum. This lateral location is more common in older children. They are typically hyperdense on CT due to dense cellularity, and show avid, homogeneous enhancement. There is usually surrounding oedema, 20% show calcification and up to 50% show necrosis/cystic change. They are highly malignant and spread occurs via the CSF in up to a third. Medulloblastoma is rarely associated with Gorlin's syndrome – an autosomal dominant disorder characterized by multiple cutaneous basal cell carcinomas during childhood with mandibular keratocysts and extensive intracranial calcification of the falx and tentorium.

At least 50% of primary brain tumours in children occur in the posterior fossa. Brainstem glioma tends to present with focal neurology due to involvement of the long tracts and cranial nerve nuclei, while the other three differential diagnoses listed present by way of mass effect and obstructive hydrocephalus with headache, vomiting and ataxia. The salient imaging features of each are listed. It is important when staging paediatric posterior fossa tumours to remember the potential for CSF spread with medulloblastoma in particular, but sometimes with ependymoma too. Post gadolinium scans should therefore include the whole spine as well as brain to pick up such deposits ('drop metastases'). A sagittal T1 MRI post-contrast (**180d**) demonstrates an enhancing medulloblastoma in the posterior fossa causing obstructive hydrocephalus. CSF spread of tumour has occurred with a metastasis in the prepontine cistern.

Practical tips

- Make sure the post contrast scan looking for drop metastases is done preoperatively as postoperative haemorrhage and granulation tissue can cause confusion.
- Haemangioblastoma is primarily a tumour of adults but can be seen in adolescents in the posterior fossa when part of von Hippel–Lindau syndrome. It is typically a cystic mass with enhancing mural nodule, so has similarities with pilocytic astrocytoma.

Further management

MRI of the spine with intravenous contrast enhancement should be undertaken to look for 'drop metastases'. Neurosurgical assessment is then clearly appropriate.

Further reading

Koeller K, Rushing E (2003). From the archives of the AFIP: medulloblastoma: a comprehensive review with radiologic-pathologic correlation. *RadioGraphics* **23**: 1613–1637.

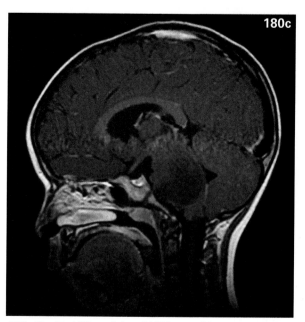

180c Sagittal T1 weighted MRI post IV contrast that shows a large pontine glioma.

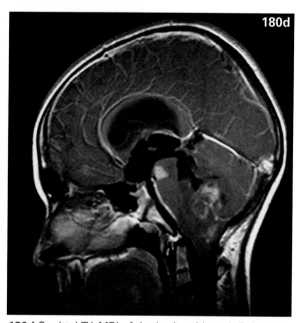

180d Sagittal T1 MRI of the brain with gadolinium showing an enhancing posterior fossa mass, which causes obstructive hydrocephalus. A metastasis is seen in the prepontine cistern. This proved to be a medulloblastoma.

ANSWER 181

Observations (181a)
There is a right sided aortic arch. The heart is boot shaped indicating right ventricular hypertrophy. The lungs are not plethoric, in fact there is a reduction in the calibre of the pulmonary vessels. Overall, the features are suggestive of Fallot's tetralogy.

Diagnosis
Tetralogy of Fallot.

Differential diagnosis
Of conditions associated with a right sided aortic arch:
- Truncus arteriosus.
- Tetralogy of Fallot.
- Transposition of great vessels.
- Pulmonary atresia.
- Ventricular septal defect (VSD).

Discussion
Tetralogy of Fallot is one of the most common causes of cyanotic congenital heart disease and is composed of the following: obstruction of right ventricular outflow, large VSD, right ventricular hypertrophy and an overriding aorta.
Radiological features on CXR are:
- Concavity in the region of the pulmonary artery, which is small.
- Enlarged aorta.
- Normal sized heart.
- Boot shaped heart due to right ventricular hypertrophy.
- Right sided aortic arch in 25% of cases.
- Decreased calibre of pulmonary vessels.

Right sided aortic arch may also be seen in patients with another cause of neonatal cyanotic congenital heart disease – transposition of the great vessels. However unlike Fallot's there is increased pulmonary vascularity and the heart has an 'egg on its side' appearance on the CXR due to the fact that the mediastinum is narrow because of the abnormal relationship of the great vessels. An example is shown (181b), though in this particular case the aortic arch is left sided.

Practical tips
- Fallot's tetralogy, pulmonary stenosis and tricuspid atresia cause cyanosis with oligaemic lungs.
- Transposition of the great vessels, truncus arteriosus and total anomalous pulmonary venous drainage cause cyanosis with plethoric lungs.

Further management
Cardiology referral for echocardiography and consideration for a palliative shunt or complete surgical repair.

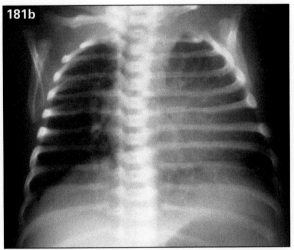

181b CXR in a child with transposition of the great vessels. There is pulmonary vascular congestion and the heart has an 'egg on its side' appearance.

CASE 182

History
An 11-month-old child with cleft palate and neurological abnormalities.

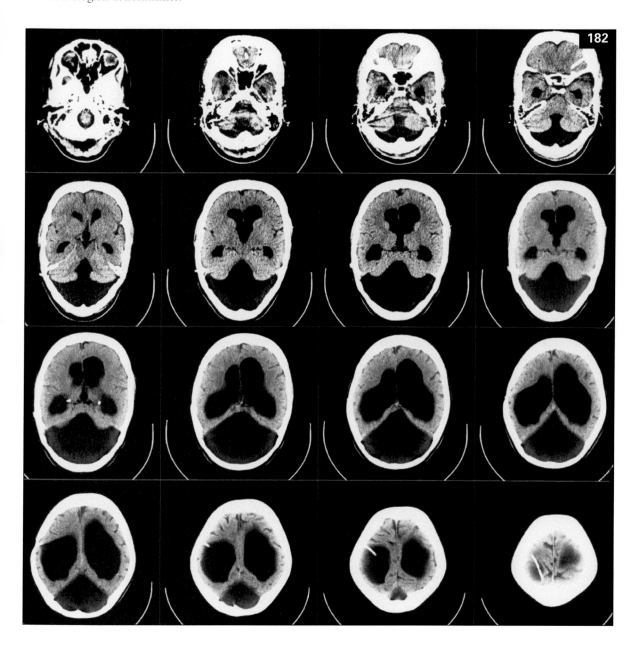

Answer 182

Observations (182)
The posterior fossa is enlarged with absence of the cerebellar vermis, hypoplasia of the cerebellar hemispheres and the presence of a large posterior fossa cyst, which is in continuity with the 4th ventricle. A ventriculoperitoneal shunt is seen in the right lateral ventricle. There is ventriculomegaly but the sulci are not effaced. The features are consistent with Dandy–Walker malformation.

Diagnosis
Dandy–Walker malformation.

Discussion
The Dandy–Walker malformation is a congenital malformation whereby the posterior fossa is enlarged and the tentorium cerebelli is elevated, however the cerebellar hemispheres are hypoplastic. Absence or hypoplasia of the cerebellar vermis is present with a posterior fossa cyst directly connected to the 4th ventricle. Ventriculomegaly and dysgenesis of the corpus callosum are associated findings. Most affected patients die in infancy. The less severe form, Dandy–Walker variant, is more common and is not associated with enlargement of the posterior fossa. The associated posterior fossa cyst is smaller and the cerebellar vermis is hypoplastic rather than absent.

There are numerous associated CNS anomalies, for example corpus callosum dysgenesis, holoprosencephaly, gyral dysplasia, grey matter migration anomalies and encephalocele. Associated anomalies outside the CNS include cleft palate, polydactyly and cardiac defects.

Practical tips
- A mega cisterna magna may mimic Dandy–Walker malformation, however there is no cerebellar vermis abnormality, continuity with or abnormality of the 4th ventricle.
- A posterior fossa arachnoid cyst may also mimic these appearances.
- If the posterior fossa is not enlarged and the cerebellar vermis is hypoplastic rather than absent, consider Dandy–Walker variant rather than malformation.

Further management
The associated CNS abnormalities can be better identified on MRI. Treatment often involves insertion of a ventricular shunt, as in this case, to relieve hydrocephalus. Genetic counselling may be appropriate for the family.

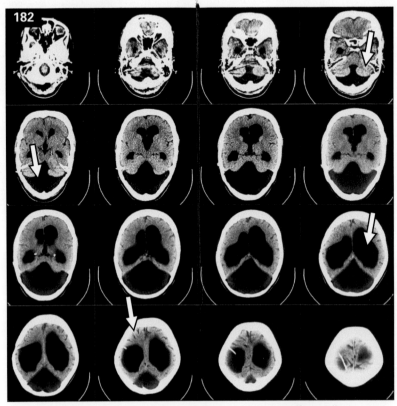

182 Absence of cerebellar vermis (left); sulci are not effaced (bottom left); ventriculomegaly (right); hypoplasia of cerebellar hemispheres (top right).

CASE 183

History
A newborn presented with bilious vomiting.

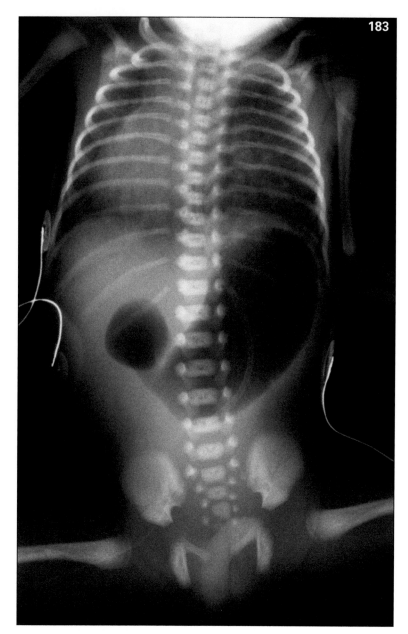

ANSWER 183

Observations (183)
Dextrocardia is present with situs solitus. A right femoral line is noted. An NG tube is present in the stomach, which is dilated with air. There is a 'double bubble' appearance of the dilated stomach and duodenal cap with no gas seen distally. The findings are consistent with duodenal atresia.

Diagnosis
Duodenal atresia, possibly part of VACTERL syndrome.

Differential diagnosis
Of 'double bubble' on abdominal radiograph:
- Annular pancreas.
- Duodenal diaphragm.
- Peritoneal band.
- Choledochal cyst.

Discussion
Duodenal atresia is due to failure of recanalization of the duodenum at around 10 weeks and is the most common cause of congenital duodenal obstruction. The other major cause is annular pancreas, and both are associated with Down's syndrome. The obstruction is just beyond the ampulla in the majority of cases and the 'double bubble' results from gas-fluid levels in the first part of duodenum and stomach. Gas may be seen more distally in the bowel if there is duodenal stenosis rather than complete atresia (though atresia is twice as common).

Duodenal atresia is associated with the VACTERL syndrome, a non-random association of congenital abnormalities affecting multiple systems, summarized by the mnemonic 'VACTERL'. Three or more of the associated defects are required to make the diagnosis. The mnemonic is as follows:
- Vertebral anomalies.
- Anorectal anomalies – imperforate anus.
- Cardiovascular anomalies – most commonly endocardial cushion defects.
- Tracheo-Esophageal fistula.
- Renal anomalies – may be associated with a single umbilical artery.
- Limb anomalies – e.g. radial dysplasia, polydactyly, syndactyly.

The characteristic cardiac abnormality is a septal defect but dextrocardia, as in this case, has been described.

Practical tips
Always check the 'double bubble' radiograph for VACTERL associations, e.g. vertebral anomalies on the film.

Further management
Fluid and electrolyte imbalance must be corrected along with decompression of the stomach via NG tube insertion. Surgical correction is then required, usually with good outcome.

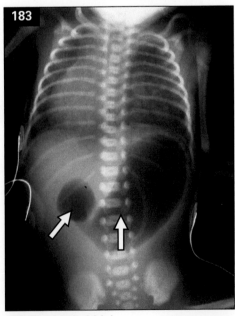

183 'Double bubble'.

CASE 184

History
A child with dwarfism.

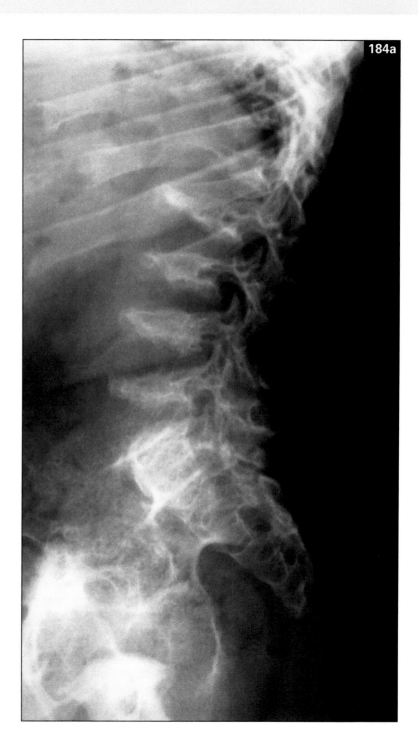

ANSWER 184

Observations (184a)
Lateral spinal radiograph shows vertebral bodies are flattened with central beaking anteriorly. There is also widening of the intervertebral disc spaces and posterior vertebral scalloping. The findings are suggestive of Morquio's syndrome.

Diagnosis
Morquio's syndrome.

Differential diagnosis
- Hurler's syndrome.
- Achondroplasia.

Discussion
Morquio's syndrome is a rare metabolic disorder classified as one of the mucopolysaccharidoses. It is autosomal recessive and presents in childhood with characteristic skeletal deformity and dwarfism. Patients also have deafness and cardiac dysfunction, however they may well live to adulthood. Atlantoaxial subluxation is a feature and there may be absence of the odontoid peg. Radiograph of the cervical spine in the same patient (**184b**) shows multiple flattened vertebral bodies and absence of the peg.

Hurler's syndrome (another of the mucopolysaccharidoses) and achondroplasia can have similar radiological features; in particular, both may cause posterior vertebral body scalloping and anterior vertebral body beaking.

The radiological features of Morquio's syndrome are described below:
- Spine:
  - Posterior vertebral scalloping.
  - Widening of intervertebral disc spaces.
  - Congenital flattening of the vertebral bodies (platyspondyly).
  - Anterior beaking of vertebral bodies.
  - Atlantoaxial subluxation.
  - Kyphoscoliosis.

- Pelvis:
  - Fragmentation and flattening of femoral heads (**184c**).
  - Flared iliac wings (**184c**).

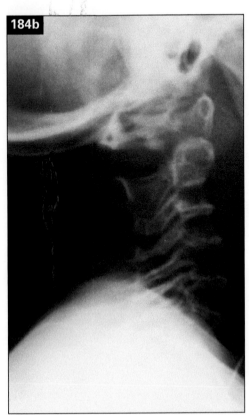

184b Lateral cervical spine demonstrating absence of the peg with flattening and posterior scalloping of the vertebral bodies.

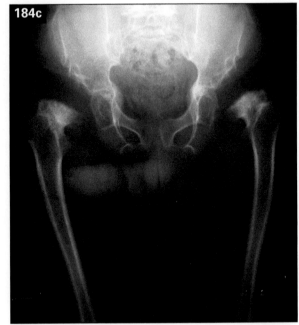

184c AP radiograph of pelvis showing fragmentation and flattening of the femoral heads with flaring of the iliac wings.

Answer 184 — Paediatric Imaging

- Lower limbs:
  - Sloping of superior margin of tibial plateau laterally (**184d**).
  - Genu valgus deformity (**184d**).
- Hands and feet:
  - Proximal tapering of the metacarpal bones producing 'bullet-shaped' metacarpals (**184e**).
  - Short widened tubular bones with metaphyseal irregularity (**184e**).

Practical tips
It may be very difficult on imaging to differentiate Morquio's from achondroplasia or the other mucopolysaccharidoses. Some features may help radiological differentiation:
- Caudal narrowing of the spinal canal is not a feature of the mucopolysaccharidoses however it is present in achondroplasia; therefore assess the interpedicular distance on the AP of the spine.
- The anterior vertebral body beaks in Morquio's tend to be in the Middle of the vertebral body whereas in Achondroplasia and Hurler's syndrome they are Anteroinferior.
- If the spine radiograph includes the craniocervical junction always assess the peg as this may be absent in Morquio's and there may be atlantoaxial subluxation.
- On a pelvic radiograph flaring of the iliac wings will be seen in achondroplasia and the mucopolysaccharidoses, however in achondroplasia the sacrum may be horizontal in orientation therefore appearing absent (see Case 151).

Further management
Mortality/morbidity are related to atlantoaxial instability due to odontoid peg hyperplasia. In addition, respiratory complications are common due to chest wall deformity.

Further reading
Wakely S (2006). The posterior vertebral scalloping sign. *Radiology* **239**: 607–609.

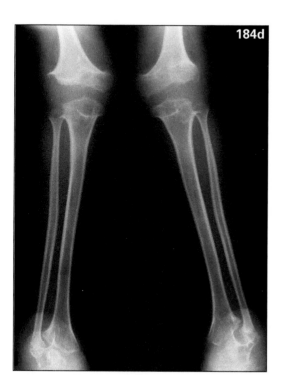

184d AP radiograph of both knees shows genu valgum with sloping of the superior margins of the tibial plateau.

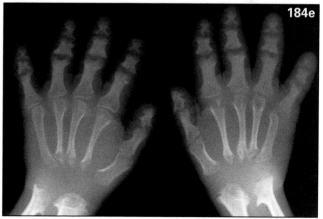

184e Radiograph of both hands shows 'bullet shaped' metacarpals.

Chapter 6

BREAST IMAGING

The breast can be evaluated with a number of different imaging modalities: the main ones utilized in diagnosis are mammography, ultrasound and MR imaging. Image-guided biopsies from specific areas in the breast can be obtained using any of these techniques to aid diagnosis and treatment of breast diseases/conditions.

With the development of more complex surgical procedures and oncological treatments, many breast cancer cases are often assessed by multiple imaging modalities including mammography, ultrasound, CT, MRI and nuclear medicine, incorporating PET/CT. This chapter focuses on a few salient breast imaging cases – complex multimodality staging is not discussed.

MAMMOGRAPHY

Until recently, most mammographic images were obtained as hard film copy. Today, many breast imaging departments have full-field digital mammography (FFDM) equipment enabling electronic storage and image manipulation to aid interpretation. In standard mammography two views of each breast are taken: the mediolateral oblique (MLO) projection and the craniocaudal (CC) or superioinferior (SI) projection. Particular care is taken with image acquisition in mammography – inadequate positioning may result in suboptimal images and missed diagnoses. During image acquisition the breast is compressed to even out the tissue thickness and hold the breast still in order to minimize blurring of the image caused by motion.

When viewing bilateral mammograms, both sides are assessed at the same time in a 'back-to-back' or 'mirror image' format, as shown opposite. By convention, the CC views are arranged with the lateral (outer) aspect at the top of the image and the medial (inner) at the bottom of the image. On the MLO view the inferior extent of the pectoral muscle should be at least at nipple level. Small densities and areas of asymmetry may be more apparent when viewing both sides simultaneously. In addition to a global overview, specific inspection of all areas is required. The examination may be evaluated by dividing each image into thirds and going back and forth between the right and left sides looking specifically for global and focal asymmetry, distortion, possible masses and calcification. Other signs to assess for are skin and nipple retraction, skin thickening, trabecular thickening and axillary lymphadenopathy. Small masses and areas of microcalcification should be looked at under magnification, using workstation tools with digital images or a magnifying glass with conventional analogue films. Previous mammograms may aid interpretation and assessing the significance of focal findings.

As in other aspects of imaging with ionizing radiation, there is always a slight chance of cancer from excessive exposure to radiation. However, the benefit of an accurate diagnosis far outweighs the risk. The effective radiation dose from a mammogram is about 0.7 mSv; about the same as the average person receives from background radiation in 3 months.

The proportion of glandular tissue to fatty tissue within the breast changes with age – there is more glandular tissue in younger women and as a result the background density on mammograms is generally dense. The glandular tissue tends to involute with age; the background density of mammograms in older women is generally lucent.

Mammography plays a central part in the early detection of breast cancers. Screening mammograms lead to early detection of cancers, when they are most curable and breast-conservation therapies suitable management options. In the UK, the NHS Breast Screening Programme saves over 1,400 lives per year. Currently, women in the UK are invited every 3 years for bilateral two-view mammography between the ages of 50 and 70 years. The screening

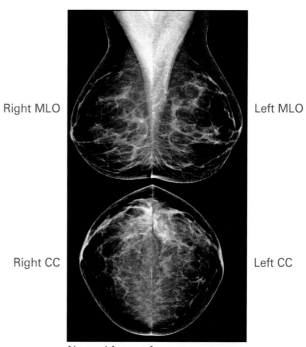

Normal format for mammograms.

programme in the UK is due to be extended to include women between ages 47 and 73.

Diagnostic mammography is used to evaluate a patient with abnormal clinical findings and may also be done after an abnormal screening mammography in order to evaluate the area of concern on the screening examination. Initial mammographic images themselves are not usually enough to determine the existence of a benign or malignant disease with certainty. And while mammography is the best screening tool for breast cancer available today, mammograms do not detect all breast cancers. Also, a small proportion of mammograms indicate that a cancer could possibly be present when it is not (a false-positive result). Between 5 and 15% of screening mammograms are equivocal and further evaluation with additional mammograms or ultrasound may be required. In addition to standard views, spot compression views which may merge out background tissue from a lesion and magnification views to further assess calcification may be undertaken. Most of these tests turn out to be normal. If there is an abnormal finding, a follow-up or biopsy may have to be performed. Most of these biopsies result in a benign diagnosis.

BREAST ULTRASOUND

Breast ultrasound is used to characterize abnormalities detected by physical examination or potential abnormalities seen on mammography. Ultrasound imaging can help to determine if an abnormality is solid (which may be a malignancy, a benign tumour such as a fibroadenoma or other nonmalignant tissue) or fluid-filled (such as a benign cyst). As ultrasound provides real-time images, it is often used to guide biopsy procedures.

BREAST MR IMAGING

MR imaging of the breast is not usually a replacement for mammography or ultrasound imaging but rather a supplemental tool for detecting and staging breast cancer and other breast abnormalities. MR imaging of the breast may be performed to:
- Identify early breast cancer not detected through other means, especially in women with dense breast tissue and those at high risk for the disease.
- Evaluate abnormalities detected by mammography or ultrasound in equivocal cases.
- Assess multiple tumour locations, especially prior to breast conservation surgery.
- Assess the effect of chemotherapy.
- Determine the integrity of breast implants.

Dynamic contrast enhanced MRI to evaluate the breast parenchyma for cancer has a high sensitivity (~90%), with a lower variable specificity (40–80%) – a relatively high number of false-positive results can be generated. Close attention to scanning technique, full standard breast imaging workup and integration of all breast imaging findings during scan interpretation increases diagnostic yield.

COMPUTER-AIDED DETECTION

Computer-aided detection (CAD) uses pattern recognition software to help read medical images. Such techniques bring features on medical images to the attention of the film reader and may decrease false-negative readings when films are single read. The use of CAD has been evaluated in both mammography and breast MRI, but has not been used widely in the UK, where screening mammograms are interpreted by two human readers.

IMAGE GUIDED INTERVENTION

Lumps or abnormalities in the breast are often detected by physical examination, or by mammography or other imaging studies. However, it is not always possible to tell from these imaging tests whether a growth is benign or cancerous. Usually the preferred modality for intervention is ultrasound, from both the operator's perspective and that of the patient's (breast compression is not required as is the case with a mammographic stereotactic biopsy or MRI biopsy).

Image guidance may be used in four biopsy procedures:
- Fine needle aspiration (FNA): rarely used in isolation when evaluating breast lesions; it may be the method of choice when sampling axillary nodes.
- Core biopsy: uses a hollow needle, usually 14G, to remove one sample of breast tissue per insertion. This process is usually repeated three to six times.
- Vacuum assisted device (VAD): where vacuum pressure is used to pull tissue from the breast through the needle, often 11G, into the sampling chamber. The device rotates positions and collects a greater volume of tissue than standard core biopsy. Small benign lesions such as fibroadenoma may be excised by this method. The diagnostic yield from sampling calcification is usually greater using this technique than standard core biopsy. A small marker coil may be placed at the site so that it can be located in the future if necessary.
- Wire localization: in which a guide wire is placed into a nonpalpable lesion/suspicious area or at the site of a marker coil to enable surgical excision biopsy. This may be undertaken when the diagnosis remains uncertain after a breast biopsy procedure.

EVALUATION OF IPSILATERAL AXILLA

Once a breast cancer is suspected or confirmed, the ipsilateral axilla may be staged clinically or with ultrasound: the area between the axillary vein, latissimus dorsi muscle and medial border of the pectoralis minor muscle is carefully inspected. Any nodes of suspicious configuration (signs include loss of uniform reniform shape, loss of echogenic fatty hilum and eccentric cortical thickening) should undergo FNA or core biopsy to assess for metastatic spread. If the axillary FNA or core biopsy histology is negative in proven cases of breast malignancy then combined aniline blue dye and scintigraphic sentinel node surgical biopsy is usually performed.

Professor Iain D Lyburn, BSc, MRCP, FRCR
Gloucestershire Breast Screening Service

CASE 185

History
Screening mammograms in a 61-year-old woman.

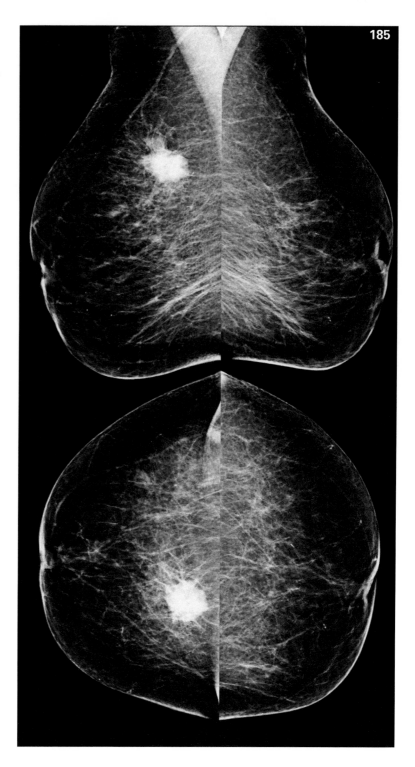

ANSWER 185

Observations (185)
There is a semi-spiculate microlobulated dense mass in the upper inner quadrant of the right breast. The remainder of the right breast is normal. The left breast is normal. The suspicious mass in the upper inner right breast likely represents a unifocal carcinoma.

Diagnosis
Breast carcinoma (invasive ductal carcinoma; IDC).

Differential diagnosis
For stellate lesion:
- Malignancy.
- Postsurgical scar (ask about a history of previous surgery).
- Fat necrosis (often post-trauma or surgery).
- Radial scar (a lesion with central scar formation and radiating hyperplastic ducts).

Discussion
The most common mammographic sign of an invasive breast cancer is a mass: a space-occupying lesion that is seen in at least two mammographic projections. The typical features on mammography of a mass due to an invasive cancer are irregular shape, ill-defined or spiculate margins and high radiographic density. In about 40% of cases the mass is associated with calcification of malignant configuration – pleomorphic and irregular.

Mammographic ill-defined masses require further evaluation. Ultrasound will often demonstrate a hypoechoic irregular mass with ill-defined borders. Image guided core biopsy should be performed – if not possible with ultrasound then under mammography guided stereotaxis.

In such cases, ultrasound of the ipsilateral axilla should be performed and any nodes of suspicious configuration should undergo fine needle aspiration (FNA) or core biopsy to assess for metastatic spread (see introduction to this chapter).

Invasive ductal carcinoma is the most common indistinctly marginated carcinoma. IDC may be divided into various specific subtypes: the majority of ductal malignancies fall into the generalized category of lesions that are undifferentiated and have no particular distinguishing histological features; these are termed not otherwise specified (NOS) and account for 65% of invasive breast cancers.

Practical tips
- Look closely for associated microcalcification in the lesion.
- Avoid satisfaction of survey: once one lesion/abnormality is identified, continue searching for multifocal (other lesions in the same quadrant, same duct system or within 4 cm of the affected breast), multicentric (other lesions in a different quadrant, different duct system or separated by >4 cm in the affected breast) or contralateral disease.
- Look in the axilla for nodes – malignant involvement cannot be diagnosed, but the presence of large nodes should be commented upon and the suggestion of ultrasound guided sampling made.

Further management
Recall for clinical examination, ultrasound +/- further mammographic views with the intention to proceed to image guided core biopsy.

CASE 186

History
A 56-year-old woman with a firm mass in the central left breast.

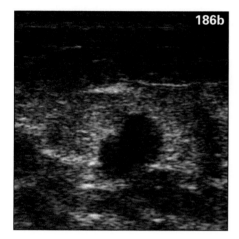

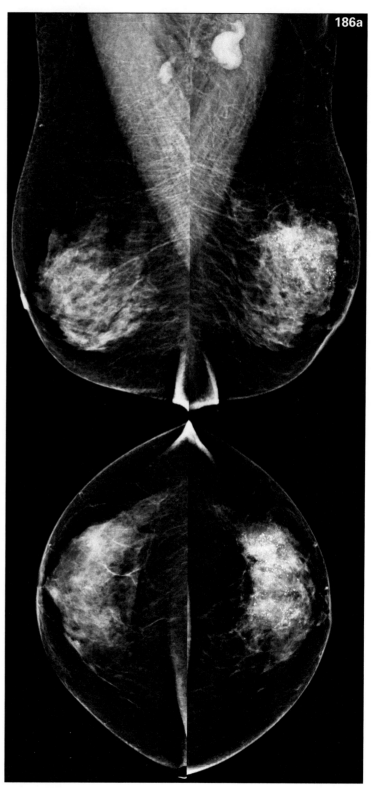

Answer 186

ANSWER 186

Observations (186a, 186b)
Bilateral mammograms show that in the upper central and lateral aspects of the left breast there is extensive pleomorphic microcalcification. Within the left axilla there is a 21 mm diameter rounded node. The right breast appears normal. Ultrasound of the superior central left breast demonstrates an irregular solid mass.

The extensive microcalcification is of a configuration suspicious for malignancy in the central left breast. There is possible metastatic spread to the large axillary node. The ultrasound demonstrates a probable malignancy. Further investigation with urgent biopsy of the lesion is required.

Diagnosis
Ductal carcinoma *in situ* (DCIS) with involved axillary nodes.

Differential diagnosis
For pleomorphic calcification on mammograms:
- DCIS.
- Atypical ductal hyperplasia.
- Fat necrosis.
- Fibrocystic change.

For enlarged axillary nodes:
- Ipsilateral breast malignancy.
- Infection/inflammation of ipsilateral breast or arm.
- Collagen vascular disease/rheumatoid arthritis.
- Lymphoproliferative diseases: lymphoma and leukaemia.
- Metastases (melanoma, lung, contralateral breast).
- HIV adenopathy.

Discussion
Pleomorphic microcalcification may be defined as irregular calcifications of varying sizes and shapes, usually <0.5 mm in size. Orthogonal mammographic views may clarify the characteristics – for instance, linear and segmental distributions suggest that the calcification is ductal in origin, whereas regional or diffuse multiple bilateral groups are less likely to represent a ductal process.

A small percentage of malignant lesions arise from the stromal elements of the breast. Ninety per cent of breast cancers have cellular features that are similar to ductal epithelium and are consequently classified as ductal cancers. When confined to the duct they are termed ductal carcinoma *in situ* (DCIS). When the cells have breached the basement membrane around the duct and invaded the surrounding tissues, they are termed invasive ductal carcinoma (IDC).

The diagnosis of DCIS is associated with the possibility of associated invasive disease. If no invasive focus is identified on mammography further assessment with ultrasound and possibly MR imaging with a view to potentially finding an invasive component may be performed.

Practical tips
- Not infrequently, microcalcification is of equivocal configuration – if there is doubt there is a low threshold to proceed to biopsy.
- Look carefully for signs of an invasive focus within the calcification – search for a spiculate mass or stromal deformity. If not identified, assess further with ultrasound and possibly MR imaging.

Further management
Further imaging assessment is suggested: mammographic magnification orthogonal views (typically craniocaudal and mediolateral) may evaluate morphology and distribution of the microcalcification. Ultrasound guided biopsy of the solid lesion and mammographic stereotactic biopsies to obtain a sample containing calcification should be performed. The suspicious node should be sampled under ultrasound guidance. In this case, the biopsies showed: ultrasound solid lesion – invasive carcinoma; stereotactic cores – DCIS; axillary node – malignant cells.

Once a diagnosis of malignancy has been established, surgical referral is required. In this case the patient underwent a mastectomy and axillary lymph node clearance. Histological findings were of a 12 mm IDC in the superior central breast with extensive (7 cm) intermediate grade DCIS; 4 out of 15 axillary nodes were involved with tumour.

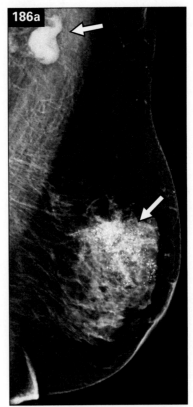

186a Left MLO: axillary lymph node (upper arrow) and extensive microcalcification (lower arrow).

Breast Imaging

CASE 187

History
A 33-year-old woman with a soft mobile smooth left breast lump.

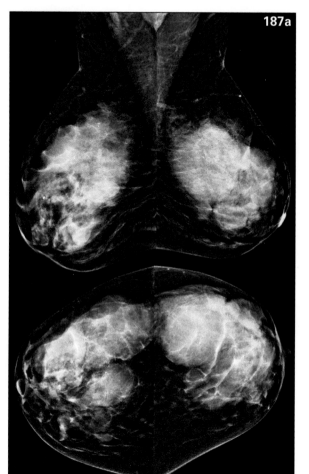

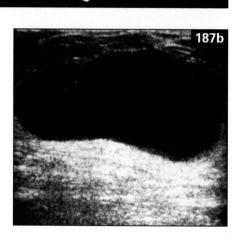

CASE 188

History
A 64-year-old woman with a swollen erythematous right breast.

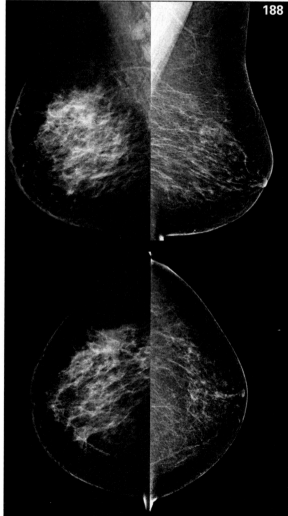

ANSWER 187

Observations (187a, 187b)
The breasts are heterogeneously dense. There are semi-ovoid low-density opacities in both breasts. There is a large dominant lesion in the upper outer left breast.

Ultrasound of the left breast lump demonstrates a well defined smooth margined anechoic mass with through transmission. The appearance of the lesion assessed with ultrasound is in keeping with a benign simple cyst.

Diagnosis
Benign simple cysts.

Differential diagnosis
Of a smooth low-density lesion on mammography:
- Simple cyst.
- Oil cyst.
- Fibroadenoma.
- ~1.5% of circumscribed round lesions may be malignancies.

Of an echoic lesion on ultrasound:
- Simple cyst.
- Complicated (proteinaceous) cyst.
- Duct ectasia.
- Intraductal/intracystic papilloma – look carefully on ultrasound for a mural lesion.

Discussion
Cysts are asymptomatic in many women. Presentation is variable. A palpable mass or masses may develop rapidly and is/are associated with tenderness. They develop perimenopausally in many women, but can be found in women of all ages. Cysts may develop after commencing oestrogen (hormone) replacement therapy.

On mammography, cysts appear as semi-ovoid masses with variable margins and density. There may be a peripheral halo and/or rim egg shell calcification. On ultrasound, cysts usually appear as well defined, anechoic masses with posterior acoustic enhancement. In some, high specular echoes shift in position as gain is increased ('gurgling' cysts). Posterior enhancement is not always demonstrable, particularly if the cyst is small or close to the chest wall. If there is any question as to the cystic nature of a lesion, aspiration is recommended. On occasion lesions appear cystic on ultrasound, but aspiration is unsuccessful – thick proteinaceous fluid may be too gelatinous to be aspirated.

Practical tips
- Avoid satisfaction of survey: look for other, more suspicious lesions.
- Cysts often recur after aspiration.
- If the lesion is clearly a simple cyst, aspiration is not required unless the symptoms of the mass are distressing.
- If there is any doubt as to the nature of the cystic lesion, core biopsy is suggested.

Further management
If there is any doubt about the mammographic appearances, further evaluation with ultrasound should be undertaken.

ANSWER 188

Observations (188)
There is diffuse trabecular prominence throughout the right breast which is of generalized increased density. The skin is thickened. There are enlarged nodes in the right axilla. The left breast is normal.

Diagnosis
Probable inflammatory right breast cancer with axillary nodal involvement.

Differential diagnosis
For diffuse trabecular/skin thickening:
- Post radiotherapy change.
- Progressive systemic sclerosis.
- Obstruction of the superior vena cava.
- Lymphoma.
- Infection/inflammatory mastitis – most common in lactating women.
- Trauma.
- Generalized oedema due to causes such as congestive heart failure or nephritic syndrome.

Discussion
Ultrasound or MR imaging may be used to find a discrete invasive focus which could be biopsied. The diagnosis could also be obtained from skin punch biopsy or from image guided core biopsy of an axillary node.

Inflammatory breast cancer may be defined by clinical diagnosis dependent on findings of oedema, erythema and 'peau d'orange' or on histological findings of metastatic breast cancer in dermal lymphatics. The definition is debatable: not all women with clinical findings suggestive of inflammatory breast cancer have involved dermal lymphatics and not all patients with tumour cells in the dermal lymphatics present with signs of inflammation. Inflammatory malignancies account for 1% of all breast cancers and up to 40% of locally advanced breast cancers.

The differentiation between mastitis and inflammatory carcinoma may be difficult.

Practical tips
- Patients often undergo neoadjuvant chemotherapy prior to mastectomy.
- Consider inflammatory breast cancer when an inflamed breast fails to respond to a brief course of antibiotics.

Breast Imaging

CASE 189

History
A 42-year-old man with a soft mobile tender left breast lump.

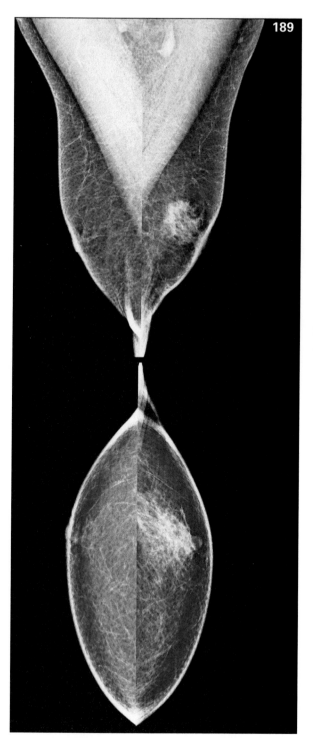

CASE 190

History
Screening mammograms in a 57-year-old woman.

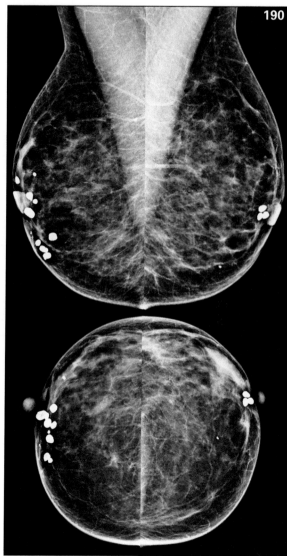

ANSWER 189

Observations (189)
In the left breast there is a fan shaped density emanating from the nipple which gradually blends into surrounding fatty tissue. The right breast appears normal.

Diagnosis
Gynaecomastia.

Differential diagnosis
Of a breast lump in a male:
- Gynaecomastia.
- Male breast cancer (circumscribed or spiculate mass usually evident; often eccentric to the nipple).
- Pseudogynaecomastia (fatty enlargement with no ductal or stromal proliferation; secondary to obesity).
- Diabetic mastopathy (firm mass in patient with longstanding type 1 diabetes mellitus).
- Abscess (erythema; acute history).

Discussion
Gynaecomastia usually appears as a fan shaped density emanating from the nipple, gradually blending into surrounding fat. Three mammographic patterns of gynaecomastia have been described: nodular, dendritic and diffuse. There may be prominent extensions into the surrounding fat and, in some cases, an appearance similar to that of a heterogeneously dense female breast. Although there are characteristic mammographic features that allow breast cancer in men to be recognized (round/spiculate subareolar mass typically eccentric to the nipple), there is substantial overlap between these features and the mammographic appearance of benign lesions. Male breast cancer is rare, accounting for <1% of all male cancers.

Gynaecomastia is characterized by hyperplasia of ductal and stromal elements of the male breast. It manifests clinically as a soft, mobile, tender mass in the retroareolar region. Gynaecomastia has been associated with an increased serum level of oestradiol and a decreased level of testosterone – this may occur with physiological changes at puberty and senescence and be caused by endocrine disorders, systemic diseases, neoplasms and certain drugs including anabolic steroids, cimetidine, spironolactone and marijuana.

Further management
On the diagnosis of gynaecomastia it is important to correlate the imaging findings with the clinical history.

Many cases of gynaecomastia are idiopathic but underlying causes should be investigated – serum hormone levels should be taken. Ask for a drug history and the presence of signs of chronic renal insufficiency, cirrhosis and a testicular mass; other imaging investigations pertaining to the patient may raise one of these possibilities.

ANSWER 190

Observations (190)
In the anterior aspects of both breasts there are smooth well defined spherical calcifications with lucent centres. No abnormal masses or distortion are seen.

Diagnosis
Bilateral calcification of benign configuration.

Differential diagnosis
For benign calcification:
- Vascular – usually secondary to medial atherosclerosis. May be associated with diabetes and hyperparathyroidism. Often demonstrates a characteristic 'train track' configuration.
- Fat necrosis – peripheral calcification in a lucent mass; history of trauma or surgery.
- Fibroadenoma involution – 'popcorn-like' calcifications usually beginning at the periphery and then involving the central portion.
- 'Milk of calcium' – a benign process that can be diagnosed with magnification views of orthogonal projections: on the CC view, calcifications appear poorly defined and smudgy; when imaged on the MLO view, the calcifications are seen as sharply defined and crescent shaped or linear.
- Plasma cell mastitis and duct ectasia – large rod-like calcifications oriented along the axes of the ductal system. These calcifications tend to be coarser and larger (usually >1 mm in diameter) than malignant calcifications.
- Skin or dermal – usually spherical and lucent-centre calcifications at the periphery of the breast.
- Suture – usually seen at a known surgical site. The calcifications may be linear or tubular.

Discussion
Calcification is a frequent finding on mammograms. The arrangement of calcification aids categorization as to whether it is benign or malignant. Clustered (occupying a volume <1 µl of tissue), linear and segmental calcification may be secondary to benign or malignant processes. Regionally and diffusely distributed calcifications are most likely due to benign processes. These calcifications are scattered in a large volume of the breast and do not necessarily conform to a ductal distribution.

Practical tips
If calcification is of equivocal configuration, there is a low threshold to proceed to biopsy.

Further management
No intervention required. Routine recall for screening.

Breast Imaging

CASE 191

History
A 44-year-old woman with fullness in the medial left breast on clinical examination. There is no discrete mass.

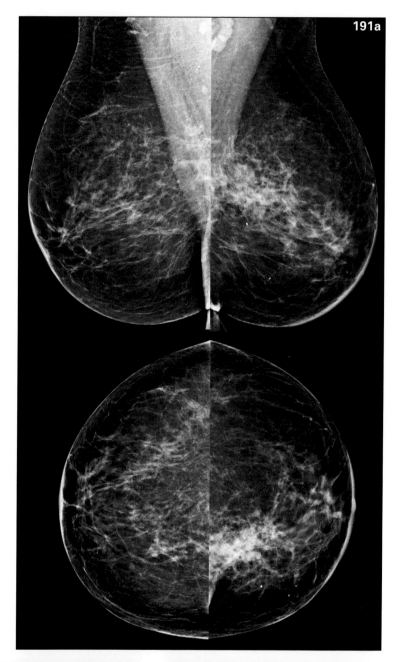
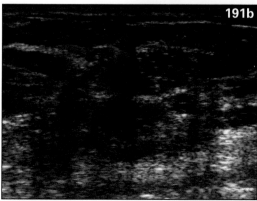
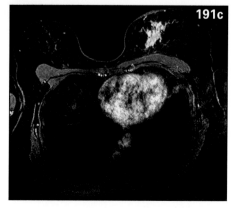

ANSWER 191

Observations (191a, 191b, 191c)
Bilateral mammograms show fibroglandular densities scattered in both breasts. There is general increased density in the medial left breast. The right breast appears normal.

Ultrasound of the upper inner left breast (**191b**) shows ill-defined architectural distortion with indistinct margins and posterior shadowing. Appearances are suspicious of an invasive malignancy and further imaging with breast MR imaging is suggested to assess extent of disease.

The single axial view of a T1 fat saturation gadolinium enhanced scan (**191c**) demonstrates extensive ill-defined microlobulated inhomogeneous enhancement within the upper inner/central left breast, which would be consistent with an invasive carcinoma.

Diagnosis
Invasive lobular carcinoma (ILC).

Differential diagnosis
For mammographic asymmetry:
- Normal variant – dominant glandular tissue (stable compared to previous mammograms, usually nonpalpable).
- Summation artefact – due to superimposed normal structures (thins on spot compression mammograms; ultrasound normal).
- Hormone influences – between 20% and 40% of women commenced on hormone replacement therapy (HRT) develop increased density which may be focal or generalized.
- Malignancy (invasive ductal carcinoma [IDC], invasive lobular carcinoma [ILC], ductal carcinoma *in situ* [DCIS]) – this must be considered when there is asymmetrical density that is newly developed when compared to previous mammograms, and that persists on spot compression mammograms; and/or when encountering a hypoechoic mass on ultrasound.

Discussion
Invasive lobular carcinoma accounts for 8–12% of invasive breast malignancies.

ILC most commonly presents as a spiculate mass on mammography, but not infrequently may manifest as isolated architectural distortion or focal asymmetry. Asymmetrical density refers to a relative increase in the volume of density as compared with the corresponding area in the other breast. Such asymmetry usually represents a normal variation in distribution of fibroglandular tissue. Occasionally, asymmetrical density is a sign of breast cancer. ILC may be difficult to detect mammographically due to the insidious growth pattern. Ultrasound may help depict mammographically subtle or occult ILC, but often underestimates the size of the lesion and multifocality/multicentricity – many centres now stage the breast with MRI prior to making a decision on the type of surgical management (breast conserving technique or mastectomy).

Practical tips
Check thoroughly for multicentric and contralateral malignancies, which are of a high proportion in ILC.

Further management
Please refer to the introductory section in this chapter for indications for breast MRI.

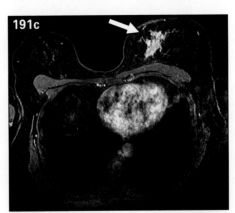

191c T1 weighted fat saturated image post gadolinium enhancement shows an ill-defined area of hyperenhancement.

Further Reading

Aids to Radiological Differential Diagnosis
Stephen Chapman, Richard Nakielny
WB Saunders, 4th edn, 2003

Clinical Imaging: An Atlas of Differential Diagnosis
Ronald L Eisenberg
Lippincott Williams and Wilkins, 4th edn, 2002

Diagnostic Imaging Head and Neck
Ric Harnsberger
Amirsys, 2004

Fundamentals of Diagnostic Radiology
William E Brant, Clyde A Helms
Lippincott Williams and Wilkins, 3rd edn, 2006

Grainger and Allison's Diagnostic Radiology: A Textbook of Medical Imaging
Ronald G Grainger, David J Allison, Adrian K Dixon
Churchill Livingstone, 4th edn, 2001

Imaging of Diseases of the Chest
David M Hansell, Peter Armstrong, David A Lynch, H Page McAdams
Mosby, 4th edn, 2004

Magnetic Resonance Imaging of the Brain and Spine
Scott W Atlas
Lippincott-Raven, 2nd edn, 1996

Neuroradiology – The Requisites
Robert I Grossman, David M Yousem
Mosby, 2nd edn, 2003

Paediatric Neuroimaging
A Barkovich
Lippincott Williams and Wilkins, 4th edn, 2005

Radiology Review Manual
Wolfgang Dahnert
Lippincott Williams and Wilkins, 6th edn, 2007

Self-Assessment Colour Review of Neuroimaging
Kirsten Forbes, Sanjay Shetty, Michael Lev, Joseph Heiserman
Manson Publishing Ltd, 2008.

Self-Assessment Colour Review of Thoracic Imaging
Sue Copley, David M. Hansell, Nestor L. Müller
Manson Publishing Ltd, 2005

Textbook of Radiology and Imaging
David Sutton, Rodney Reznek, Janet Murfitt
Churchill Livingstone, 7th edn, 2002

Index of Differential Diagnoses

Figures refer to case numbers

achalasia 57
  secondary 57
achondroplasia 184
acro-osteolysis (SHARTEN) 152
ankylosing spondylitis 143
anterior mediastinal mass 10
anus, imperforate 173
aortic arch, right sided 181
aphthous ulceration 54
arthropathy
  erosive 143
  nonerosive deforming 132
atlantoaxial subluxation 120
atypical medulloblastoma 104
avascular necrosis (AVN) (DRIED HIP) 139
axillary nodes, enlarged 186

basal ganglia
  calcification 166
  low-density 166
Behçet's disease 38
bladder
  calcification 62
  pear shaped (HELP) 70
  radiolucent filling defects on IVU 56
  small 60
bone lesions, permeative 118
bone within bone appearance (SHARPS POOL) 145
bony sclerosis 140
bowel (small), smooth thickened folds 59
bowel, obstruction 46, 47
brain, white matter lesions 97
breasts
  anechoic lesion 187
  benign calcification 190
  enlarged axillary nodes 187
  lump in male 189
  mammographic asymmetry 191
  pleomorphic calcification 186
  skin thickening 188
  smooth low-density lesion 187
  stellate lesion 185
  trabecular thickening 188
Brodie's abscess 134

calcaneus, lucent lesion in 146
calcification
  basal ganglia 166
  bladder wall 62
  breast: benign 190
  fingertip 152
  gall bladder 82
  hilar 1

calcification (*continued*)
  liver metastases 52
  ocular 91
  periarticular soft tissue 121
  pleomorphic: breast 186
  popcorn, of lymph nodes 25
  spleen 25
calcified liver lesion 40
Candida oesophagitis 38
Caroli's disease 80
cavitating lesion, solitary 13
central nervous system (CNS)
  lesions, ring enhancing 90
central pontine myelinolysis 105
centrilobular nodules 2
cerebellopontine (CP) angle, lesions in 94
cerebral atrophy, diffuse 105
cerebral territory infarct 113
Chagas' disease 57
children, osteosclerosis in 119
chondrosarcoma 141
clavicle, lateral end erosion 6
congenital diaphragmatic hernia (CDH) 164
congenital pseudarthrosis 127
congenital thoracic outlet syndrome 28
consolidation and lymphadenopathy 2
corpus callosum, lesions 110
Crohn's disease 38
cystic adenomatoid malformation (CAM) 164
cystic lung disease 27
cystic mandibular lesions 95
cysts: breast 187

double bubble on abdominal radiograph 183
double density sign 148
dysplasia, lethal neonatal 161

eosinophilic granuloma 148, 158
epiphyseal lesions 133
epiphyses, irregular 135
Erlenmeyer flask deformity (Lead GNOME) 178
erosive arthropathy 143
Ewing's sarcoma 125
extraosseous osteosarcoma 136

fallen fragment sign 115
fibrous dysplasia 127, 158
fingertip calcification 152
'flitting' pneumonia 21
fractures, nonunion of 127

gallbladder, calcification 82

gastric folds, thickened 42, 54
gastric varices 42
gastrointestinal haemorrhage 39
giant cell tumour (GCT) (in child) 134
ground glass opacity 29

haemangioblastoma 104
hair on end sign (STAN) 129
HELP (pear shaped bladder) 70
hemithorax
  complete opacification of 4, 14
  veil-like opacification of 14
hepatic lesions
  calcified 40
  with central scar 85
  hyperechoic 71
herpes simplex (HSV) encephalitis 113
hilar calcification 1
hilar enlargement, bilateral 1
Hirschsprung's disease 173
Hurler's syndrome 184
hyperdensity, unilateral 31
hyperechoic hepatic lesions 71
hypertransradiancy, unilateral 31
hypophosphatasia 176

ileal atresia 173
imperforate anus 173
inferior rib notching 32
inguinal hernia 173
interlobular septal thickening 29
intrasellar/suprasellar mass lesion 106
irregular epiphyses 135
ivory vertebra sign (Mets...LP HIM) 137

juvenile pilocytic astrocytoma 104
juxtacortical haematoma 136

Kerley B lines 12

large bowel obstruction 46
lethal neonatal dysplasia 161
leukaemia 158
linitis plastica appearance (CALM RAGE) 76
lipidoses 178
liver
  calcified lesion 40
  calcified metastases 52
  hyperechoic lesions 71
  lesions, with central scar 85
liver disease, polycystic 80
lung disease, cystic 27
lung nodules
  centrilobular 2

Index of Differential Diagnoses

lung nodules (*continued*)
  miliary 4
  multiple 8
  multiple cavitating 5
  perilymphatic 1
  pin-point high-density 20
  pulmonary 8, 33
  solitary pulmonary 11
  subpleural 12
lungs
  cavitating lung nodules 5
  high-density opacification 20
  multiple nodules 8
  pin-point high-density nodules 20
  pulmonary fibrosis 17, 18
  solitary nodule/mass 11
lymph nodes, popcorn calcifications 25
lymphadenopathy and consolidation 2
lymphangitis, tumours causing 12
lymphoma 141, 158
lytic lesion in digits (SEGA GAME F) 144
lytic/sclerotic destructive lesion 141

Madelung deformity (TILDti) 153
male breast lump 189
mandible: cystic lesions 95
meconium ileus 173
mediastinal mass
  anterior 10
  posterior 10
medulloblastoma, atypical 104
melorheostosis 122
metacarpal, short 4th 147
metastases
  brain 104
  hemipelvis 141
  lung 24
  sclerotic 122, 137
metatarsal, short 4th 147
middle mediastinal mass 10
miliary nodules 4
miliary opacities, increased density 25
Morquio's syndrome 184
myositis ossificans 136

neonatal dysplasia, lethal 161
nephrogram, persistent dense 58
neuroblastoma 174
neurofibromatosis 127
neuropathic joint 138
nonerosive deforming arthropathy 132

ocular calcification 91
oesophageal mass lesion 34
oesophageal strictures 38
oesophageal varices 42

opacification
  ground glass 29
  high-density 20
  over hemithorax 14
ophthalmic vein (superior)
  distension 103
optic nerve thickening 99
orbital pseudotumour 88
osteochondritis dissecans 131
osteochondroma 136
osteogenesis imperfecta 127
osteoid osteoma 148
osteomyelitis 158
osteonecrosis, spontaneous 131
osteopoikilosis 122
osteosarcoma 125, 134, 136
osteosclerosis
  in adults 140
  in children 119, 145

pancreas, annular 44
parosteal osteosarcoma 136
pear shaped bladder (HELP) 70
pencil in cup deformity 143
periarticular soft tissue calcification 121
perilymphatic nodules 1
periosteal reaction, diffuse bilateral 157, 175
periventricular white matter 97
permeative bone lesions 118
persistent dense nephrogram 58
pilocytic astrocytoma, juvenile 104
pineal region mass 92
platyspondyly 154
pleomorphic calcification: breast 186
pleural lesions 9
pleural thickening, diffuse 2
pneumoconiosis, mass lesion with 7
pneumomediastinum, causes of 34
pneumonia, flitting 21
pneumoperitoneum, causes of 75
polycystic liver disease 80
polydactyly, causes of 177
pontine glioma 105
posterior fossa tumour 180
posterior mediastinal mass 10
posterior vertebral scalloping 151
primary sclerosing cholangitis (PSC) 45
pseudarthrosis, congenital 127
pseudotumour, orbital 88
psoriatic arthropathy 143
pulmonary fibrosis
  lower zone 17
  upper zone 18
pulmonary nodules 8, 33
Pyle's disease 178

radiolucent bladder filling defects on IVU 56

radiolucent filling defects in the ureters 77
renal papillary necrosis (SAD ROPE) 78
rheumatoid arthritis 143
ribs, notching 32
rickets 176

sacroiliitis 116
sclerosis (dense), and cortical thickening 148
sclerotic metastases 122, 137
sclerotic/lytic destructive lesion 141
septal (Kerley B) lines 12
septal thickening
  nodular interlobular 29
  smooth interlobular 29
skull, hair on end 129
splenomegaly 140
small bowel
  obstruction 47
  smooth thickened folds 59
solitary cavitating lesion 13
spleen, calcification 25
spontaneous osteonecrosis 131
stellate lesion: breast 159
subluxation, atlantoaxial 120
subpleural nodules 12
superior ophthalmic vein distension 103
superior rib notching 32
superscan, causes of a 156
suprasellar/intrasellar mass lesion 106
suture diastasis (TRIM) 162
syndactyly, causes of 177

target lesions 64
terminal ileal disease 53
thoracic outlet syndrome, acquired 28
thumb-printing 53
thyroid ophthalmopathy 88
Trypanosoma cruzi infection 57
tumours, causing lymphangitis 12

unilateral hyperdensity 31
unilateral hypertransradiancy 31
ureters, radiolucent filling defects 77
urinary tract, gas in 63

varices, gastric 42
ventricular lesion 89
vertebra, posterior scalloping 151
vertebra plana 154

white matter lesions on MRI 97
Wilms' tumours, bilateral 174
wormian bones (PORKCHOPSI) 168, 179

General Index

Figures refer to case numbers

achalasia 57
achondroplasia 151, 184
acoustic neuroma 94
acromegaly 98
acro-osteolysis 152
adamantinoma 95
adenomyosis 81
adrenal adenoma 67
air bronchogram, hyaline membrane disease 165
air trapping, meconium aspiration syndrome 170
albendazole 40
alcohol consumption/alcoholism 105
  erosive gastritis 54
  pancreatitis 72
allergic bronchopulmonary aspergillosis (ABPA) 21, 36
alveolar microlithiasis 20
ameloblastoma 95
amputation, lymphoma recurrence 118
aneurysmal bone cyst 95, 115
angiodysplasia 39
angiography
  arteriovenous malformations 33
  coarctation of the aorta 32
  focal nodular hyperplasia 85
  mesenteric 39
angiomyolipoma 48
angiotensin converting enzyme (ACE) serum levels 1
ankylosing spondylitis 18, 116, 120, 127
anterior cruciate ligament 159
antinuclear antibodies (ANA) 17
anus, imperforate 44, 173
aorta, coarctation 32
aortic aneurysms, thoracic 10
aortic arch, right sided 26, 181
aortic stenosis, angiodysplasia association 39
aortic valve, bicuspid 32
aortitis, ankylosing spondylitis 18
Apert's syndrome 177
aphthous ulcers, Crohn's disease 53
arachnoid cyst 89, 94
arteriovenous malformations 102
arthropathy of haemochromatosis 50
asbestosis 3, 15
Aspergillus
  allergic bronchopulmonary aspergillosis 21, 36
  cystic fibrosis 36

secondary infection 7
upper lobe segment 18
aspiration pneumonia 171
asthma
  allergic bronchopulmonary aspergillosis 21
  global cerebral anoxia 114
atelectasis
  meconium aspiration syndrome 170
  rounded 15
atherosclerotic disease
  coronary artery 30
  renal artery stenosis 58
  subclavian steal syndrome 19
atlantoaxial subluxation 120, 184
atrial fibrillation 23
Auerbach's plexus degeneration 57
autonephrectomy, renal tuberculosis 74
avascular necrosis of femoral head 117, 135, 139

balloon occlusion, pulmonary arteriovenous malformation 33
balloon angioplasty, subclavian steal syndrome 19
bamboo spine 18, 120
barium aspiration 20
basal ganglia, low-density 166
biliary stasis, Caroli's disease 80
biliary tree
  gas 41, 47
  hepatic cysts 80
biopsy
  core 185
  ultrasound guided 186
bird's beak sign 46, 57
bladder
  calcification 62
  cancer 62
  neurogenic 60
  pear shaped 70
  squamous cell carcinoma 62
  stones 56
  trabeculation 172
  tuberculosis 62, 74
bladder tumour, pseudoureterocele 56
blood transfusion, iron overload 50
bone
  achondroplasia 151, 184
  acromegaly 98
  aneurysmal cyst 95, 115
  Caffey's disease 175
  chondrosarcoma 141
  diaphyseal aclasis 130
  Ellis–van Creveld syndrome 177

bone (*continued*)
  enchondroma 144
  Ewing's sarcoma 125
  fibrous dysplasia 149
  growth plate widening 176
  intraosseous lipoma 146
  ivory osteoma 96
  Madelung deformity 147, 153
  melorheostosis 122
  osteochondritis dissecans 131
  osteogenesis imperfecta 179
  osteoid osteoma 134, 148
  osteomalacia 126, 176
  osteopetrosis 119, 140, 145
  osteopoikilosis 122
  osteosclerosis 119, 140
  parosteal osteosarcoma 136
  polysyndactyly 177
  Pyle's disease 178
  resorption 160
  simple cyst 115
  slipped upper femoral epiphysis 117
  trabeculation 124
bone within bone appearance 140, 145
bowel
  ischaemia 167
  see also large bowel; small bowel
bowel loop displacement 84
bowel obstruction, endometrioma 83
bowel strictures 167
bow tie sign, meniscal 159
brain abscess 33
brain damage, irreversible 163
brainstem glioma 180
brainstem infarction 100
brainstem tumours 180
breast
  benign calcification 187, 190
  gynaecomastia 140, 189
breast cancer
  ductal carcinoma *in situ* 186
  inflammatory 188
  invasive ductal carcinoma 185, 186
  invasive lobular carcinoma 191
  metastatic spread 115, 185
  microcalcification 185, 186
  miliary metastases 4
  recurrence 31
  sclerotic bone metastases 31, 137, 140
breast cysts, benign 187
breast fibroadenoma, calcified 11
Brodie's abscess 134
bronchi, mucous-filled 21

General Index

bronchiectasis
  airway walls 27
  cystic in allergic bronchopulmonary aspergillosis 21
  traction 1
bronchioles, mucoid impaction 21
bronchogenic carcinoma
  metastatic 24
  miliary metastases 4
bronchogenic cyst, intrapulmonary 13
brown tumours 160
bucket handle tear, meniscal 159
bulla, right sided 35
butterfly glioblastoma multiforme 110

caecal volvulus 46
Caffey's disease 175
calcification
  ankylosing spondylitis differential diagnosis 18
  atrial 23
  basal ganglia 166
  benign breast 190
  benign breast cysts 187
  bladder in schistosomiasis 62
  breast cancer 185, 186
  breast fibroadenoma 11
  chondrosarcoma 141
  enchondroma 144
  gall bladder 82
  intraosseous lipoma 146
  ivory osteoma 96
  ligamentous insertion 119
  liver lesions 40
  liver metastases 52
  lung 7, 8, 11, 20
  mammography 185, 186
  microcalcification in breast cancer 185, 186
  myositis ossificans progressiva 123
  obstructing gallstone 41
  optic drusen 91
  ovarian dermoid cysts 84
  peritoneal 167
  pleural 15
  pleural pseudotumour 11
  popcorn of lymph nodes 25
  scleroderma 152
  spleen 25
  testicular microlithiasis 73
  tumoral calcinosis 121
  ureters in schistosomiasis 62
  vascular 138
calvaria, wormian bones 168
Calvé–Kummel–Verneuil disease 154
Candida 63, 79
Caplan's syndrome 6
capsule endoscopy, Crohn's disease 53

cardiac granulomas 22
cardiac sarcoid 22
cardiomegaly, pulmonary arterial hypertension 16
cardiothoracic ratio
  pleural pseudotumour 11
  pulmonary oedema due to heart failure 29
Caroli's disease 80
caroticocavernous fistula 103
carpal tunnel syndrome 150
cavernoma 102
cavernous haemangioma 71
cavernous sinus, caroticocavernous fistula 103
central nervous system (CNS) tumours 89
central pontine myelinolysis 105
cerebral abscess 90
cerebral anoxia, global 114
cerebral hemispheres, schizencephaly 169
cerebral injury, global 114, 166
cerebrovascular accident 33
cervical ribs, bilateral 28
cervical spine 120
Charcot joint 138
chemotherapy, nephroblastoma 174
chest wall
  abnormalities 31
  lipoma 9
chocolate cyst 83
cholangitis 80
cholecystectomy, porcelain gallbladder 82
chondroblastoma 133
chondrocalcinosis 50
chondrosarcoma 141
cigarette smoking, asbestos exposure 15
circumferential resection margin (CRM) 52
cirrhosis risk with haemochromatosis 50
Claude's syndrome 100
cleidocranial dysostosis 127
  multiple wormian bones 168
coal workers
  progressive massive fibrosis 7
  rheumatoid arthritis 6
coarctation of the aorta 32
Codman's triangle 125
coeliac disease 44, 69
colectomy 49
colloid cyst 89
colon
  adenocarcinoma 65
  metastases 61
  pneumatosis 66
  polyps 49
  strictures 65
  vascular ectasia 39
colorectal carcinoma 52

computed tomography (CT) angiography
  angiodysplasia association 39
  coarctation of the aorta 32
congenital anomalies
  coarctation of the aorta 32
  neuronal migration 169
congenital diaphragmatic hernia (CDH) 164
congenital oesophageal atresia with tracheo-oesophageal fistula 171
continuous diaphragm sign 34
cor pulmonale, cystic fibrosis 36
coronary artery atherosclerotic disease 30
corpus callosum
  agenesis 107
  butterfly lesions 110
Cowden's syndrome 49
cranial suture diastasis 162
craniometaphyseal dysplasia 178
craniopharyngioma 106
CREST syndrome 17
crocidolite 15
Crohn's disease 53
  erosive gastritis 54
  primary sclerosing cholangitis association 45
  ulcerative colitis differentiation 65
Cronkhite–Canada syndrome 49
cystic adenomatoid malformation (CAM) 164
cystic fibrosis 36
  allergic bronchopulmonary aspergillosis 21
  meconium ileus 36, 173
cystitis, schistosomiasis 62
cytomegalovirus (CMV) oesophagitis 79

Dandy–Walker malformation 182
dentigerous cyst 95
dermatomyositis 121
dermoid cyst 89
  ruptured 112
detrusor muscle denervation 60
diabetes mellitus
  cerebral abscess 90
  emphysematous pyelitis 63
  neuropathic foot 138
  renal papillary necrosis 78
diaphragmatic hernia, congenital 164
diaphyseal aclasis with sarcomatous transformation 130
double bubble sign 44, 183
double density sign 148
double PCL sign 159
Down's syndrome
  annular pancreas association 44, 183
  duodenal atresia 183
drug-induced conditions, pulmonary fibrosis 18

General Index

ductal carcinoma *in situ* (DCIS) 186
duodenal atresia 44, 183
dwarfism, thanatophoric 161
dyspnoea
 Langerhans cell histocytosis 27
 left upper lobe tumour with lymphangitis carcinomatosa 12
 right sided bulla 35

Echinococcus granulosus 40
Ehlers–Danlos syndrome 132
Eisenmenger's syndrome 16
Ellis–van Creveld syndrome 177
embolization, arteriovenous malformations 33
emphysematous pyelitis 63
emphysematous pyelonephritis 63
encephalitis, herpes simplex virus 113
enchondroma 144
endometrioma 83
endometriosis 81, 83
endoscopic retrograde cholangiopancreatography (ERCP)
 annular pancreas 44
 primary sclerosing cholangitis 45
endotracheal tube position 14
enlarged vestibular aqueduct syndrome 86
eosinophilic granuloma 154, 158
eosinophils, pulmonary infiltration 21
ependymoma 89, 180
epidermoid cyst 94
epilepsy
 haemoangioblastoma 104
 tuberous sclerosis 101
Erlenmeyer flask deformity 119, 140, 178,
Escherichia coli, emphysematous pyelitis 63
Ewing's sarcoma 125
extra-corporeal membrane oxygenation (ECMO) 164
extrinsic allergic alveolitis (EAA) 17
eyes
 optic drusen 91
 thyroid ophthalmopathy 88

18 fluoro-2-deoxyglucose (FDG) 24
fallen fragment sign 95
Fallot's tetralogy 181
familial adenomatous polyposis (FAP) 49
feline oesophagus 38
femoral epiphysis, slipped upper 117
femoral head
 avascular necrosis 117, 135, 139
 congenital multicentric ossification 135

femur
 congenital pseudarthrosis 127
 parosteal osteosarcoma 136
fibrodysplasia ossificans progressiva 123
fibromuscular dysplasia 58
fibrous dysplasia 149
figure of 3 sign 32
fine needle aspiration (FNA) 185
fistulae, Crohn's disease 53
fluorosis 119, 140, 157
focal nodular hyperplasia (FNH), hepatic 85
Fong's disease 128
fontanelle, tense 162
football sign 75, 167
fracture, slipped upper femoral epiphysis 117
frontal sinus osteoma 96
fungal infections
 Candida 63, 79
 Pneumocystis carinii pneumonia 37
 see also allergic bronchopulmonary aspergillosis (ABPA); *Aspergillus*

gadolinium BOPTA 85
gallbladder, porcelain 82
gallbladder carcinoma 82
gallstone ileus 41, 47
gallstones
 annular pancreas association 44
 Crohn's disease 53
 ectopic 41
 pancreatitis 72
Gardner's syndrome 44, 49
gastric adenoma 49
gastric carcinoma, linitis plastica 76
gastric leiomyoma 64
gastric lipoma 64
gastric varices 42
gastritis, erosive 54
Gastrograffin 173
gastrointestinal mucosa, cobblestone 53
gastro-oesophageal reflux 38
gastro-oesophageal sphincter, pneumatic dilatation 57
Gaucher's disease 119, 178
germ cell tumours 92
giant cell tumour 115, 133, 134
glioblastoma multiforme, butterfly 110
glomus jugulotympanicum tumour 108
gluten-free diet 69
gluten-sensitive enteropathy 69
gouty arthropathy 143
granulomatous disease
 Crohn's disease 53
 Langerhans cell histiocytosis 27
 Wegener's granulomatosis 5

grey matter
 basal ganglia density 166
 heterotopic 169
groin, hernial orifices 47
ground glass density lesion 149
gynaecomastia 140, 189

haemangioblastoma 104, 180
haemangioma 129, 137
haemochromatosis 50
haemoptysis, cystic fibrosis 36
haemosiderosis, pulmonary 23
hair on end sign 129, 155
hearing loss
 acoustic neuroma 94
 enlarged vestibular aqueduct syndrome 86
 glomus jugulotympanicum tumour 108
heart failure 29
hepatic abscess 80
hepatic adenoma 85
hepatocellular carcinoma
 focal nodular hyperplasia differential diagnosis 85
 risk with haemochromatosis 50
hepatocytes, focal nodular hyperplasia 85
herpes oesophagitis 79
herpes simplex virus (HSV) encephalitis 113
high resolution computed tomography (HRCT)
 interstitial lung disease 17
 primary tuberculosis 2
 pulmonary sarcoidosis 1
hip joint, primary tuberculosis 2
Hirschsprung's disease 173
Histoplasma capsulatum (histoplasmosis) 25
HIV infection
 oesophagitis 79
 Pneumocystis carinii pneumonia 37
horizontal meniscal tear 159
humeral head, avascular necrosis 6, 18, 53, 65
Hurler's syndrome 184
hyaline membrane disease (HMD) 165, 170
hydatid disease 40
hydrocephalus 106, 180
hydronephrosis
 horseshoe kidney 51
 posterior urethral valves 172
 renal obstruction 68
hypercalcaemia, pancreatitis 72
hyperparathyroidism 152, 160
 renal medullary nephrocalcinosis 43
hypertension
 nephroblastoma 174
 neurofibromatosis 58
 systemic 58

General Index

hypertrophic pulmonary osteoarthropathy (HPOA) 36, 157
hypothyroidism, multiple wormian bones 168
hypoxic-ischaemic injury 163
  low-density basal ganglia 166
hysterectomy, adenomyosis 81

ileum, jejunalization 69
iliac horns, bilateral posterior 128
immunocompromised patients, oesophagitis 79
imperforate anus 44, 173
infantile cortical hyperostosis 175
infections
  pancreatitis 72
  renal scarring 68
  see also fungal infections
infertility
  adenomyosis 81
  endometrioma 83
inflammatory bowel disease
  primary sclerosing cholangitis 45
  see also Crohn's disease; ulcerative colitis
inflammatory malignancy 188
inguinal hernia 47
intracranial pressure, raised 162
intraosseous lipoma 146
intraperitoneal gas, free 75
intussusception, coeliac disease 69
invasive ductal carcinoma (IDC) of breast 185, 186
iron overload 50
ivory osteoma 96
ivory vertebra sign 137

Jaccoud's arthritis 132
jejunum folds 69
joints
  primary tuberculosis 2
  see also knee joint
juvenile pilocytic astrocytoma 104, 180
juvenile recurrent parotitis 87

Kerley B lines 12
kidneys
  horseshoe 51
  medullary sponge 43
  multicystic dysplastic 172
  partial duplex 78
  Wilms' tumour 51, 174
Klebsiella, emphysematous pyelitis 63
Klein's lines 117
knee joint
  osteochondritis dissecans 131
  tumoral calcinosis 121
knee instability 159
Kupffer cells, focal nodular hyperplasia 85

kyphosis, ankylosing spondylitis 18

lamda sign 1
Langerhans cell histiocytosis 27, 158
large bowel
  obstruction in sigmoid volvulus 46
  occult bleeding 39
lead poisoning 178
left atrial apical enlargement 23
left ventricular infarct 30
leontiasis ossea 149
Leri–Weil disease 153
ligamentous insertion calcification 119
light bulb sign 71
linitis plastica 76
lipoma
  chest wall 9
  gastric 64
  intraosseous 146
lissencephaly 169
liver
  calcified metastases 52
  Caroli's disease 80
  cavernous haemangioma 71
  focal nodular hyperplasia 85
  hydatid disease 40
  transplantation 45
liver overlap sign 46
loose body formation 138
Looser's zones 126, 176
lung(s)
  ground glass opacity 165
  left upper lobe tumour with lymphangitis carcinomatosa 12
  lobar collapse 14
lung calcification 7, 8
  alveolar microlithiasis 20
  pleural pseudotumour 11
lung cancer
  miliary metastases 4
  pulmonary asbestosis 15
lung cavitation 7, 8
  Aspergillus fungus ball 18
  pleural pseudotumour 11
  pulmonary metastases 14
lung disease, interstitial 17
lung nodules
  alveolar microlithiasis 20
  cavitating 5
  histological characterization 8
  metastases with underlying osteosarcoma 8
  pleural pseudotumour 11
  Pneumocystis carinii pneumonia 37
lymph nodes
  breast cancer spread 185, 186
  inflammatory breast cancer 188
  popcorn calcifications 25

lymphadenopathy
  primary tuberculosis 2
  pulmonary sarcoidosis 1
lymphangioleiomyomatosis 27
lymphangitis carcinomatosa, with left upper lobe tumour 12
lymphoma 110, 140
  osteoblastic response 137
  recurrence following amputation 118
  staging 24

Madelung deformity 147, 153
  see also pseudo-Madelung deformity
Maffucci's syndrome 144
magnetic resonance angiography (MRA), coarctation of the aorta 32
magnetic resonance cholangiopancreatography (MRCP)
  annular pancreas 44
  primary sclerosing cholangitis 45
magnetic resonance imaging (MRI), cardiac 30
malabsorption, coeliac disease 69
malignant mesothelioma 3, 15
mammography 185, 186
  benign breast cysts 187
  calcifications 185, 186, 190
  gynaecomastia 189
  invasive lobular carcinoma 191
marble bone disease 119
mastectomy, previous breast cancer 31
mastocytosis 137, 140
McCune–Albright syndrome 149
mebendazole, hydatid disease 40
meconium aspiration syndrome 170
meconium ileus 36, 173
meconium peritonitis 167
mediastinal mass
  bronchogenic cyst 13
  thoracic aortic aneurysm 10
medullary sponge kidney 43
medulloblastoma 104, 180
mega-oesophagus 57
melorheostosis 122
meningioma 89, 94
meningitis, chemical 112
meniscus sign 40
meniscus, tears 159
mesenteric angiography, angiodysplasia association 39
mesenteric desmoid tumour, with familial adenomatous polyposis (FAP) 49
mesenteric ischaemia 59
mesenteric metastases 61
mesentery, tumour spread 61

General Index

metacarpals
  head flattening 50
  idiopathic shortening of 4th 147
metastases
  adrenal adenoma differentiation 67
  breast cancer 115, 185
  bronchogenic carcinoma 24
  colonic 61
  colorectal carcinoma 52
  drop 180
  lung 8
  nephroblastoma 174
  osteoblastic 137
  pelvic 115
  prostate carcinoma 140
  pulmonary 130
  sclerotic 122
  sclerotic bone from breast cancer 31, 137, 140
  superscan 156
metastatic calcinosis 20
Meyer's dysplasia 135
microcolon 173
microlithiasis, testicular 73
midbrain infarction 100
middle cerebral artery (MCA)
  aneurysm 114
  infarct 113
miliary nodules 25
MISME syndrome 94
mitral valve disease 23
mitral valvotomy 23
Morquio's syndrome 120, 135, 184,
Moulage sign 69
mucocele, sphenoid sinus 109
mucopolysaccharidoses 184
multiple endocrine neoplasia (MEN) 108
multiple epiphyseal dysplasia 135
multiple sclerosis 97
myelofibrosis 140
myocardial fibrosis, cardiac sarcoid 22
myometrial hyperplasia 81
myositis ossificans 121
  progressiva 123

nail–patella syndrome 128
nasal region, Wegener's granulomatosis 5
necrotizing enterocolitis 167
neonates
  duodenal atresia 183
  meconium aspiration syndrome 170
  meconium ileus 173
  see also prematurity
neoterminal ileum, Crohn's disease 53
nephroblastoma 174
nephrocalcinosis, renal medullary 43

neuroblastoma 174
neurofibroma 111
  mediastinal mass 10
neurofibromatosis 127
  angiomyolipoma 48
  CXR changes 27
  hypertension 58
neurofibromatosis type 1 111, 127
  optic glioma 99
  skin nodules 8
neurofibromatosis type 2 94
neurogenic bladder 60
neuronal migration, congenital anomalies 169
neuropathic foot, diabetic 138
non accidental injury (NAI) 175, 179

oblique meniscal tear 159
odontogenic keratocyst 95
odontoid peg 120
oesophageal atresia, congenital with tracheo-oesophageal fistula 171
oesophageal cancer 34
oesophageal rupture 34
oesophageal stents 34
oesophageal strictures 38
oesophageal tumour, with left lower lobe collapse and cavitating pulmonary metastases 14
oesophageal varices 42
  erosive gastritis 54
oesophagitis 79
oesophagus
  achalasia 57
  feline 38
  leiomyoma 55
oligohydramnios, posterior urethral valves 172
Ollier's disease 144
onion peel sign 40
opsoclonus, neuroblastoma 174
optic chiasm 99
  compression 106
optic drusen 91
optic nerve glioma 99
oropharyngeal candidiasis 79
Osler–Weber–Rendu syndrome 33
  multiple haemangiomas 71
osteitis condensans ilii 116
osteoarthropathy
  Crohn's disease 53
  hypertrophic 36, 157
osteochondritis dissecans 131
osteochondroma 130
osteochondromatosis, synovial 121, 135
osteochondrosis, vertebral 154
osteofibrous dysplasia 149
osteogenesis imperfecta 127, 161, 179
  multiple wormian bones 168
osteoid osteoma 134, 148
osteomalacia 126, 176

osteo-onychodysplasia 128
osteopenia 168, 176
osteopetrosis 119, 140, 145
osteopoikilosis 122
osteosarcoma 125, 134
  conventional 136
  lung metastases 8
  parosteal 136
osteosclerosis 119, 140
  diffuse 155
ovarian cancer 61
ovarian dermoid cysts 84

pachydermoperiostosis 157
pachygyria 169
Paget's disease 137, 140
pancreas
  annular 44, 183
  pseudocyst formation 72
pancreatic insufficiency, cystic fibrosis 36
pancreatitis 72
panda sign 1
paranasal sinus osteoma 96
parotitis, juvenile recurrent 87
parrot beak tear
  meniscal 159
patent ductus arteriosus 32
pectoral muscle atrophy/absence 31
pelvic haematoma 70
pelvic overlap sign 46
peptic stricture feline oesophagus 38
percutaneous valve balloon dilatation 23
pericarditis, histoplasmosis 25
peritoneal calcification 167
periventricular leukomalacia 166
Peutz–Jeghers disease 49
phakomatoses 101
pilocytic astrocytoma 104
pineal germinoma 92
pituitary macroadenoma 106
pleural calcification, asbestos exposure 15
pleural effusions
  asbestos exposure 15
  meconium aspiration syndrome 170
  primary tuberculosis 2
  pulmonary oedema due to heart failure 29
pleural fluid, oblique fissure 11
pleural lesions, chest wall lipoma 9
pleural plaques
  asbestos exposure 15
  malignant mesothelioma 3
pleural pseudotumour 11
pneumatocele, *Pneumocystis carinii* pneumonia 37
pneumatosis
  colon 66

General Index

pneumatosis (continued)
  cystoides intestinalis 66
  intestinalis 65, 167
pneumobilia 41
pneumoconiosis 6, 7
Pneumocystis carinii pneumonia (PCP) 37
pneumomediastinum 34, 165
  meconium aspiration syndrome 170
pneumonia, aspiration 171
pneumoperitoneum 34, 75
  necrotizing enterocolitis 167
pneumothorax 31
  bulla differential diagnosis 35
  cystic fibrosis 36
  endometrioma 83
  Langerhans cell histiocytosis 27
  meconium aspiration syndrome 170
  Pneumocystis carinii pneumonia 37
  positive pressure ventilation complication 165
polycystic kidney disease 48
polydactyly 177
polyhydramnios, annular pancreas 44
polymicrogyria 169
portal hypertension, oesophageal varices 42
positive pressure ventilation 165
positron emission tomography (PET), metastatic bronchogenic carcinoma 24
posterior cruciate ligament 159
  double PCL sign 159
posterior inferior cerebellar artery infarction 100
posterior urethral valves 172
Pott's disease 142
prematurity
  hyaline membrane disease 165, 170
  necrotizing enterocolitis 167
primary sclerosing cholangitis 45
primitive neuroectodermal tumour (PNET) 180
progressive massive fibrosis 7
prostate carcinoma, metastases 140
Proteus, emphysematous pyelitis 63
prune belly, posterior urethral valves 172
pseudodiverticulosis, intramural 38
pseudohyperparathyroidism 147
pseudo-Madelung deformity 130, 153
Pseudomonas, emphysematous pyelitis 63
pseudoureteroceles 56
psoas abscess 142
psoriasis 116
psoriatic arthropathy 143, 152
pulmonary arterial hypertension 16

pulmonary arteriovenous malformation 33
pulmonary asbestosis 3, 15
pulmonary embolus 31
pulmonary fibrosis
  drug-induced 18
  lower zone 15, 17
  upper zone 15, 17, 18
pulmonary haemosiderosis 23
pulmonary interstitial emphysema (PIE) 165
pulmonary malignancy
  asbestosis 15
  systemic sclerosis 17
pulmonary metastases, cavitating 14
pulmonary nodules
  follow-up 6
  mitral valve disease 23
  oesophageal tumour 14
  rheumatoid lung 6
  sarcoidosis 1
pulmonary oedema 31
  heart failure 29
pulmonary opacity
  barium aspiration 20
  ground glass 29
  left upper lobe tumour with lymphangitis carcinomatosa 12
  lung lobe collapse 14
  metastatic calcinosis 20
  pleural pseudotumour 11
pulmonary sarcoidosis 1
pulmonary venous hypertension
  mitral valve disease 23
pulmonary oedema due to heart failure 29
pyelitis, emphysematous 63
pyeloureteritis cystica 77
pyknodysostosis 119, 168
Pyle's disease 119, 178

Rathke cleft cyst 106
Raynaud's phenomenon 17
  thoracic outlet syndrome 28
rectum
  stented tumour with calcified liver metastases 52
  ulcerative colitis 65
Reiter's syndrome 116, 143
renal adenocarcinoma 51
renal artery stenosis 58
renal ectopia, crossed fused 68
renal lesions, fat 48
renal medullary nephrocalcinosis 43
renal obstruction, hydronephrosis 68
renal osteodystrophy 119, 140
renal papillary necrosis 78
renal scarring, infections 68
renal stones, horseshoe kidney 51
renal tuberculosis with autonephrectomy 74
renal tubular acidosis 43

renin–angiotensin system, overactivity 58
respiratory distress, meconium aspiration syndrome 170
reversal sign 114, 163
rheumatic heart disease 23
rheumatoid arthritis 120, 143
rheumatoid factor 17
rheumatoid lung 6
rheumatologic syndromes, histoplasmosis 25
ribs
  bilateral cervical 28
  exostoses 130
  lesions 9
  notching 32
rickets 168, 175, 176
right ventricular hypertrophy, mitral valve disease 23
Rigler sign 75, 167
Rigler's triad 41
Rokitansky nodule 84

S sign of Golden 14
sacral agenesis 173
sacroiliac joint disease
  Crohn's disease 53
  ulcerative colitis 65
sacroiliac joint fusion 139
sacroiliitis 116, 143
sandwich vertebrae 140
sarcoidosis
  cardiac sarcoid 22
  pulmonary 1
schistosomiasis 62
schizencephaly 169
scleroderma 132, 152
sclerosis
  Charcot joint 138
  diffuse 119
septal thickening, interlobular 29
sialectasis, juvenile punctate 87
sickle cell disease 129, 140, 155
siderosis, transfusion 50
sigmoid colon, displacement 84
sigmoid volvulus 46
silicosis 18
simple bone cyst 115
Sjögren's syndrome 87
skin folds, lung edge artefact 35
skin nodules, neurofibromatosis type 1 8
slipped upper femoral epiphysis (SUFE) 117
small bowel
  adenoma 49
  ischaemia 59
  loop dilatation 69
  strictures 59
  thickening in Crohn's disease 53
small bowel obstruction 41
  adhesions 47
  mechanical 41, 47

General Index

sphenoid sinus mucocele 109
spleen, calcification 25
spondyloarthropathy 143
spondylitis, tuberculous 142
Staphylococcus aureus, Brodie's abscess 134
steroid use
  avascular necrosis of femoral head 139
  avascular necrosis of humeral head 6, 18, 53, 65
  cerebral abscess 90
  Meyer's dysplasia 135
  rheumatoid disease 6
stillbirth 161
string of beads sign 47
subarachnoid haemorrhage 114
subclavian artery stenosis 19
subclavian steal syndrome 19
subependymal hamartomas 101
subependymal nodules 169
sulphur colloid scans, focal nodular hyperplasia 85
superior mesenteric vein thrombosis 59
superscan, metastases 156
surfactant therapy 165
Swyer–James syndrome 31
syndactyly 177
syndesmophytes 18, 116
synovial osteochondromatosis 121, 135
systemic lupus erythematosus (SLE) 132
systemic sclerosis 17

teeth, ovarian dermoid 84
tension pneumothorax
  intrapulmonary bronchogenic cyst 13
  positive pressure ventilation complication 165
terminal ileum
  Crohn's disease 53
  ulcerative colitis 65
testicular microlithiasis 73
tetralogy of Fallot 181
thalassemia 119, 178
  major 124, 129
thanatophoric dysplasia 161
thoracic aortic aneurysm 10
thoracic outlet syndrome 28
thyroid acropachy 157
thyroid cancer, miliary metastases 4
thyroid ophthalmopathy 88
TNM staging, colorectal carcinoma 52
total mesorectal excision (TME) procedure 52
toxic megacolon, perforation 65
tracheo-oesophageal atresia 44

tracheo-oesophageal fistula with congenital oesophageal atresia 171
transfusion siderosis 50
transitional cell carcinoma 51
transjugular intrahepatic portosystemic shunt (TIPS) 42
transposition of the great vessels 181
triangle sign 75
tuberculoma 2
tuberculosis
  bladder 62, 74
  miliary 2
  Pneumocystis carinii pneumonia 37
  primary 2
  reactive 2
  renal with autonephrectomy 74
  ureteral 74
tuberculous spondylitis 142
tuberous sclerosis 27, 101
  angiomyolipoma 48
  subependymal nodules 169
tumoral calcinosis, knee joint 121
Turcot syndrome 49
Turner's syndrome 147, 153

ulcerative colitis 53, 65
  linear gas opacity 66
  primary sclerosing cholangitis association 45
umbilical vessel catheters, hyaline membrane disease 165
upper limb ischaemia, thoracic outlet syndrome 28
urachus sign 75
ureteroceles, bilateral 56
ureteropelvic junction obstruction 51
ureters
  calcification 62
  filling defect 78
  pyeloureteritis cystica 77
  strictures 62
  tuberculosis 74
urinary calculi 56
urinary tract infection
  pyeloureteritis cystica 77
  ureteroceles 56
urine ascites, posterior urethral valves 172
urinoma, posterior urethral valves 172

VACTERL syndrome 171, 183
valvulae conniventes 47
  atrophic 59
vascular ectasia, colonic circulation 39
venous angiomas 102

venous insufficiency 157
venous sinus thrombosis 93
ventilation, mechanical 164, 165
ventricular septal defect
  coarctation of the aorta association 32
  pulmonary arterial hypertension 16
vertebra
  collapse in avascular necrosis 6
  ivory 137
  plana 154
  posterior scalloping 151
  sandwich 140
vertebral osteochondrosis 154
vertebrobasilar insufficiency, subclavian steal syndrome 19
vertebroplasty 137
vesicoureteric reflux
  horseshoe kidney 51
  schistosomiasis 62
vestibular aqueduct, enlarged 86
villous atrophy, coeliac disease 69
viscus, perforated 75
visual loss
  sphenoid sinus mucocele 109
  thyroid ophthalmopathy 88
vitamin D deficiency 126, 176
vomiting, annular pancreas 44
von Hippel–Lindau syndrome 104, 180

Wallenberg's syndrome 100
water lily sign 40
Wegener's granulomatosis 5
Wilms' tumour
  bilateral 174
  horseshoe kidney association 51
wormian bones, multiple 119, 168, 179